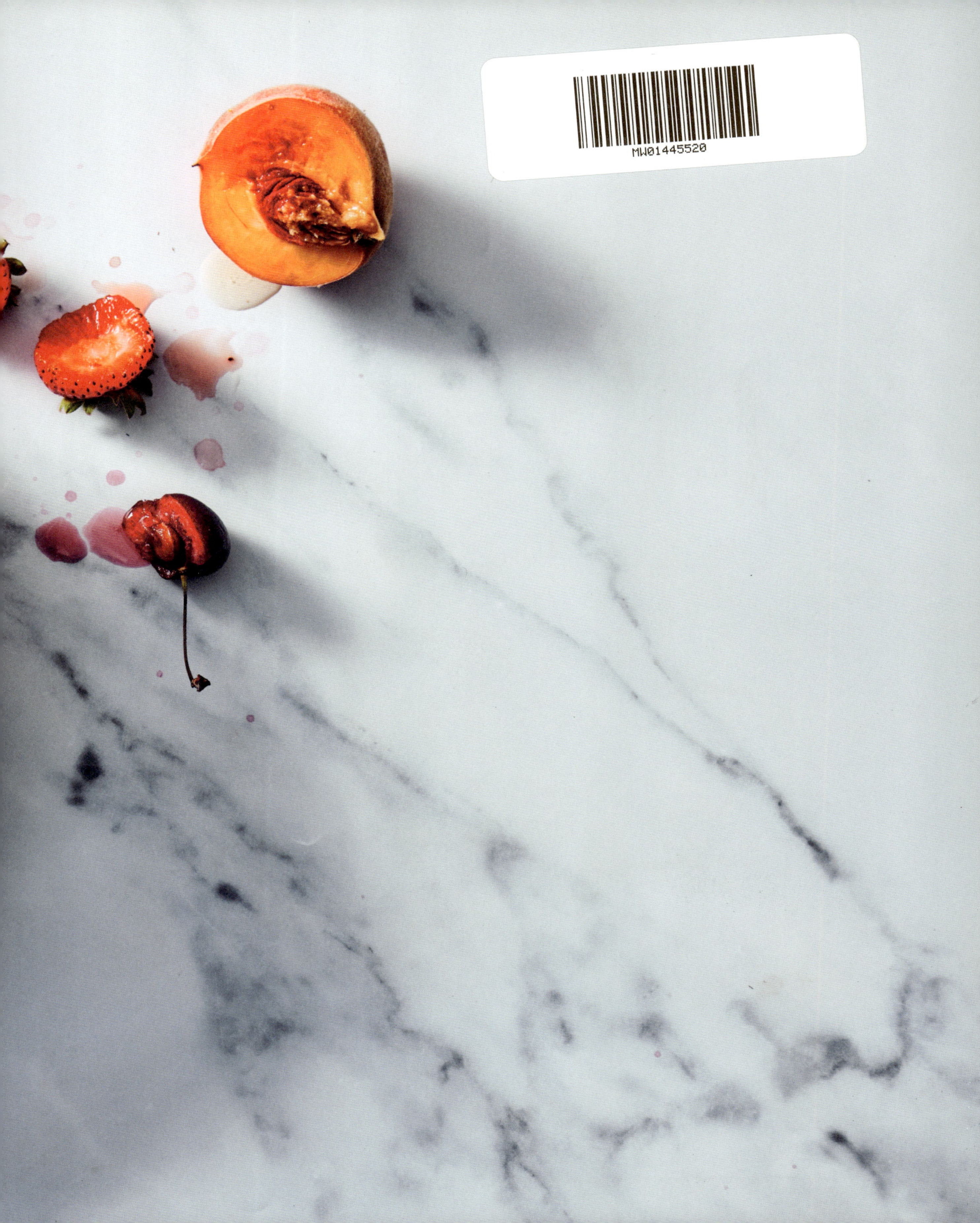

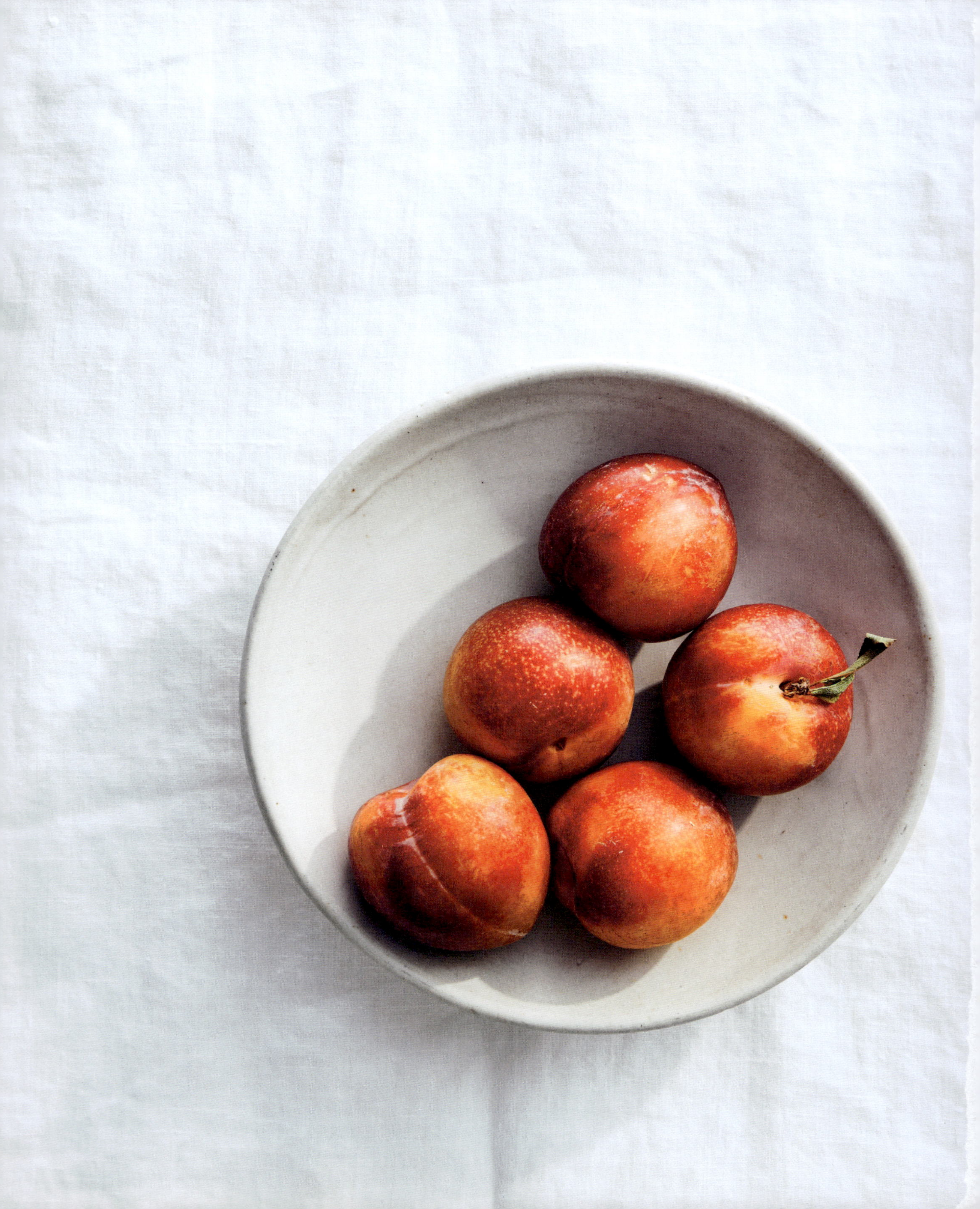

IN GOOD HEALTH

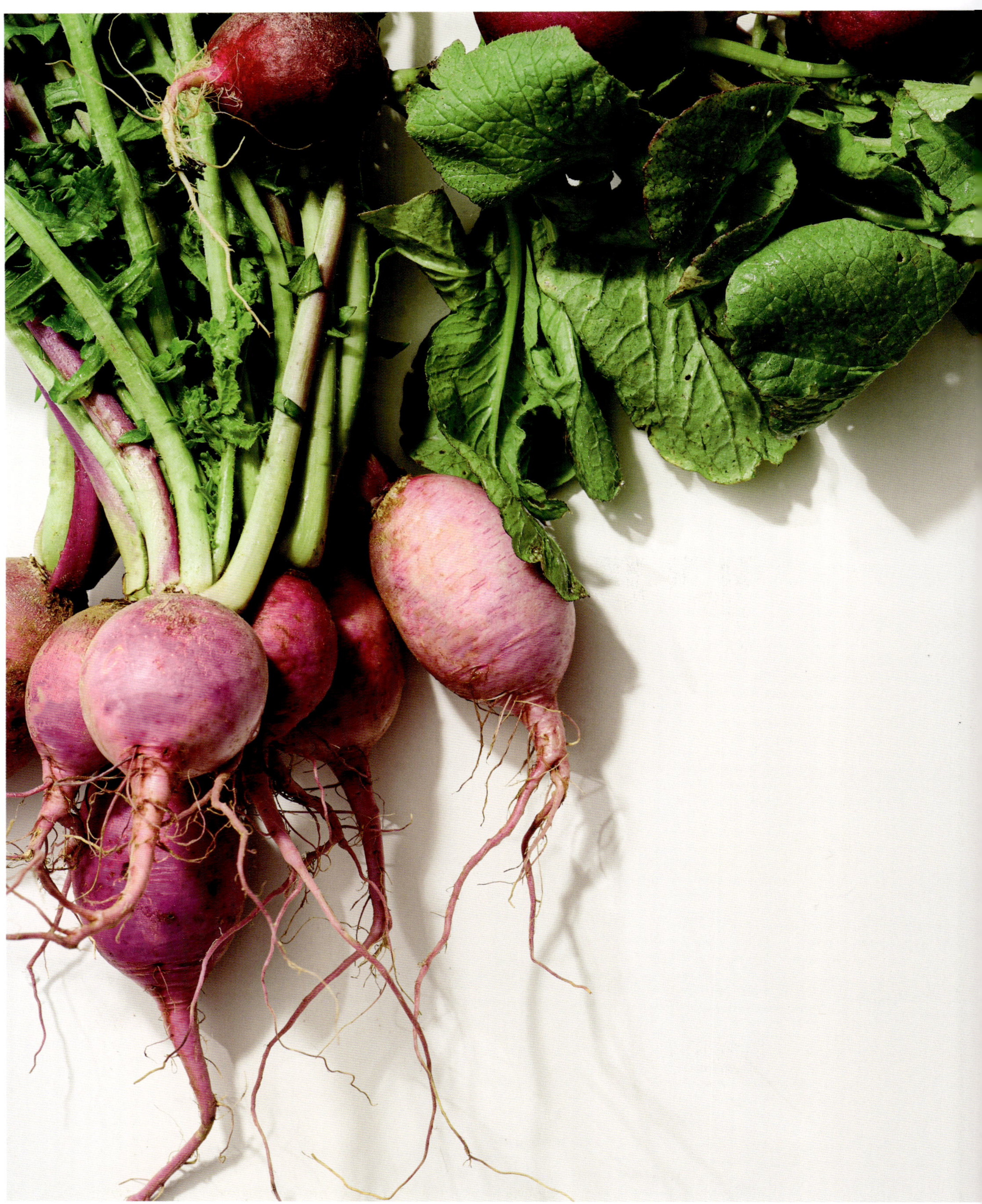

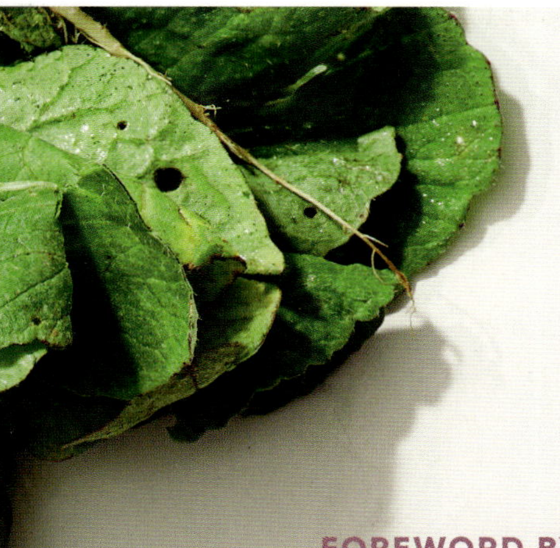

FOREWORD BY DR. TERRY WAHLS RACHEL RIGGS

IN GOOD HEALTH

UNCOMPLICATED, ALLERGEN-AWARE RECIPES FOR A NOURISHED LIFE

Figure.1
Vancouver/Toronto/Berkeley

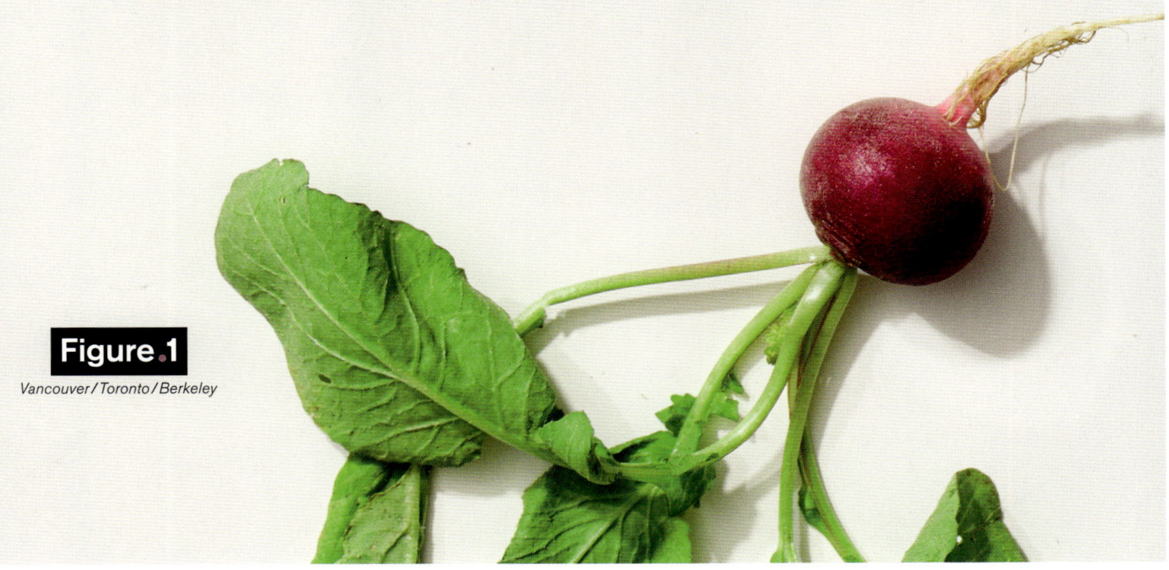

Recipes have been tested by a team of home cooks.

25 26 27 28 29 5 4 3 2 1

This book is intended for informational purposes only and should not be construed as medical advice. The content provided here is based on general knowledge and research, and while it may be helpful in understanding health and wellness, it is not a substitute for professional medical guidance. Always consult a qualified health care provider before making any changes to your diet, exercise routine, or lifestyle. The author and publisher are not responsible for any adverse effects or consequences arising from the use of the information presented in this book.

Cataloguing data is available from Library and Archives Canada
ISBN 978-1-77327-278-8 (hbk.)

Design by Jessica Sullivan | DSGN Dept.
Photography by Colin Price and styled by Marian Cooper Cairns except on pages 2–3, 4–5, 26, 30–31, 35, 40, 50, 87, 128, 145, 146–47, 157, 190, 197, 209 by Megan Morello and styled by Rachel Riggs. Pages 46–47 styled by Haley Hazell.

Editing by Michelle Meade
Copy editing by Christine Rowlands
Proofreading by Anastasia Organ
Indexing by Iva Cheung

Printed and bound in China by Shenzhen Reliance Printing Co., Ltd.

Figure 1 Publishing Inc.
Vancouver BC Canada
figure1publishing.com

Figure 1 Publishing is located in the traditional, unceded territory of the xʷməθkʷəy̓əm (Musqueam), Sḵwx̱wú7mesh (Squamish), and səlilwətaɬ (Tsleil-Waututh) peoples.

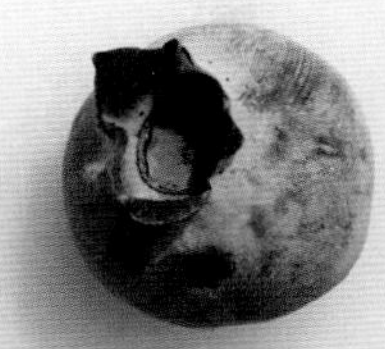

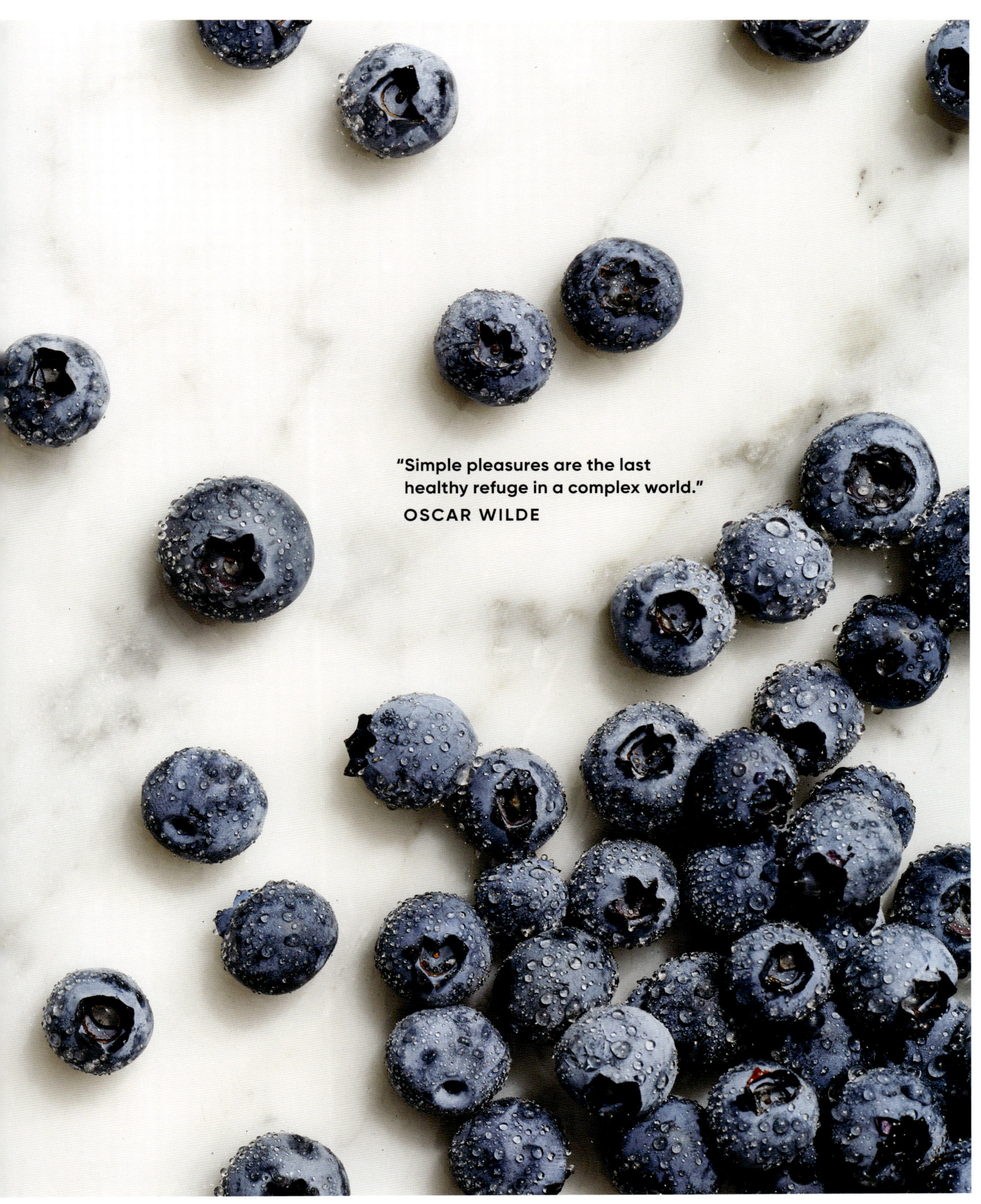

"Simple pleasures are the last healthy refuge in a complex world."
OSCAR WILDE

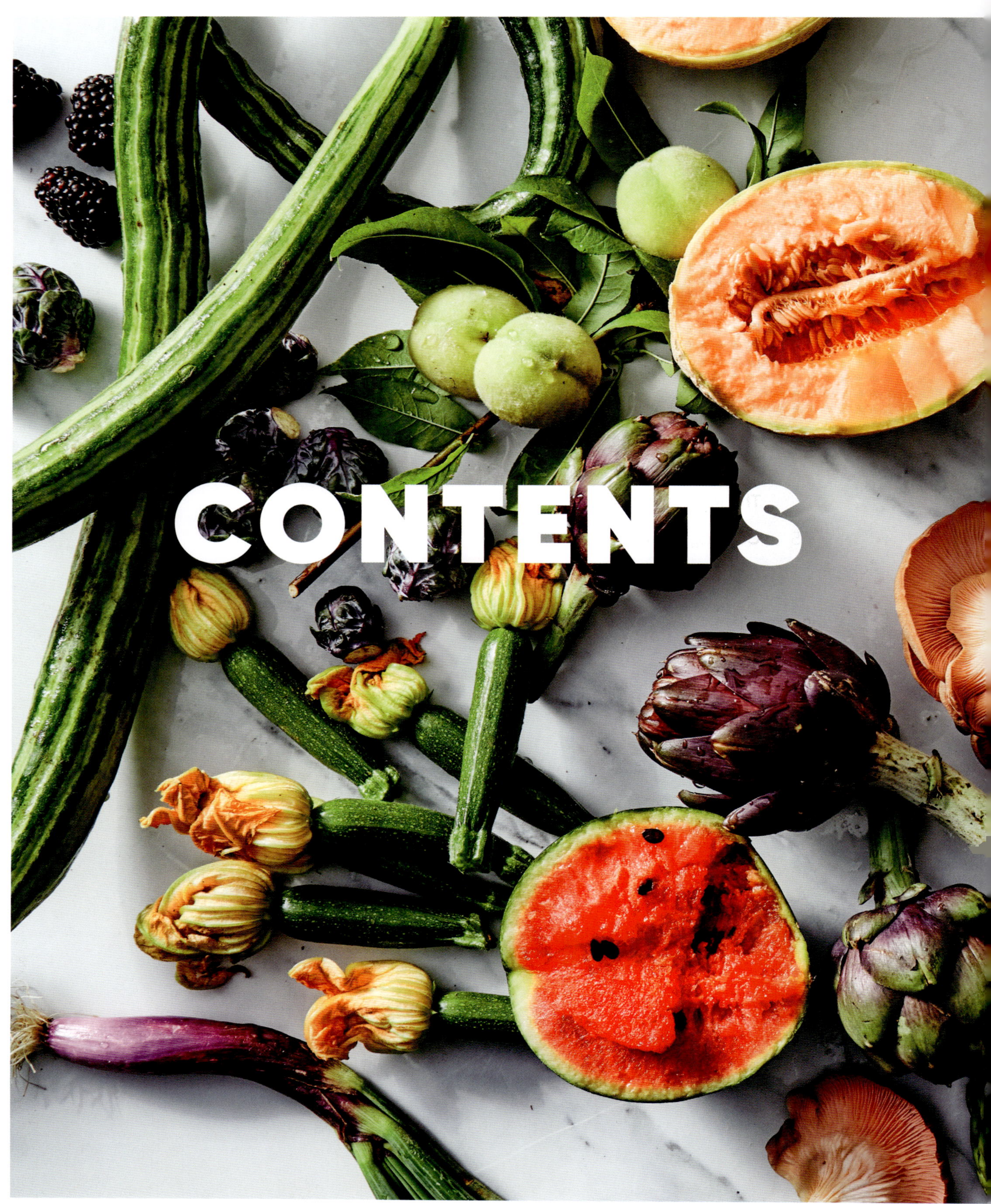

CONTENTS

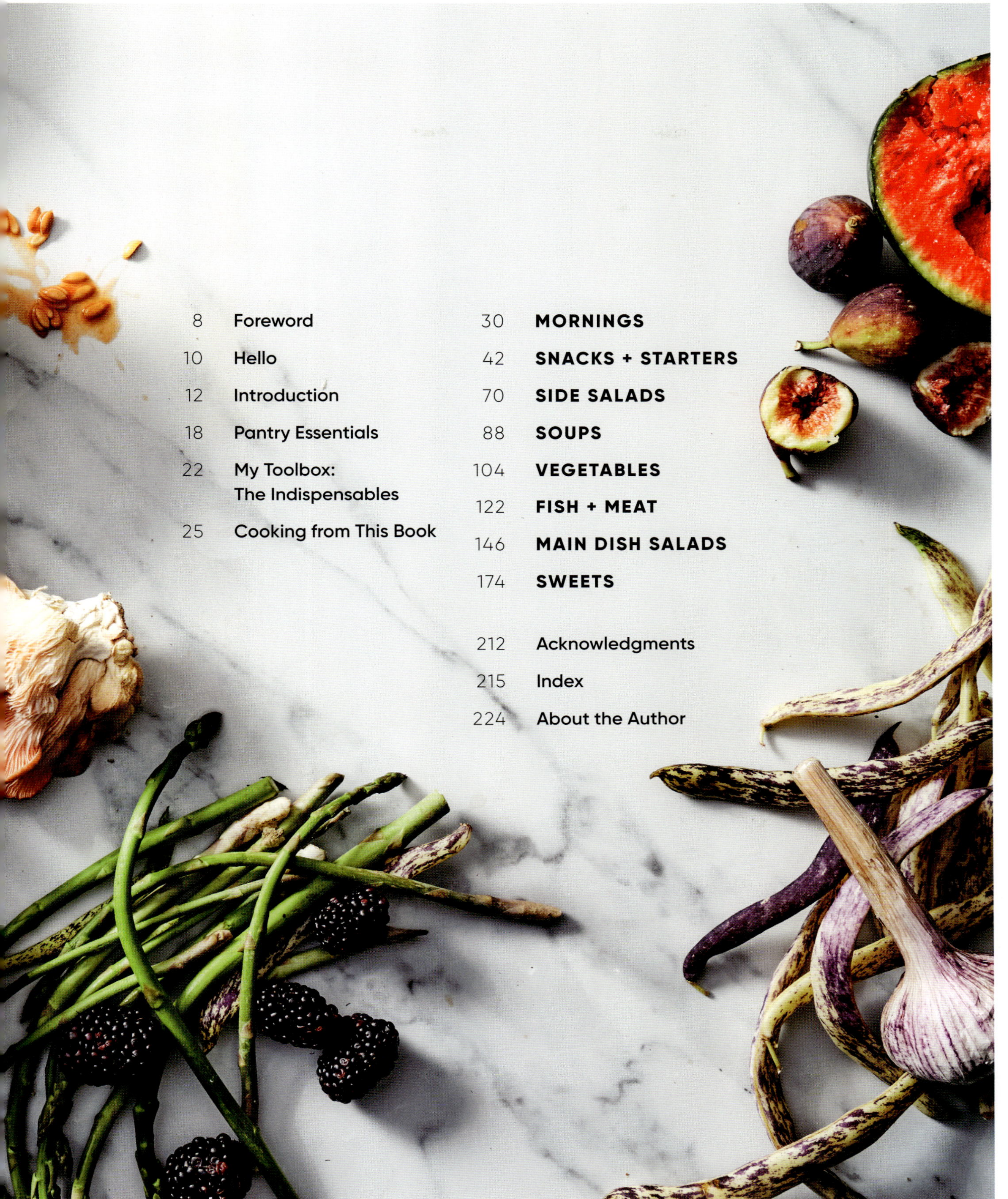

8 Foreword

10 Hello

12 Introduction

18 Pantry Essentials

22 My Toolbox: The Indispensables

25 Cooking from This Book

30 **MORNINGS**

42 **SNACKS + STARTERS**

70 **SIDE SALADS**

88 **SOUPS**

104 **VEGETABLES**

122 **FISH + MEAT**

146 **MAIN DISH SALADS**

174 **SWEETS**

212 Acknowledgments

215 Index

224 About the Author

FOREWORD

When I first experienced electrical face pain in medical school, I had no idea where the path would lead. Over the next twenty years, my health deteriorated due to trigeminal neuralgia and a diagnosis of multiple sclerosis (MS). Eventually, I found myself in a tilt/recline wheelchair. This turning point sparked my determination to find solutions. I began exploring the role of mitochondrial dysfunction in my disease and created a supplement regimen to support my mitochondria. Though it helped alleviate some fatigue, I knew I had to dig deeper.

In 2007, I discovered the Institute for Functional Medicine and redefined the Paleolithic diet I had been following for years. This new approach, now known as the Wahls Paleo™ diet, was designed to optimize mitochondrial function and brain health. I added daily meditation and electrical muscle stimulation to my routine. The results were nothing short of astonishing. Within a year, I went from being unable to sit up to riding 18.5 miles on my bike with my family.

As I applied these principles at the Iowa City VA Medical Center, my patients began experiencing remarkable improvements—reduced autoimmune symptoms, increased energy, and a decreased reliance on medications. My success led to clinical trials, and in the past 15 years, I've published over a hundred peer-reviewed studies and taught thousands of clinicians how to integrate these principles into their practices.

The recipes in this book reflect the same healing principles that helped me reclaim my health. They focus on nourishing the body with foods that support mitochondrial function, reduce inflammation, and promote brain health. *In Good Health* provides a simple, accessible way to adopt a diet and lifestyle that can transform your health from the inside out.

Healing isn't just about taking the best FDA-approved treatments for your conditions. It's about understanding the interconnectedness of our bodies, our environment, and the choices we make every day. It's about improving our nutrition and self-care routines. *In Good Health* is more than a collection of recipes; it's a guide to how food can either create health or contribute to disease, depending on the choices we make. Here you can learn how to make better choices, step by step.

Ongoing research with the Wahls Research Team continues to show how diet, exercise, stress management, and environmental factors can dramatically improve quality of life, manage symptoms, and even reverse disease progression. You have more power to change the course of your health than you may realize.

I invite you to explore these recipes and begin your own healing journey.

Dr. Terry Wahls, MD, FACP, IFMCP
Author of *The Wahls Protocol: A Radical New Way to Treat All Chronic Autoimmune Conditions Using Paleo Principles*

HELLO

Hi, my name is Rachel.

I was a specialty food shop owner when my life was upended by illness. Not only did I have to sell my shop and give up my livelihood and my passion, but I also suddenly couldn't tolerate any of the foods I'd built a career and life around. I feared I'd never be able to enjoy a meal with others again, one of life's great pleasures.

It turns out my fear is shared by people with a variety of chronic conditions, food allergies or sensitivities, and energy limitations that impact the ability to prepare meals. Figuring out what to eat can be a frustratingly long learning curve. Surprisingly, people with very different conditions often end up eliminating the same foods to help them feel better.

Due to my compromised stamina, I needed to find simple dishes with short ingredient lists, making them easy to cook within my new food parameters. The recipes I was finding didn't appeal to me, so I began creating my own, drawing on the skills I'd developed throughout my food career. I never imagined my passion for food would ever return, but with every coconut milk swap and citrus squeeze, I felt the tide begin to turn.

I found that food could still be one of life's great pleasures—a delicious, full sensory experience created with everyday dishes that celebrate what's included rather than what's omitted. I could share these dishes with people I love—without apology or explanation. And I discovered that people with all sorts of conditions—multiple sclerosis, diabetes, celiac disease, mast cell activation, ulcerative colitis, rheumatoid arthritis, long

COVID, and other autoimmune conditions, as well as myalgic encephalomyelitis/chronic fatigue syndrome (ME/CFS) and Ehlers-Danlos syndrome that I have—face many of the same challenges and losses around food. They, too, needed a cookbook, not only for weeknight meals but also for holidays and family events, which can be tricky for us and for those cooking for us.

I sought to capture the effortless sophistication, freshness, and beauty of California cuisine. I wanted to make it possible for clean-eating enthusiasts, food lovers, and those who live with food sensitivities to enjoy food again. Harnessing the goodness of seasonal fruits and vegetables, I aimed to let peak produce shine with little coaxing, allowing its natural flavors to take center stage.

To that end, I've created this collection of vibrant and modern dishes, designed to be as inclusive as they are flavorful. These recipes are free from commonly triggering foods, including:

- **artificial sweeteners**
- **cashews**
- **dairy**
- **gluten**
- **grains and pseudo-grains**
- **legumes**
- **nightshades (eggplant, tomatoes, peppers, and potatoes)**
- **peanuts**
- **pork**
- **refined sugar**
- **shellfish**
- **soy**

These recipes are not just for people with chronic illness—anyone who cares about health and nutrition will find them indispensable. Short ingredient lists and minimal prep time are *universal* desires!

Rachel

INTRODUCTION

I never imagined I would find myself housebound by illness.

I've now been mostly housebound for over ten years. Prior to becoming ill, I had no awareness that this space even existed: the space in between life and death, which can persist in perpetuity for people who live with myalgic encephalomyelitis/chronic fatigue syndrome (ME/CFS). There are hundreds of thousands (millions, actually) of us who are missing from our careers, our families, our social lives.

I had been healthy my whole life. And I live in San Diego, where I was able to rollerblade and hike and lead an active outdoor lifestyle year-round. I never saw this coming.

How I Got Here

In 2003, my health first faltered after having a common virus. By 2012, I didn't know what was wrong. I just knew I was sick and getting worse and began searching for answers.

In 2015, I received a definitive diagnosis at the Mayo Clinic in Rochester, Minnesota. I was diagnosed with hyperadrenergic POTS (postural orthostatic tachycardia syndrome), a condition that disrupts the body's autonomic nervous system, and ME/CFS. Later, I was diagnosed with Ehlers-Danlos syndrome (I have the COL1A1 mutation), a genetic condition that affects connective tissues, and mast cell activation syndrome (MCAS), which leads to abnormal reactions in the body's immune system. And just when I thought it couldn't worsen, I developed craniocervical instability (CCI), which impacts the stability of my neck, a consequence of Ehlers-Danlos syndrome.

Receiving these diagnoses was both a relief and an emotional challenge. While they provided much-needed answers, they also brought the difficult realization that I would have to live with multiple chronic conditions.

My quest to regain my health eventually led me to an elimination diet and, ultimately, a paradigm shift in how I approached food. In the beginning it wasn't a choice but a survival strategy. I've found that, though my illnesses are debilitating and, likely, lifelong, when my body is unburdened and supported with good nutrition, they take less of a toll.

Eating Your Veg

Once, it was enough to eat like our grandparents: real, natural, and (mostly) unprocessed foods that were free of additives and made in the home kitchen. Today, that is no longer true. Even a diet consisting primarily of natural foods may lack enough nutrients due to the industrial food production practices that deplete our soils and strip nutrients from our foods.

This cookbook offers a path around the reality of a declining food supply. Malnutrition does not only affect the developing world. Every industrialized country now faces imbalanced nutrition from the consumption of too many "empty calories"—processed foods rich in fats and carbs but low in essential micronutrients. Good nutrition is ever more critical for fueling health.

Not surprisingly, an increasing number of people worldwide are affected by chronic conditions such as type 2 diabetes, cardiovascular disease, cancer, and autoimmune disorders. Unhealthy diets, sedentary lifestyles, and environmental toxins—in concert with underlying genetics—contribute to the high prevalence of chronic diseases, many of which leading researchers believe can be reversed or forestalled with better nutrition.

Fatigue, lethargy, weight gain, poor sleep, bloating, allergies, and more can trick people into thinking these symptoms are part of normal aging. I assure you they are not. Convenient hyper-processed foods often are the culprits. If you're not feeling your best and can't pinpoint why, adjusting your diet is one of the most powerful and accessible tools we have in seeking optimal health.

Eschewing hyper-processed "Frankenfoods" may seem complicated at first. But over time, you will find they will lose their appeal. As you shift to a healthier diet, cravings for processed foods will diminish, and your palate will adapt. Eventually, these foods will lose their power over you.

Food can be our medicine... or our undoing. In this book, I present a collection of delicious recipes that seek to fill nutrient gaps in our diet while avoiding common foods that can trigger sensitivities and allergies. I wanted to keep the ingredient lists short, the flavors accessible, and the preparation time reasonable. My goal was to create everyday dishes that feel bountiful rather than restrictive.

Getting Back to Our Kitchens

I hope you embrace the process of cooking as the ultimate form of self-care and the whole sensory experience it is. It's a creative and therapeutic outlet for many—plus, preparing nutrient-rich food for the people in your life is a generous gift and a wonderful expression of love.

For many, cooking is a daunting prospect. So many of us lack the time and experience to feel confident in the kitchen. In this book, I help demystify the art of cooking by providing helpful tips on stocking your pantry and highlighting the kitchen gadgets you need to succeed. I offer step-by-step guidance on preparing the recipes, including time-saving steps, and point to efficiencies, such as batch cooking.

Anyone can eat "clean" for a day or even a few weeks, but what if you had to (or wanted to) do it forever? What if the difference between a good day at work and a bad day in bed was on your plate? By getting into the habit of cooking fresh whole foods in your own home kitchen, you will eventually crowd out the bad stuff, like ultra-processed foods. I hope this collection of recipes helps make healthful eating—even while living with numerous dietary restrictions—a sustainable endeavor.

Dark Chocolate (yep, I said chocolate!)

You'll notice an abundance of dessert recipes in this book that feature dark chocolate. If you're not on board with dark chocolate, try thinking of it as its own entity instead of comparing it to milk chocolate. Tap into the part of your palate that loves coffee! Rich in healthy compounds such as catechin, epicatechin, and flavonoids, dark chocolate is a superfood with cardiovascular and mitochondrial benefits. Dark chocolate contains theobromine, which is like caffeine's gentler cousin. It has the same positive effects on our mood but has fewer unwanted effects than caffeine. I hope you discover new opportunities here to fall in love with it!

The many cakes found in the Sweets chapter are nutritiously balanced, can be whipped up with a single bowl and whisk, and are totally scrumptious. While many flour alternatives are available, I mostly stick to the nutritious option that is teeming with protein and micronutrients: almond flour (see page 18 for more on this). I hope you'll enjoy them with abandon. You know that three o'clock snack that sort of wipes you out? These cakes won't do that to you.

If the cookies, cakes, brownies, and truffles here won't satiate your sweet tooth, consider this a barometer of sugar still hijacking your tastebuds. Sweets like these with a more balanced macronutrient profile should be super satisfying, without provoking cravings that cause you to overeat in the way traditional baked goods made with sugar and flour might.

The *In Good Health* Approach

In Good Health heartily embraces the trending shift from weight to wellness and recognizes that more and more people are intrinsically motivated to lose weight for health purposes rather than vanity. This transition away from diet culture is a welcome change.

Though whole foods are the foundation, these recipes go well beyond that. They can help identify and eliminate foods that trigger ill health. You may find that certain foods exacerbate autoimmune conditions, create inflammation, cause migraines, and worsen other health challenges.

Ultimately, there's no perfect blueprint—clean eating requires personalization. But the key principles are built around packing a nutritional punch through whole, organic, and unprocessed plants and animals that your body needs to thrive, while removing the chemicals, artificial preservatives, and toxins standing in the way of better health.

Other important principles involved in achieving balance and feeling your best include combining fat, carbohydrates, fiber, and protein in each meal; drinking eight+ glasses of water daily; and eating regular meals to keep blood sugar levels in check. Working intermittent fasting into your routine where possible is highly advised. The 16/8-hour rotation is easy enough to adhere to, and I've been doing it for years, primarily to give my digestion a rest.

The recipes in this book are free of gluten, grains and pseudo-grains, dairy, soy, nightshades (eggplant, tomatoes, peppers, and potatoes), legumes, squash, spinach, pork, shellfish, refined sugar, artificial sweeteners, cashews, and peanuts. I have swapped shellfish and processed and cured meats in favor of organic, grass-fed, or pasture-raised chicken, beef, lamb, organ meats, and bison. Wild salmon, halibut, and wild-caught canned tuna are staples. Organic and pasture-raised eggs are a great source of complete proteins.

Fresh fruits and vegetables, particularly the "Dirty Dozen,"* should be organic when that's an option. These foods offer optimal macro- and micronutrients.

I choose mostly extra-virgin olive oil (and occasionally coconut oil) over canola, corn, and other highly processed oils. Olive oil is rich in polyphenols, which help prevent cellular damage and reduce the risk of chronic diseases. I steer clear of soy and ditch refined table salt in favor of Himalayan pink salt for its mineral content. I avoid nightshades—eggplant, tomatoes, peppers, and potatoes—because they can trigger inflammation, particularly in people with certain autoimmune diseases. As for sweeteners, I eschew all artificial sweeteners and stick to the judicious use of raw honey, maple syrup, and dates. Food triggers are highly individual, but the recipes here avoid many of the common ones.

*The "Dirty Dozen" is an annual list highlighting fruits and vegetables most commonly found with pesticide residues. Compiled by the Environmental Working Group (EWG), this list is based on data from the U.S. Department of Agriculture (USDA) and the Food and Drug Administration (FDA). Foods on this list typically have thin skins or are consumed unpeeled, making them harder to thoroughly clean of pesticides.

Shifting from processed foods to a diet rich in nutrients helps foster clear and glowing skin, strengthened immunity, better sleep, increased energy and muscle mass, weight loss, improved cholesterol, reduced inflammation, stabilized blood sugar levels, better mood, and increased mental clarity. Other benefits include lowering the risk of cardiovascular disease and certain cancers and improving metabolism, digestive health, and overall well-being.

I fervently hope this cookbook will become a valuable and trusted resource in your quest for optimal health.

Radical Acceptance

These days, my body is a veritable shit show and a lot to navigate. Living in a constant state of uncertainty is hard. Despite all of that, I am so grateful. Grateful for the functions it still gets right, and grateful for each day.

I've learned that I can create a rich life within four walls. A simpler life. It has required radical acceptance. I bring a keen awareness and appreciation of my surroundings, and I celebrate each small victory. I protect myself from indifference. And I go to bed dreaming of the cake I plan to bake the following day, even if I've baked it a billion times. And though grief is not a linear process, somehow, I always find my way back to a place of equanimity.

It's as though I've lost one of my senses and the others have become heightened. As someone who is food-obsessed, my indoor life hinges on a deep embrace of each changing season and a celebration of its bounty.

I love spring's cheerful awakening and the way it announces itself with birds chirping and leaves budding. Asparagus is fresh and abundant, chive blossoms make a brief appearance, and there's the promise of sweet summer berries around the next bend. By mid-April I'm on salmon watch, stalking the Costco meat department by phone, eagerly awaiting the first wild Alaska king salmon of the season.

Before you know it, summer is in full bloom, and I've had my first strawberries of the season. Soon cherries and blackberries will be at peak ripeness—their fleeting availability being part of their charm. Long days and the sounds of children playing late into the afternoon, the wafting scent from our neighbors' grills, peaches so juicy they need to be enjoyed over the kitchen sink... it all makes my heart leap with appreciation.

As summer gives way to shorter, cooler days, it's my chance to snag some figs at their finest. Fall's arrival means I can say goodbye to the mealy apples from last year's harvest and sink my teeth into a crisp, bright Honeycrisp—likely slathered in almond butter.

Winter is my friend. It's when everyone retreats to their indoor spaces, and we embrace all that is cozy. It's a celebratory time with holidays, hearty winter greens, and endless reasons to bake treats. It's a time when being indoors is normalized, a shared experience rather than one of the things that separates us. Each season brings something to savor, and as one season slips away, I greet the next with anticipation.

My husband of over twenty years is a self-proclaimed "turbo introvert." A real indoor enthusiast. Even though I lament his gaming habits, I admit it's one of the keys to our success, as he's quite happily parked in front of his computer most of the time. We joke that my illness cramps my style *way* more than his.

I build some structure into each day by starting with a morning ritual of supporting my circadian rhythm. I stand on my front balcony looking into the sunlight while performing gentle lymph massage. Then, I'm off to the kitchen to assess the dinner situation. Dinner is the bane of my existence, if I'm honest. It requires the most of my stamina—if there are greens to wash or dressings to make, I do it first thing. These small acts may seem mundane, but they make me happy, as it's never lost on me that having fresh organic food and the ability to create something with my own hands is a privilege.

PANTRY ESSENTIALS

Here, I aim to take the guesswork out of brand choices. Over time, I've found certain brands to be more reliable, flavorful, and affordable, or to contain better ingredients. They are listed here not because of any brand loyalty or personal relationship, but simply to make your life easier—particularly if you're making profound changes to your diet. Some of these ingredients may be unfamiliar to you. Please note that vendors can change over time; these suggestions reflect my choices at the time of print.

ALMOND BUTTER

Check the ingredient list to be sure it's free of additives and sugar and made with roasted almonds rather than raw. Costco's Kirkland Signature brand is good quality and an economical option. Be sure to stir each new jar well. That can be easily accomplished by inserting a single electric beater into the jar and blending. Make sure you have a solid grip on the jar when you do it!

ALMOND FLOUR

Bob's Red Mill is my preferred brand because of its fine grind. I often wait until it goes on sale and stock up. Store it at room temperature and not in the fridge, or it will absorb moisture. A one-pound bag of almond flour contains less than five cups, so you'll go through it quickly if you bake regularly. All the recipes in this book use blanched almond flour, rather than natural almond meal.

ANCHOVIES

It's not necessary to use expensive anchovies. I like the small tins of Cento anchovies at Trader Joe's. It's so nice to have a single-use option because once anchovies packed in olive oil are refrigerated, the oil solidifies, making it harder to fish them out.

BAKING CHOCOLATE

Guittard 100% cacao baking bars are my favorite, by a mile. They have depth of flavor and contain only cacao beans and come as a box of three 2-ounce (57-g) bars. Wait for them to go on sale and load up! This San Francisco-based, family-owned company also omits soy from all of its products.

BLACK PEPPER

When pepper is ground, the oils begin to dissipate and taste less vibrant over time. Always opt to use a pepper mill for the freshest cracked black pepper. All the recipes here call for coarsely ground pepper, and a pepper mill also allows you to dial up or down to vary the grind from fine to coarse. In my opinion, black pepper is overused and doesn't belong in every dish.

COCOA POWDER

I prefer Dutch process cocoa and use Valrhona cocoa exclusively because of its deep, rich flavor and velvety hue. It can be found packaged in bulk tubs at Whole Foods or online. Guittard Cocoa Rouge (not its organic natural) is my next choice.

COCONUT AMINOS

Coconut aminos is a soy-free, gluten-free seasoning sauce made from the sap of coconut trees and is often used as a substitute for soy sauce in cooking. Whatever brand you choose, the only ingredients should be coconut nectar, water, and salt. My favorites are from Trader Joe's or Big Tree Farms.

COCONUT CREAM

Seek out thick and additive-free coconut cream, such as Savoy, which can be found in select grocery stores, Asian markets, and online. I also like Let's Do Organic's Organic Heavy Coconut Cream, but it contains more liquid and will only net about half the amount of whipped cream compared to the Savoy brand. It also has a looser texture once whipped. If you plan to make coconut whipped cream, refrigerate the can for a minimum of twenty-four hours in advance.

COCONUT MILK

Canned coconut milk, which I use throughout this book, is very different than boxed coconut milk and should only contain coconut milk (or coconut extracts) and water. I like to shake the can of coconut milk well to combine the liquids and solids, and once opened, give it a stir before measuring. All the recipes in this book were developed using Trader Joe's organic coconut milk—full fat rather than reduced fat.

COCONUT OIL

I purchase unrefined virgin coconut oil in large tubs from Costco. It has a long shelf life, so don't worry about the larger container.

EXTRA-VIRGIN OLIVE OIL

This incredibly healthful oil serves as my primary cooking and finishing oil. Olive oils are notoriously not always pure, so find one you like and trust to be your kitchen staple. Costco's Kirkland Signature organic olive oil is my go-to. It's tested for purity, well balanced, and very affordable. Store it away from heat and light.

FLAX SEEDS

Buying whole flax seeds and grinding them yourself in a blender is less expensive than pre-ground—and it's more nutritious. A fresher, finer grind makes for better absorption of the nutrients. Store it in an airtight container in the fridge to maintain freshness.

HIMALAYAN PINK SALT

I use pink salt because of its trace mineral content and as a matter of utility because its grind is fairly universal, making for consistent measuring. Kosher salt measures very differently depending on brand (e.g., Morton versus Diamond Crystal). To achieve the balance of seasoning as intended, please use pink salt when specified.

MALDON SALT

Maldon salt is my flake salt of choice! Ordering the large tub online is the most economical way to go—and it makes a fantastic gift.

MAPLE SYRUP

Maple syrup is my preferred sweetener—be sure you're using pure maple syrup. Costco's Kirkland Signature brand is my go-to for quality and affordability.

MAYONNAISE

I avoid seed oils for the most part, but sometimes rely on aioli and mayo-based dressings to maximize my vegetable consumption. (It's a strategy.) The dressing and aioli recipes here will only be as good as the mayonnaise you use. Sir Kensington's organic mayonnaise is my preferred choice.

MEDJOOL DATES

Look for fresh, moist, and plump organic Medjool dates—I like the ones from Costco. I double-wrap them and store them in the fridge. I do not recommend using pitted dates because they dry out more quickly.

NUTS

I make my life easier by purchasing pre-toasted nuts when possible. If you're toasting them yourself, it's easiest to do the full bag at once. I like to toast them at 325°F within an inch of their life for maximum crunch and flavor—but keep a watchful eye on them because they can go from perfectly golden to scorched in seconds. Almonds are best stored in the pantry, but Brazil nuts, pecans, hazelnuts, and walnuts go rancid more quickly. Wrap them well and store in the fridge to extend their freshness.

ORGANIC PRODUCE

I use organic produce, when possible, but do not specify organic produce in my recipes because that's an individual choice and may be a matter of affordability. Consider using the Environmental Working Group's annual "Dirty Dozen" and "Clean Fifteen" lists as your guide. They can be found online.

PASTURED EGGS

Eggs from hens that are pastured (i.e., those allowed to roam outside and forage for food, as opposed to being confined in cages or indoor systems) are more nutritious. They contain higher levels of omega-3s, beta-carotene, and vitamins A, D, and E. And they're lower in cholesterol and saturated fat than eggs from hens raised on traditional feed.

RED BOAT FISH SAUCE

Red Boat brand fish sauce is the most flavorful and considered to be the "cleanest." It's widely available, but when you can find it at Trader Joe's, it's a steal. Once open, store it in the fridge.

SHERRY VINEGAR

Sherry vinegar has more depth and complexity than most other vinegars. Look for Spanish brands labeled as *vinagre de Jerez*. This designation of origin indicates that it's been aged for at least six months.

TAHINI

For maximum flavor choose a product made from toasted, not raw, sesame seeds. (After all, their flavor comes from toasting!) Whatever brand you use (I use 365 by Whole Foods Market), mix well, then refrigerate once opened.

TOASTED SESAME OIL

Toasted sesame oil is incredibly fragrant and flavorful. Be sure to use one made with toasted sesame seeds and store it in the fridge to preserve its freshness.

MY TOOLBOX: THE INDISPENSABLES

From high-speed blenders that effortlessly whip up smoothies and soups to the precision of a digital scale or a chef's knife that makes slicing and chopping a breeze, these essentials are designed to support your efforts. I find them essential for my cooking. By investing in these trusted tools, you'll streamline your process, achieve better results, and enjoy a more satisfying cooking experience from start to finish.

BLENDERS

I understand the sticker shock associated with a high-speed blender such as a Vitamix, but it will change your life. I use an immersion blender to blend my morning smoothie right in the same large tumbler I drink it from. A quick swish in soapy water and it's ready for the following day. An immersion blender is also a no-fuss way to blend soups right in the pot, though keep in mind the texture may not be quite as smooth as when using a traditional blender.

CAKE PANS

I use 6-inch (15-cm) round pans for all my layer cake recipes because cakes made with almond flour are dense and have some heft. The pans will remain nonstick unless you scratch the surface, so treat them with care. My favorites are the Goldtouch Pro nonstick pans from Williams Sonoma.

CHEF'S KNIFE

A quality knife is a worthwhile investment that will dramatically impact the ease and efficiency of preparing meals. The workhorse in my kitchen is the Global Classic 7-inch (18-cm) hollow-ground santoku knife (G-80). I own several of them. Each time I get a new one, I keep a rubber band around the handle for the first couple months to remind me that it's sharper than the other ones.

CITRUS REAMER

I use a good bit of citrus in these recipes, and the easiest way to extract all the juice is with a citrus reamer. I prefer the non-porous plastic versions that are dishwasher-safe, rather than one made of wood.

CUTTING BOARDS

I order 8 × 11-inch (20 × 28-cm) white plastic cutting boards online and keep eight on hand. They are non-porous, dishwasher-safe, lightweight, and perfect for smaller tasks. Plus, they take up the same amount of space as a dinner plate in your dishwasher, making them incredibly practical.

DIGITAL SCALE

A digital scale is an affordable and invaluable tool, especially when measuring ingredients like chocolate or ensuring precise vegetable weights for a recipe. And, even if you're not yet using it for your baked goods, it's helpful in many other ways. (See "Baking with a Kitchen Scale" on page 25).

INSTANT-READ THERMOMETER

My go-to thermometer for speed and accuracy is the Thermapen ONE by ThermoWorks. It's perfect for ensuring your meats and seafood are cooked to perfection. Why invest in high-quality meats and seafood, only to risk overcooking them?

MANDOLINE

I keep my full-size mandoline mostly tucked away because it feels clunky, but I use the OXO Good Grips handheld mandoline slicer regularly. It's inexpensive, lightweight, compact, and ideal for quick, even slicing of onions, cucumbers, radishes, and more. Plus, it's dishwasher-safe, so cleanup is a breeze.

METAL TONGS

Metal tongs are essential in my kitchen for tasks like flipping fish, chops, and steaks, and transferring hot vegetables. The OXO 9-inch (23-cm) stainless steel locking tongs are my favorite.

MICROPLANE

I shudder to think of a time before the Microplane grater existed. It's essential for zesting citrus, grating garlic and ginger, or creating a fine dusting of nutmeg. If you use one regularly, be sure to replace it every few years to maintain its sharpness.

MINI FOOD PROCESSOR

A mini food processor is a lightweight and easy-to-use tool that's indispensable for small jobs such as making salad dressings.

PARCHMENT PAPER

Spending a little extra on pre-cut sheets and rounds of parchment paper has made my life easier. No more wrangling the roll! Also, parchment paper acts as a barrier between your food and aluminum, which is a toxic metal that can accumulate in your body. Liberate yourself. The easier the process, the more cakes you'll bake!

RIMMED BAKING SHEETS

A half sheet pan (18 × 13-inch) is generally the standard for home use. It's a versatile workhorse, and I can never have too many. The Nordic Ware half sheet pan is my favorite for all-around durability and heat conduction. I have a few quarter sheet pans (13 × 9-inch) for smaller tasks.

RUBBER SPATULAS

Rubber spatulas are essential for folding ingredients and scraping batter from bowls. I love the OXO silicone spoon spatula for its one-piece design and durability. Smaller spatulas are perfect for getting every last bit out of jars or mixing bowls.

SALAD SPINNERS

Salad spinners help extend the life of your produce and make it easy to wash, spin dry, and store leafy greens in one vessel. I use the OXO large spinner for salad greens and the OXO small spinner for parsley, cilantro, and other herbs. They stack nicely in the fridge.

SPRINGFORM PAN

I love a springform pan. Cakes made with almond flour and maple syrup can be trickier to get out of a cake pan. Also, many of the cakes in this book have nut toppings, which require extra care if using a standard cake pan. So, for ease of removal, most of the cake recipes here use a 9-inch (23-cm) nonstick springform pan. I recommend hand washing them because they tend to rust in the dishwasher.

STAINLESS STEEL COOKWARE

I use All-Clad cookware exclusively for its unbeatable quality and durability. It's commercial-grade, oven-safe, and will last a lifetime with proper care. Each year, I add one piece to my collection, as it's definitely an investment.

WECK JARS

Glass Weck jars with plastic lids are perfect for storing leftovers or smaller portions in the fridge and freezer. They're stackable and airtight, and they protect against odors and freezer burn. I use the 743 for soups and energy balls and the 900 for coconut milk, cooked proteins, and concentrated chicken stock. The plastic lids must be ordered separately.

WHISKS

I don't use standard balloon whisks—I prefer slimmer-profile whisks for greater control and efficiency. For dressings, vinaigrettes, and small amounts of ganache, I use a mini 6-inch (15-cm) whisk, while for cake batter, I opt for an 8-inch (20-cm) whisk. A whisk with more tines makes mixing faster and easier. French whisks also have a slimmer profile and more tines than a standard balloon whisk.

COOKING FROM THIS BOOK

Cooking with efficiency and ease is all about setting yourself up for success with smart preparation and the right tools. Here are strategies to streamline your cooking process, from measuring ingredients accurately to prepping proteins in advance, allowing you to spend less time in the kitchen and ensuring each recipe turns out as intended.

Ingredient Handling & Measurement

INGREDIENTS MATTER

The recipes here rely on fresh, well-sourced ingredients rather than fancy techniques. I recommend sourcing the best produce and meats available to you and saving recipes like the Fresh Strawberry Pie and the Black Forest Cake for when strawberries and cherries are in season and at their peak ripeness.

SUBSTITUTIONS

I'm sure you've heard that baking is a science, and it's true. All the baked goods contained in this book have been thoughtfully crafted and made a billion times in my home kitchen to ensure they turn out perfectly for you. I've cut the clutter and abbreviated as many steps as possible, but the ingredients listed and the steps involved are important to the success of each recipe. Each ingredient plays a key role in the structure, moisture balance, and flavor, so I recommend not making any substitutions. The ingredients used in these recipes (almond flour, maple syrup, coconut flour, etc.) *are* the substitutions!

BAKING WITH ALMOND FLOUR

Almond flour is dense and moist, and therefore less forgiving than other gluten-free flours. Be sure to measure accurately and avoid making substitutions. Using a scale to weigh the almond flour is the most accurate method of measurement. You can also achieve consistent results using the fluff, dip, and sweep method for measuring almond flour: Pour the almond flour into an airtight storage container and give it a little shake to fluff the contents. Dip your measuring cup directly into the bag or container, overfilling the cup. Then use the flat edge of a knife to sweep the excess off the top and level it. Do not pack almond flour or use your finger to level it, or you might end up with a dense cake.

BAKING WITH A KITCHEN SCALE

I was late to the kitchen scale party, but it has changed my life. By using a scale, I'm able to get cakes and muffins into the oven in about ten minutes. You don't have to understand metric measurements to save time and energy by using a digital kitchen scale for your baking. Simply set the bowl on the scale, tare it (zero it out), and spoon or pour the ingredients into the bowl, zeroing it out before you add each new ingredient. No more scraping sticky ingredients like honey, maple syrup, or almond butter out of measuring cups, and no more washing dirty measuring cups. Baking tutorials can be found in the "highlights" on my Instagram account (@the.rachel.riggs).

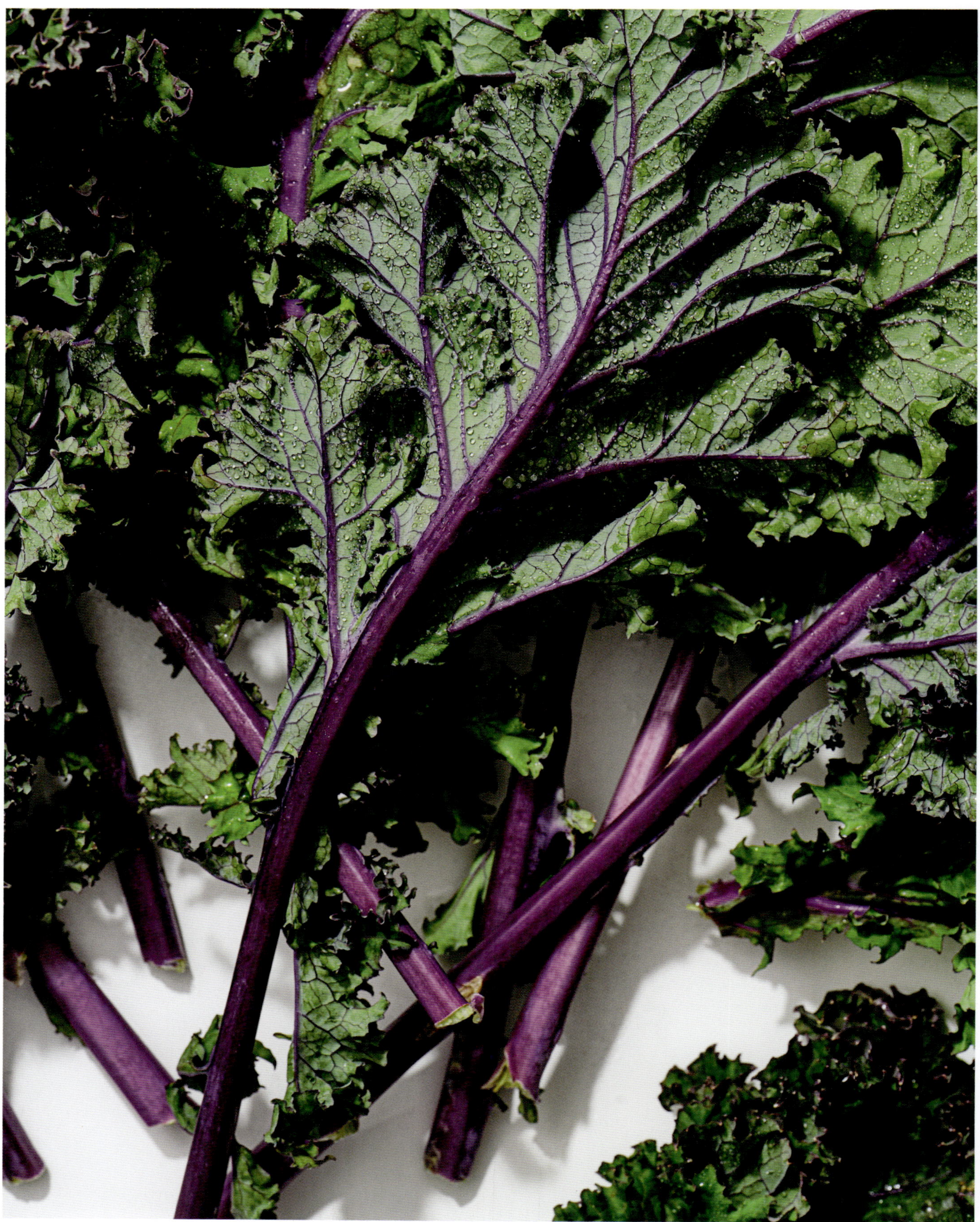

MEASURING COCONUT FLOUR

Coconut flour is hyper-absorbent, so I use strategic amounts of it in my baking to add moisture balance. For accuracy, be sure to level it with a knife when measuring it, instead of using your finger.

USING FRESH GINGER

Storing fresh ginger in the freezer means you'll always have some when you need it, and frozen ginger grates up nice and fluffy instead of the fibers gumming up your Microplane. Make sure the ginger is well wrapped, and use a vegetable peeler to freshen up the exposed surfaces before each use.

ZESTING CITRUS

Grating citrus zest is best accomplished while holding the fruit in your non-dominant hand and the Microplane in your dominant hand. Position the Microplane above the fruit, rather than under it. This allows you to see the area being zested and prevents you from zesting the bitter pith. Aim for a single pass with the Microplane—additional passes end up zesting the pith. You can find a demo of this in the "highlights" on my Instagram account (@the.rachel.riggs).

Meal Prep Strategies

READING THROUGH EACH RECIPE IN ADVANCE

Reading each recipe all the way through before beginning ensures there are no surprises and gives you a sense of the time commitment and kitchen tools involved. You will notice that I suggest making many of the dips, dressings, and aioli a few hours in advance so the flavors can develop.

WASHING GREENS IN ADVANCE

Washing your greens in advance, when possible, ensures they are cool and crisp rather than wilted and waterlogged. Wet greens will dilute your dressing. Use a large salad spinner to submerge the greens and agitate gently. If the water is dirty or there's a lot of sediment at the bottom, repeat the process. Spin dry, line the bowl with paper towels to wick away any excess moisture, and store in the fridge until use.

MEAL-PREPPING PROTEINS

Having pre-cooked chicken available for recipes puts you ahead of the game. Here are some easy options.

Rotisserie chicken: Grab a ready-made chicken, remove the chicken from the bone, pack it in glass jars, and refrigerate.

Baked chicken breasts: Bake bone-in, skin-on chicken breasts until an instant-read thermometer inserted into the meat registers an internal temperature of 165°F.

Roasted whole chicken: I suggest roasting two chickens, side by side, on a rimmed baking sheet so there are lots of leftovers. Cook the chickens to an internal temperature of 160°F because carryover cooking during the resting period will bring the temperature up to 165°F.

For the best texture, I prefer cooking whole chickens and chicken breasts that have never been frozen, but the most critical step is to not overcook them. Remove the chicken from the bone, discard the skin, refrigerate some, and freeze the rest. My favorite strategy is to pack the chicken tightly into glass Weck 900 jars (with plastic lids), which hold two 4-ounce servings (8-oz/227-g total) of cooked chicken. Thaw it as needed for salads and other recipes; reheating is not necessary. I do the same with fresh salmon because I find previously frozen salmon to be mealy. Cook fresh salmon to an internal temperature of 130°F, then pack it into Weck 900 jars (with plastic lids) and freeze it. It thaws beautifully and doesn't require reheating.

BREAKING UP YOUR MEAL PREP

Rinsing greens and spinning them dry in the salad spinner in the morning allows them to cool down and crisp up by dinnertime. All the dressings, vinaigrettes, and relishes in this book will benefit from being made in advance. It gives the flavors a chance to develop and reach their potential. When dinner rolls around, it will be a speedier process and an assembly-only situation.

FOOD WASTE & AFFORDABILITY

It's important to acknowledge that nutritious whole foods—particularly if you don't consume grains and legumes—are more expensive than packaged and processed foods. The best way to manage this is to avoid throwing food away. Meal planning is key: Rather than leaving the grocery store with a random collection of items, I have a list and a plan. Then every ten days or so, we have what we call "bit and bob" night where all the leftover bits get rounded up and turned into dinner. Sometimes it's surprisingly tasty, and other times not so much, but it's deeply satisfying to achieve a nearly zero waste situation.

Shopping for food more often—usually twice per week—helps ensure freshness and allows for switching gears mid-week if cravings lead in another direction. I wait for more expensive pantry items like almond flour and baking chocolate to go on sale and then stock up. The other way to manage costs is keeping proteins (fish, bison, chicken) at 4 ounces (114 g) per serving and avoiding overeating in general. And if I spot something in the fridge that will not be consumed by its best-before date, I get it into the freezer. Taking control where you can helps the planet and your pocketbook, and it feels really good.

Cooking Techniques & Tools

GETTING TO KNOW YOUR OVEN

It's not unusual for oven temperatures to be inaccurate or for it to take longer to reach temperatures than the indicator bell would lead us to think. Accurate temperatures are especially important when baking with almond flour and maple syrup, as is the case here. Oven thermometers are inexpensive and will help you identify a miscalibration. If you discover a discrepancy, dial the oven temperature up or down to compensate rather than increasing the cook time.

TEMPING YOUR SPENDY PROTEINS

When it comes to cooking fish or meat of any kind, my philosophy is exceedingly simple: Start with the freshest product possible and *do not overcook*. Preventing overcooking is far more important than the cooking method or seasoning. Use an instant-read thermometer to ensure perfect results instead of leaving it to chance.

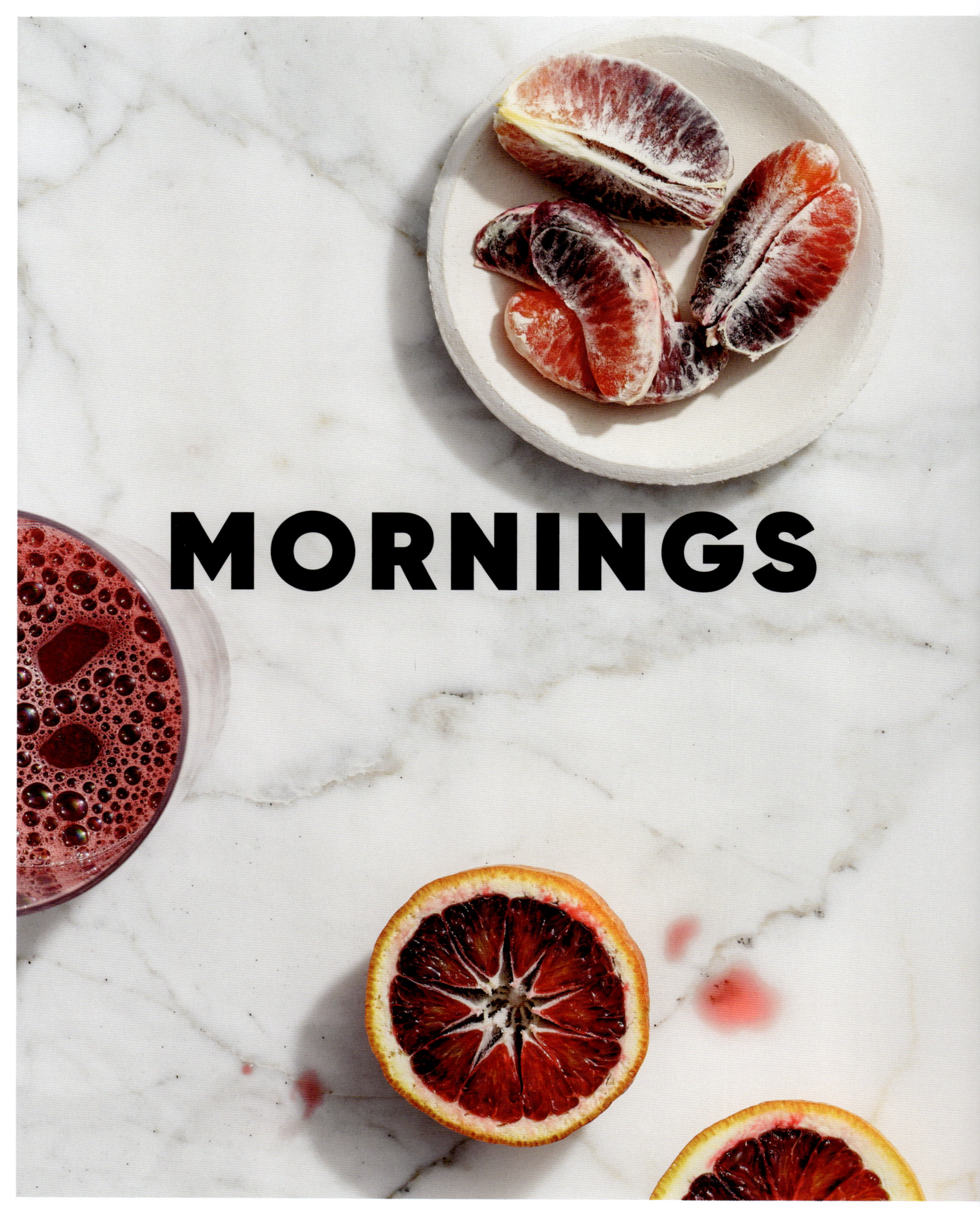

MORNINGS

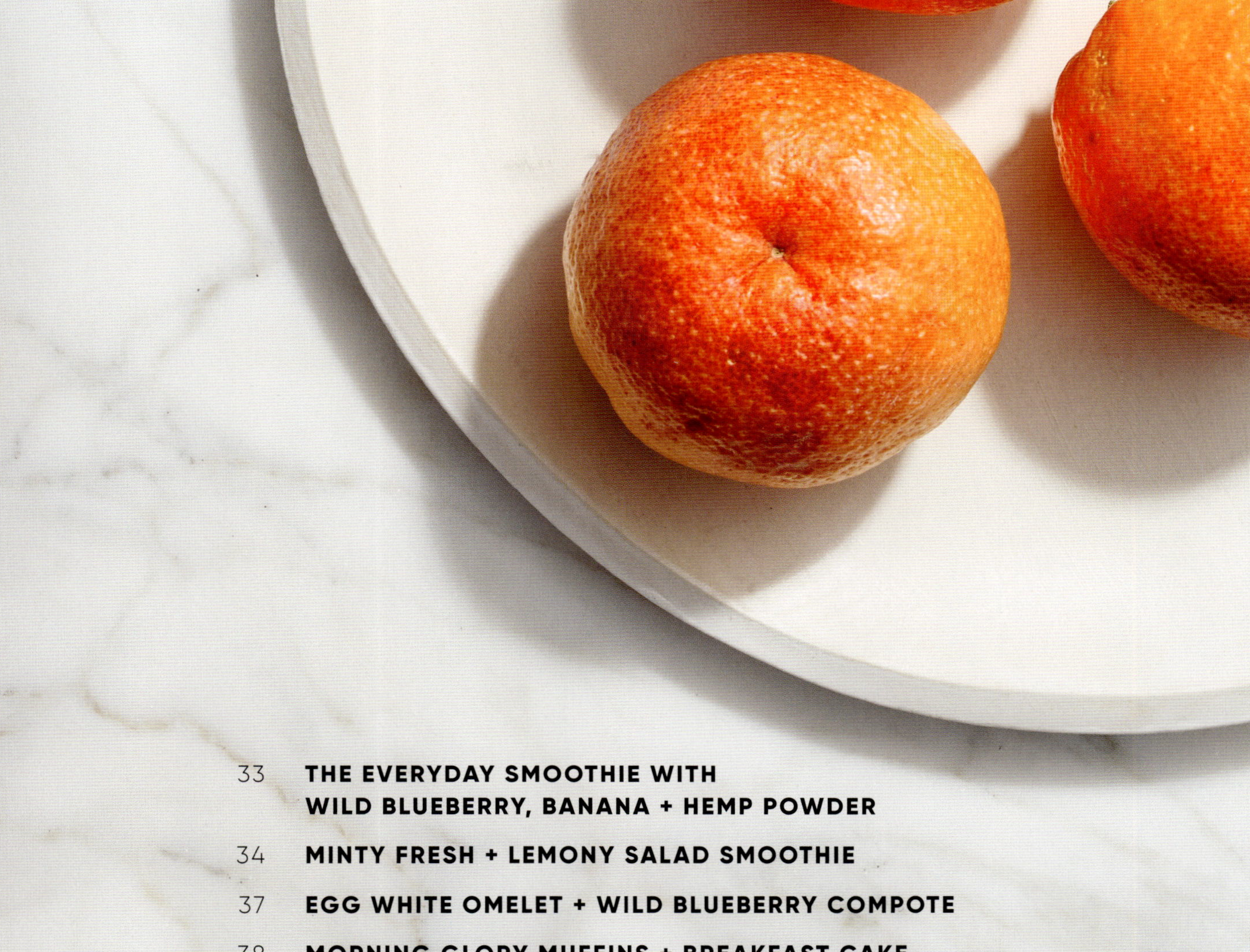

33 **THE EVERYDAY SMOOTHIE WITH WILD BLUEBERRY, BANANA + HEMP POWDER**

34 **MINTY FRESH + LEMONY SALAD SMOOTHIE**

37 **EGG WHITE OMELET + WILD BLUEBERRY COMPOTE**

38 **MORNING GLORY MUFFINS + BREAKFAST CAKE**

41 **VANILLA COCONUT YOGURT + WILD BLUEBERRY COMPOTE**

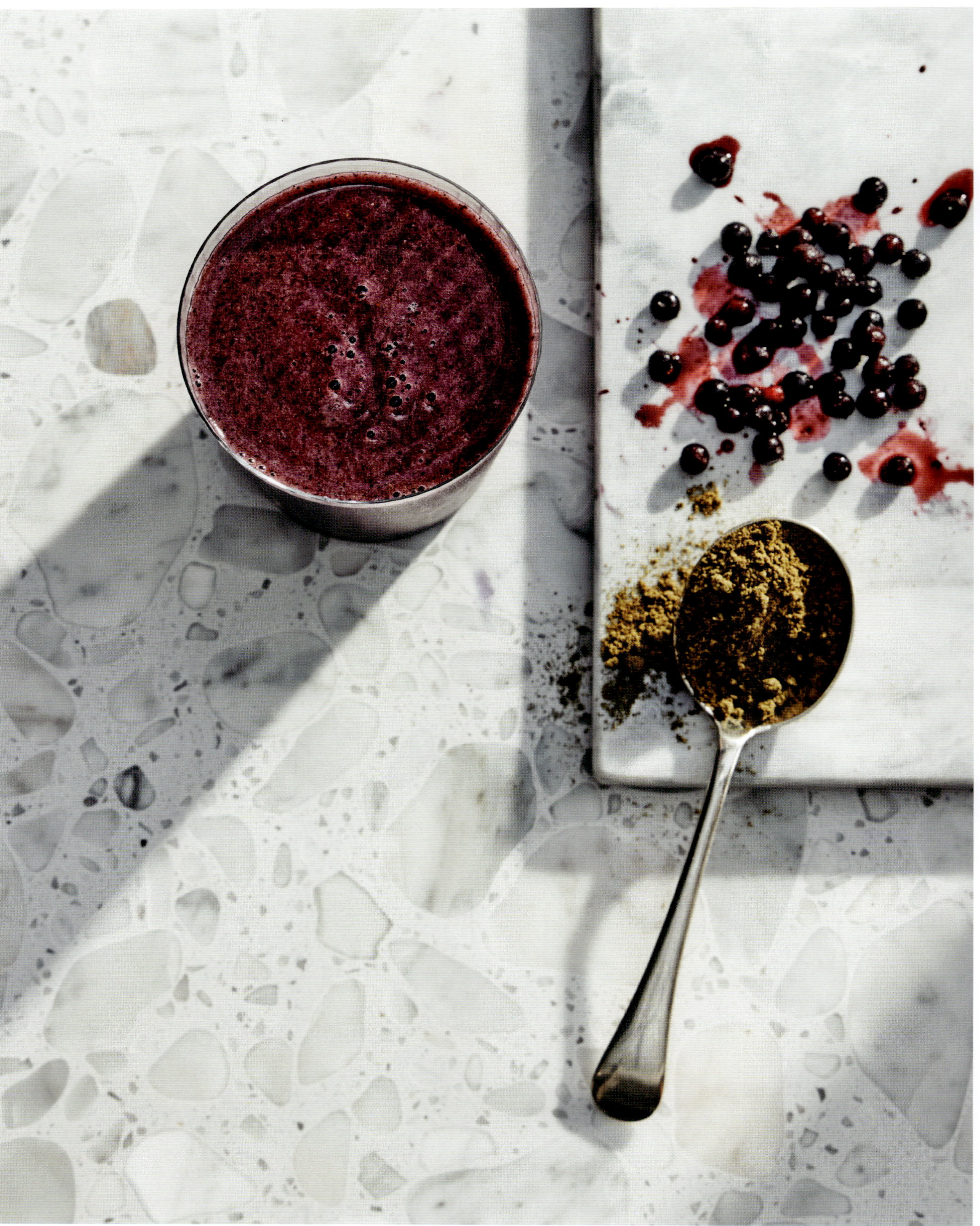

Hemp is my favorite choice of protein powder because it's a complete source of protein—meaning it provides all nine essential amino acids. It also contains a good bit of iron and is less processed than other plant proteins. When adding a ripe banana to a smoothie, its sweetness balances the subtle grassiness of the hemp. If you're unsure about the hemp flavor, you can start with the vanilla-flavored powder and graduate over time to the unflavored formula.

Wild blueberries are critical to a great-tasting smoothie. They are sweet and intensely flavored and contain nearly twice as many antioxidants as regular blueberries. These simple (but specific) ingredients provide a good balance of flavor and nutrients.

Flax seed is another great addition to your smoothie. It's rich in fiber, omega-3 fatty acids, and phytochemicals like lignans, as well as alpha-linolenic acid. Grinding whole flax seeds yourself in a high-speed blender will help you get a fresher, finer grind and therefore absorb more of the nutrients.

This delicious smoothie with wild blueberries, banana, and hemp powder has been my morning strategy for years! It's ice-free, so it comes together at lightning speed using an immersion blender directly in a 743 Weck jar (or something of similar size), which also doubles as a drinking vessel. For added convenience, I use water instead of nut milks. All you need is a steady supply of frozen wild blueberries (I find them at Trader Joe's) and fresh bananas, and you're set to start the day off right.

I usually munch on a couple Brazil nuts while I make my smoothie. They provide the recommended daily intake of selenium, and the healthy fats help slow the absorption of sugars from the fruit, while also aiding in the absorption of my morning supplements.

The Everyday Smoothie with Wild Blueberry, Banana + Hemp Powder

SERVES 1

- 1 ripe banana
- 1 cup (130 g) frozen wild blueberries
- 2–3 tablespoons pure hemp protein powder
- 1 cup (240 g) cold filtered water
- 1 tablespoon ground flax seeds (optional)

Combine all ingredients in a blender and blend until smooth. Enjoy immediately.

If you set yourself a high bar for vegetable consumption, you know that some days the thought of staring down a plate of veg is simply out of the question. This smoothie is not only refreshing and flavorful (with the most delightful verdant hue), but also a great way sneak in essential nutrients. Romaine is a powerhouse in the nutrient department—packed with minerals as well as vitamins A, C, and K to help your body function at its best.

Minty Fresh + Lemony Salad Smoothie

SERVES 1

- 4 cups (140 g) roughly chopped romaine hearts (see Note)
- 5 large fresh mint leaves (or 2–3 basil leaves)
- ½ ripe avocado, pitted and peeled
- 1 tablespoon honey
- 2 tablespoons freshly squeezed lemon juice
- A good pinch of pink salt
- 1 cup (240 g) cold filtered water
- 1 cup (135 g) ice

Combine all ingredients in a blender and blend until smooth. It's best when slightly slushy but not overly thick. If it's not icy cold, add a few more ice cubes and blend again. Serve immediately, as the avocado will discolor in time.

NOTE

Wash and spin dry the romaine lettuce in advance so it will be well chilled rather than warm and waterlogged—this makes for a better smoothie.

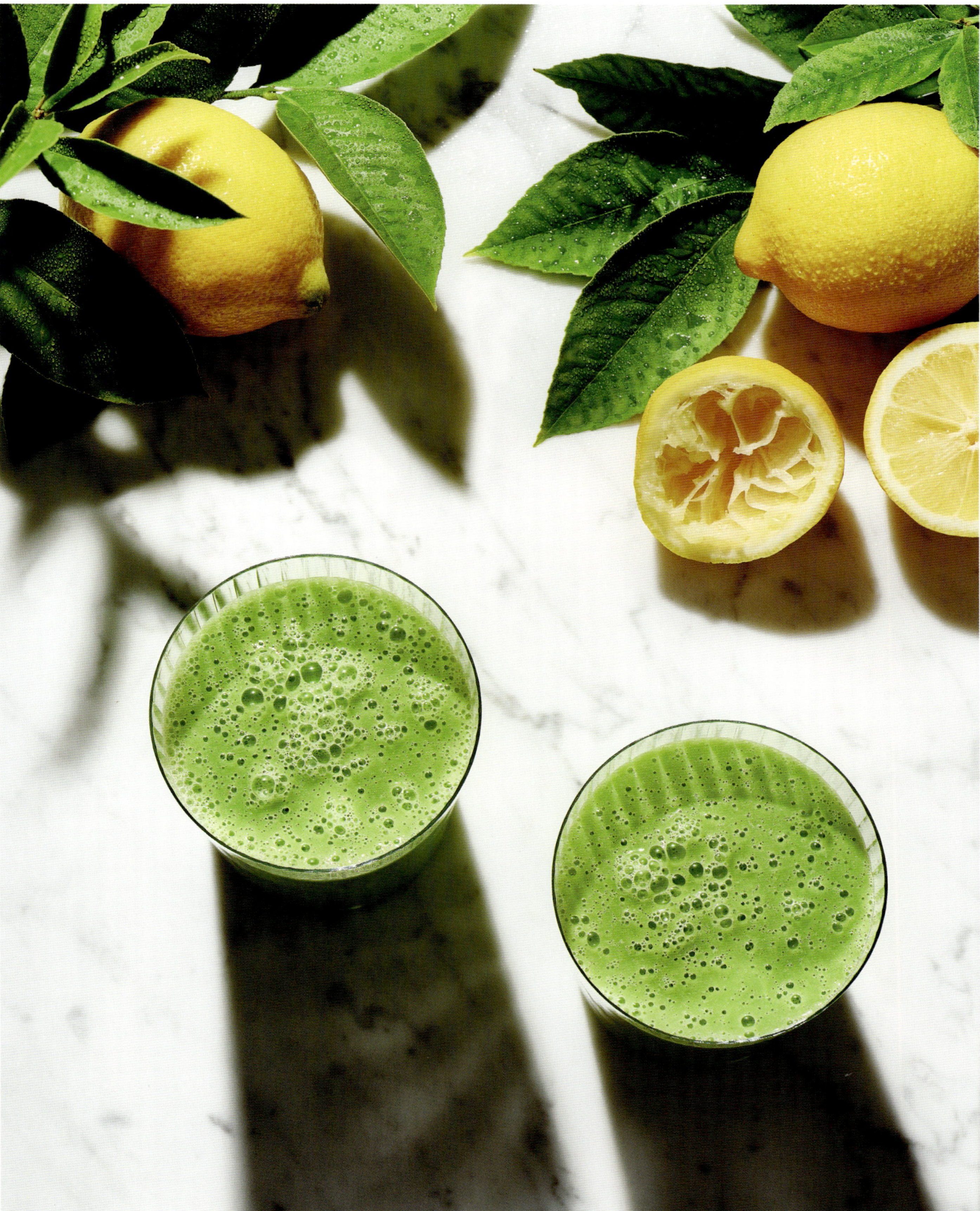

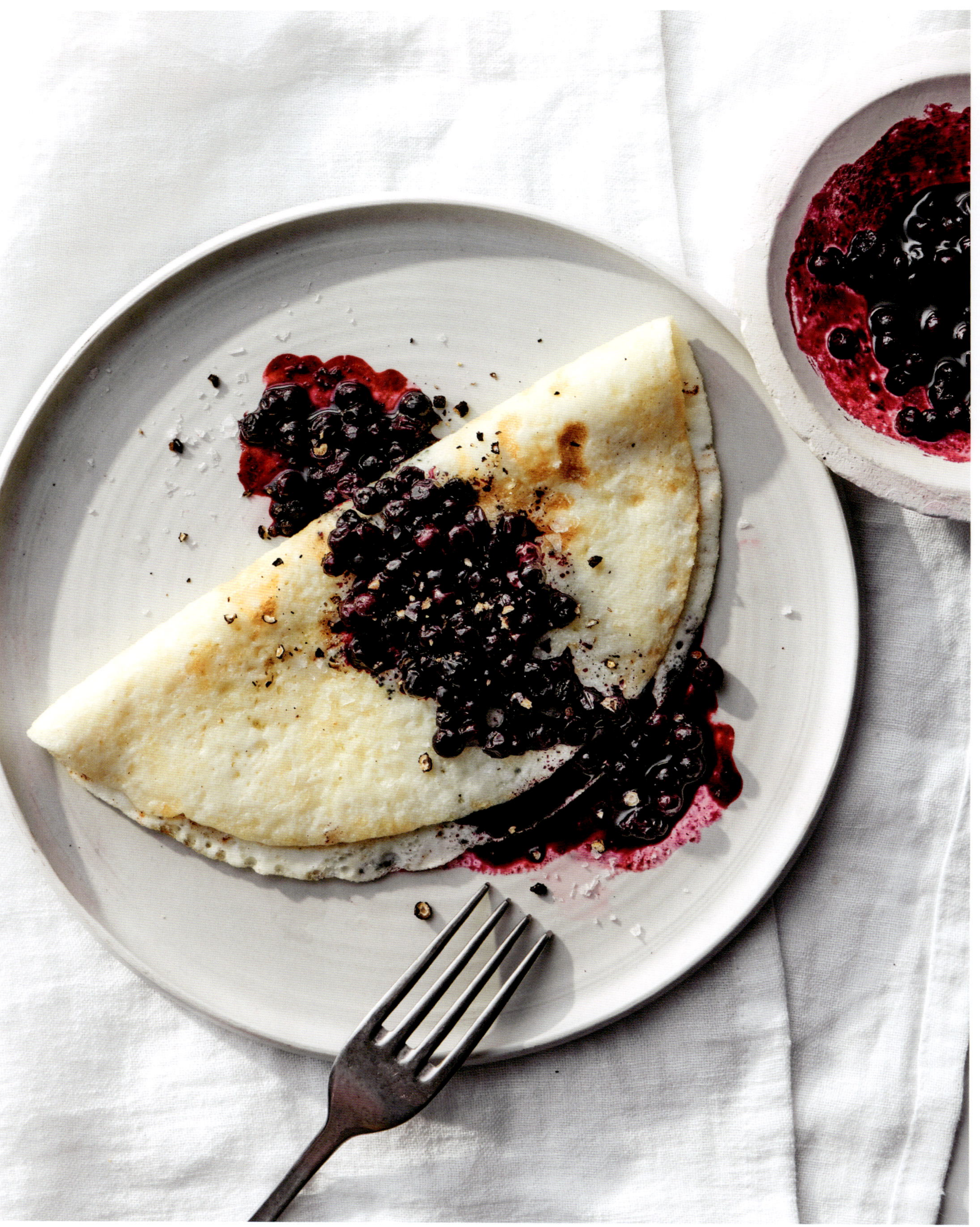

Wild blueberries are packed with nearly twice as many antioxidants as their cultivated counterparts thanks to a higher concentration of the flavonoid anthocyanin—so enjoy with abandon. This quick blueberry compote makes extra that can be spooned over coconut yogurt or used in a variety of other ways—you'll be happy to have extra!

Egg White Omelet + Wild Blueberry Compote

SERVES 4

Compote

1 (1-lb/454-g) bag frozen wild blueberries

3 tablespoons pure maple syrup

Pinch of pink salt

1 tablespoon freshly squeezed lemon juice

Omelet (per single serving)

Extra-virgin olive oil, for the pan

4 large egg whites, whisked until frothy

Maldon flake salt and freshly cracked black pepper

Ground cinnamon, for sprinkling

Compote In a medium saucepan (a small saucepan won't have enough surface area), combine the berries, maple syrup, and pink salt. Cook over high heat for 10–15 minutes—allowing it to bubble vigorously and stirring often to prevent it from sticking to the bottom—until it's reduced and slightly thickened. Remove from heat, then stir in lemon juice. Transfer to a bowl, then set it aside to cool and thicken.

Omelet Meanwhile, heat a generous splash of oil in a medium nonstick skillet (or omelet pan) over low heat. Add the egg whites and sprinkle with salt and pepper. Leave it untouched for the first minute, then cover and cook for 2 minutes. Using a rubber spatula, carefully run it along the edges and flip the entire thing. Cook for another minute, uncovered. Remove from heat.

Lightly sprinkle the omelet with cinnamon. Using the rubber spatula, fold it in half, enveloping the cinnamon. Gently slide it onto a plate for serving.

Top omelet with a few spoonfuls of blueberry compote, then season with flake salt and pepper. Repeat for additional omelets.

Leftover compote can be refrigerated for up to 5 days.

Snag one of these hearty muffins on your way out the door or enjoy as an anytime snack. They're nutritionally dense, loaded with fruit and nuts, and just sweet enough! The raisins and coconut provide important moisture balance, so please don't omit them. See the tip below to bake the batter as a breakfast cake!

Morning Glory Muffins + Breakfast Cake

MAKES 9 MUFFINS

- 2 cups (220 g) super-fine blanched almond flour
- ⅓ cup (30 g) finely shredded unsweetened coconut
- 2 teaspoons ground cinnamon
- 1 teaspoon baking soda
- ½ teaspoon pink salt
- 4 large eggs, room temperature
- ⅓ cup (105 g) pure maple syrup
- ¼ cup (50 g) extra-virgin olive oil
- 1 teaspoon vanilla extract
- 1½ cups (136 g) grated carrots (do not pack)
- ½ cup (83 g) raisins, plus ⅓ cup (52 g) for the topping
- 1 cup (120 g) chopped walnuts (divided)
- Maldon flake salt, for sprinkling

Preheat oven to 350°F. Line a muffin pan with 9 paper liners.

The best method for measuring almond flour by the cup can be found on page 25.

In a medium mixing bowl, combine almond flour, coconut, cinnamon, baking soda, and pink salt and whisk together, breaking up any lumps. Whisk in each of the remaining ingredients, except walnuts, until combined. Add ½ cup (60 g) of walnuts and whisk again until the ingredients are well combined.

Using a spoon, divide the batter among the prepared muffin cups. (Note: Cups will be full because almond flour doesn't rise as much as all-purpose flour.) Top muffins with the remaining ½ cup (60 g) of walnuts and ⅓ cup (52 g) of raisins. Finish with a light sprinkling of flake salt.

Bake for 25 minutes on the center rack. Set aside to cool.

Leftover muffins can be covered and stored at room temperature for up to 4 days.

NOTE

To bake as a cake, line an 8-inch (20-cm) square metal baking pan with parchment paper. Prepare the batter as directed, then pour it into the pan. Tap the pan on the counter a few times to level the batter. Sprinkle the remaining ½ cup (60 g) of walnuts and ⅓ cup (52 g) of raisins over the top, with the goal of covering all the batter. Finish with a light sprinkling of flake salt. Bake for 30 minutes on the center rack.

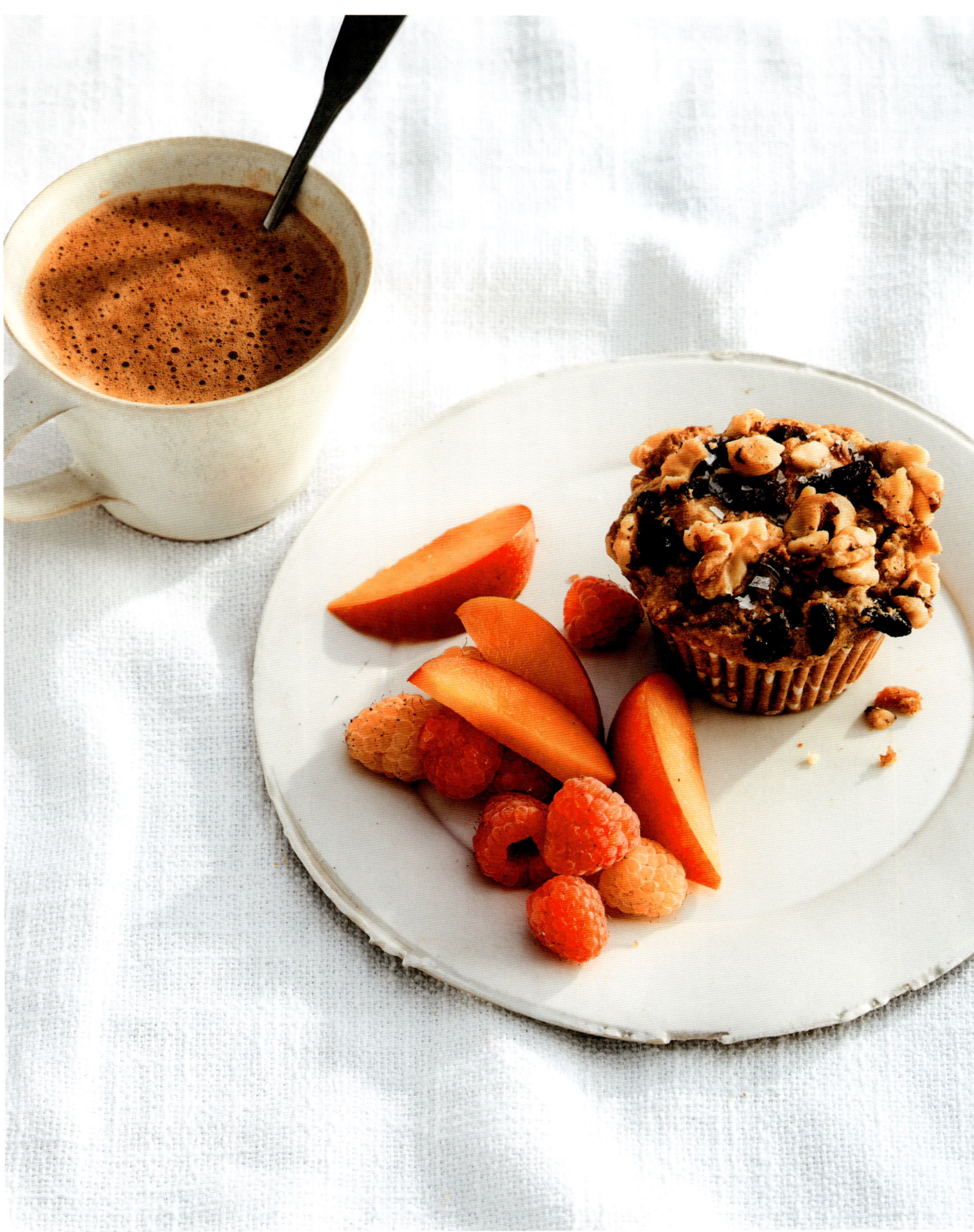

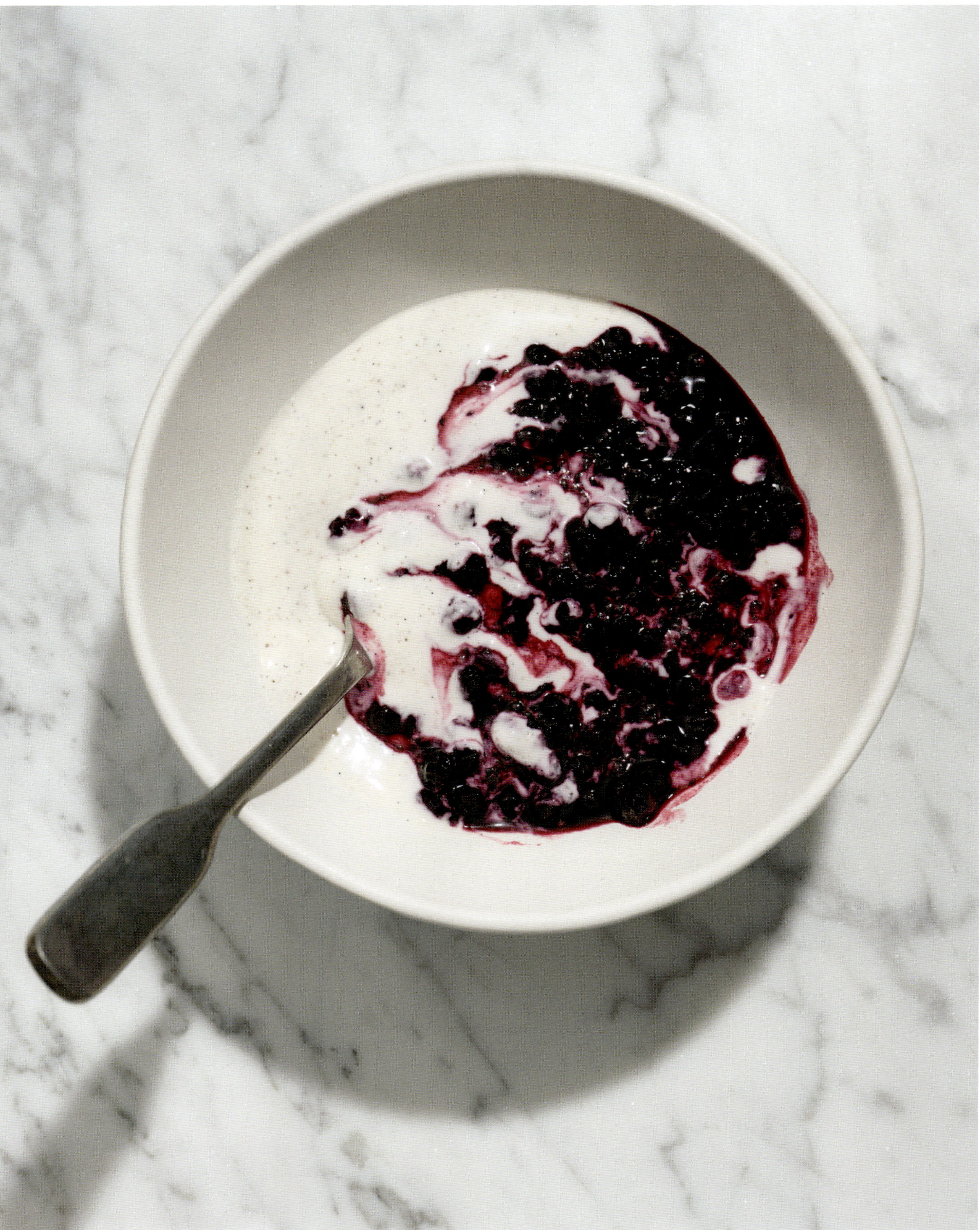

Cool, creamy coconut yogurt paired with sweet fruity compote is an easy way to begin your day. Vanilla bean paste has become ubiquitous, but most brands contain gums and additives. Once you make your own, you'll never go back! The quick blueberry compote is loaded with antioxidants and serves double duty, as it's also used for the Egg White Omelet on page 37.

Vanilla Coconut Yogurt + Wild Blueberry Compote

SERVES 4

Vanilla bean paste

¼ cup (80 g) pure maple syrup

2 teaspoons ground vanilla bean powder (see Note)

Yogurt

1 (16-oz/454-g) container unsweetened coconut yogurt (see Note)

1 tablespoon vanilla bean paste, or to taste

Compote

1 (1-lb/454-g) bag frozen wild blueberries

3 tablespoons pure maple syrup

Pinch of pink salt

1 tablespoon freshly squeezed lemon juice

Vanilla bean paste In a small bowl, mix the maple syrup and ground vanilla bean powder until combined. Refrigerate until needed. Leftover vanilla bean paste can be kept refrigerated in a sealed container for up to a month.

Yogurt Stir vanilla bean paste into the container of coconut yogurt. Refrigerate until needed.

Compote In a medium saucepan (a small saucepan won't have enough surface area), combine the berries, maple syrup, and salt. Cook over high heat for 10–15 minutes—allowing it to bubble vigorously and stirring often to prevent it from sticking to the bottom—until it's reduced and slightly thickened. Remove from heat, then stir in lemon juice. Transfer to a bowl, then set it aside to cool and thicken.

To serve, divide the yogurt among 4 small bowls. Top each with compote. Using the tip of a knife, drag the compote slightly through the yogurt to create swirls. Serve.

Leftover compote can be refrigerated for up to 5 days.

NOTES

I use Beyond Good pure ground vanilla bean powder.

My favorite coconut yogurt brand is Cocojune.

Frozen wild blueberries can be found at Trader Joe's.

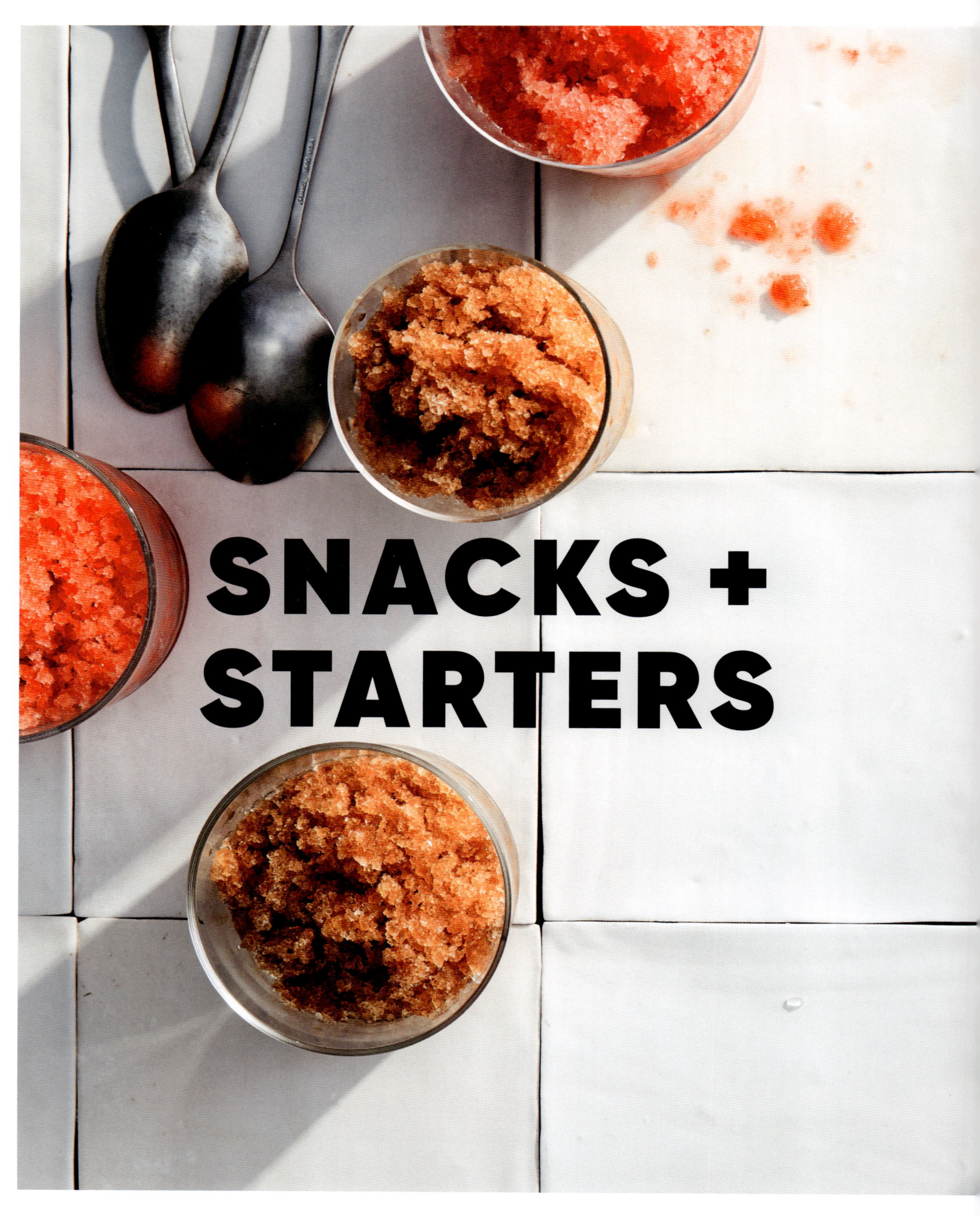

SNACKS + STARTERS

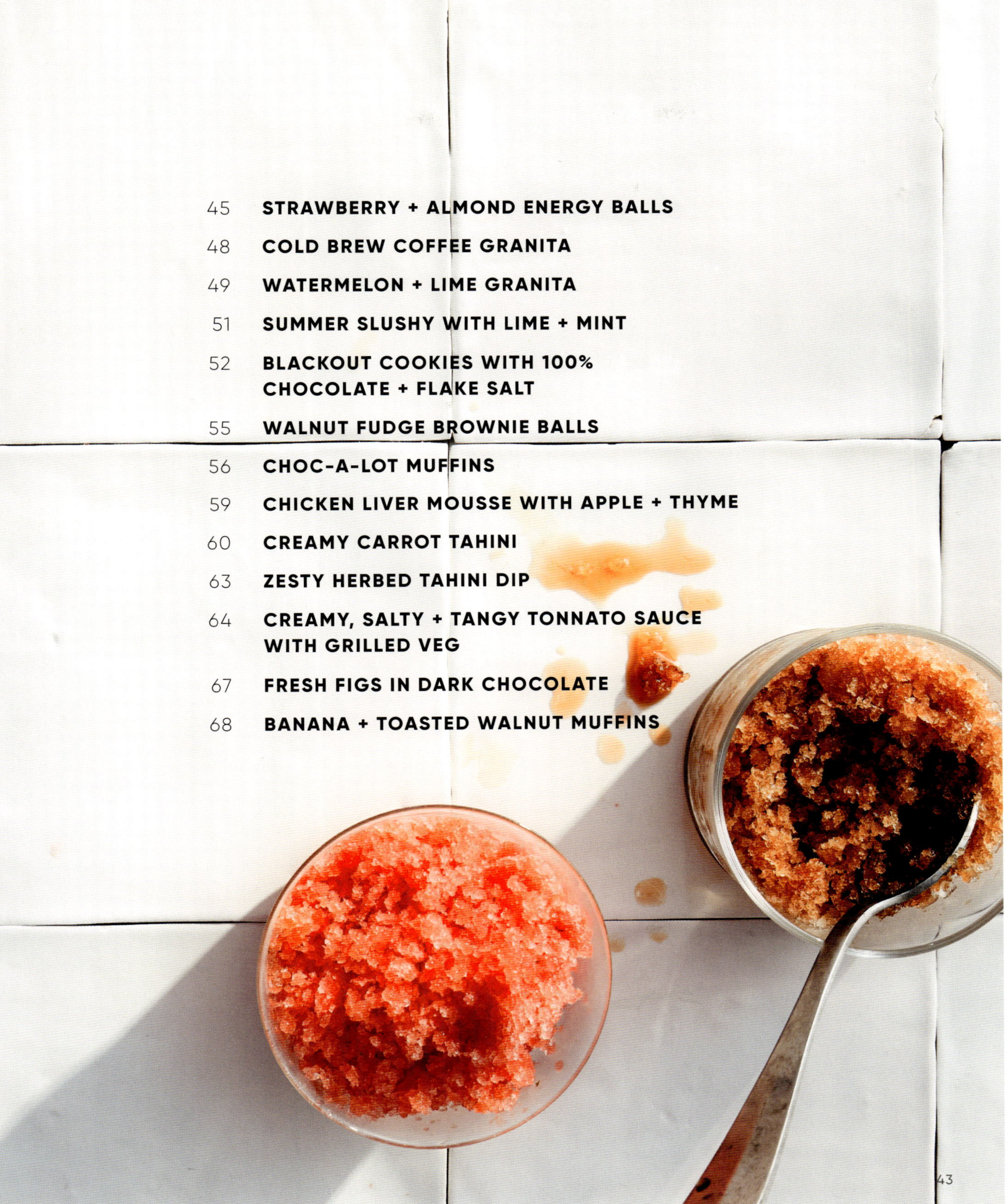

45 STRAWBERRY + ALMOND ENERGY BALLS

48 COLD BREW COFFEE GRANITA

49 WATERMELON + LIME GRANITA

51 SUMMER SLUSHY WITH LIME + MINT

52 BLACKOUT COOKIES WITH 100% CHOCOLATE + FLAKE SALT

55 WALNUT FUDGE BROWNIE BALLS

56 CHOC-A-LOT MUFFINS

59 CHICKEN LIVER MOUSSE WITH APPLE + THYME

60 CREAMY CARROT TAHINI

63 ZESTY HERBED TAHINI DIP

64 CREAMY, SALTY + TANGY TONNATO SAUCE WITH GRILLED VEG

67 FRESH FIGS IN DARK CHOCOLATE

68 BANANA + TOASTED WALNUT MUFFINS

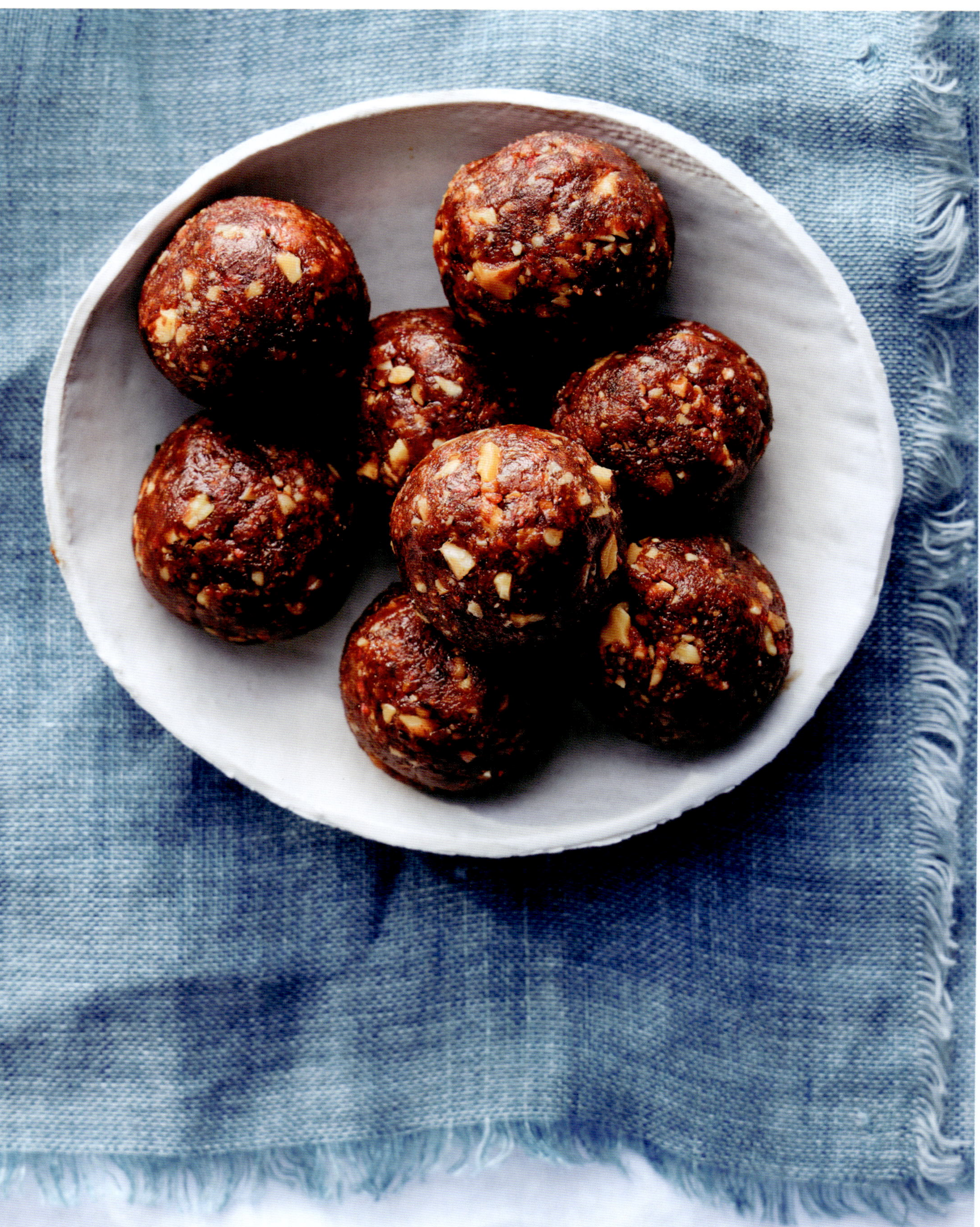

These Strawberry + Almond Energy Balls are a wholesome twist on the nostalgic PB&J and packed with natural energy and heart-healthy fats. Sweet, crunchy, and full of flavor, they're the perfect grab-and-go snack for busy days. The almonds retain their crunch the best when these balls are stored in the freezer.

Strawberry + Almond Energy Balls

MAKES 12 BALLS

- 12 large Medjool dates, pitted (see Note)
- ⅓ cup (90 g) well-stirred almond butter
- 1 cup (20 g) freeze-dried strawberries (do not pack)
- ¾ teaspoon pink salt
- 1 teaspoon vanilla extract
- ⅔ cup (80 g) unsalted dry-roasted almonds

Place dates in a food processor and process until a smooth paste forms. (It may eventually form a ball.) Add almond butter, strawberries, salt, and vanilla and pulse until everything starts to come together. Add almonds and pulse until slightly chunky. (If it's too chunky, the balls will not hold their form—see the photo for the ideal consistency.) Using a rubber spatula, scrape down the sides of the bowl really well. Pulse the mixture 1 or 2 times.

Transfer mixture to a bowl. Press dough together, then divide it into 12 equal portions and roll them into balls. Store them in an airtight container in the fridge for up to a week or in the freezer for up to a month.

NOTES

Costco has nice large Medjool dates. You may need to add an extra date or two if your dates are not plump and moist or are on the small side.

I find dry-roasted almonds and freeze-dried strawberries at Trader Joe's.

Granita is a refreshing icy treat that hails from Sicily, offering a delightful balance of sweetness and texture. Made with just a few simple ingredients, it's both light and invigorating—perfect for warm days.

Watermelon + Lime Granita

Cold Brew Coffee Granita

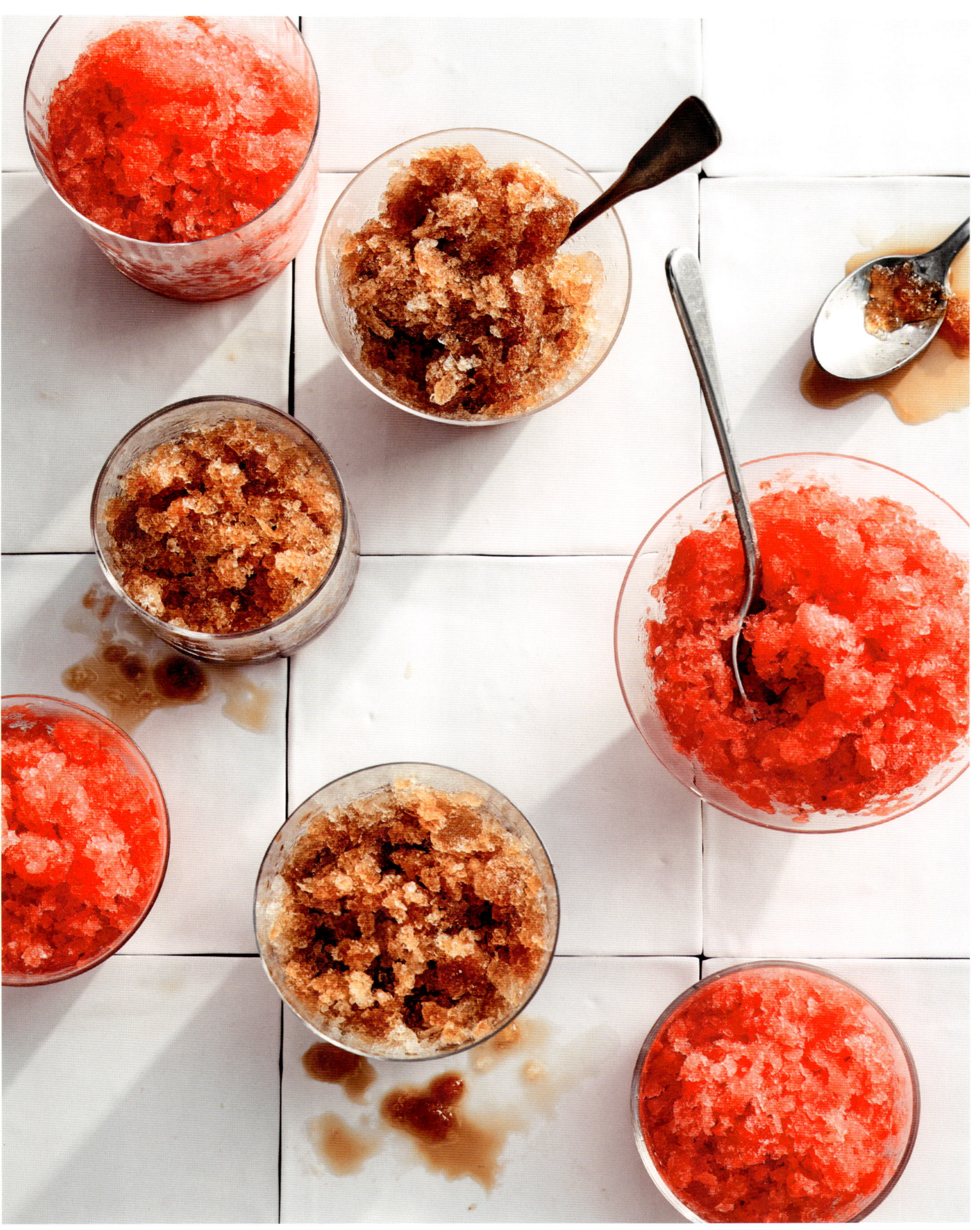

Get your coffee fix and beat the summer heat with this cool and refreshing treat! Cold brew coffee is smoother and less acidic than regular coffee because the coffee grounds are slowly steeped in cold water rather than being exposed to high temperatures. You can find cold brew at most grocery stores. I like the 32-ounce (946-ml) bottle of 100% Arabica cold brew from Trader Joe's.

Cold Brew Coffee Granita

SERVES 8

4 cups (946 ml) cold brew coffee
½ cup (157 g) pure maple syrup
Pinch of pink salt
1 tablespoon vanilla extract

First, make sure you have a level space in your freezer to accommodate the pan.

Combine all ingredients in a 9 × 13-inch (23 × 33-cm) baking dish or shallow vessel. Whisk to combine, then place it in the freezer. Every hour or so, use a fork to scrape the sides and give the mixture a quick stir. After the fourth time, cover with plastic wrap and freeze until solid.

To serve, chill 8 glasses in the freezer for 10 minutes. This will keep the granita from melting.

Scrape the surface of the granita with a fork to produce fluffy shaved ice. Scoop it into the chilled glasses and serve.

Granita can be stored for up to a month in glass jars.

Refreshing icy-cold granita is the perfect antidote to summer's heat! Watermelon is an essential summer treat, and lime gives it that extra something special.

SERVES 8

Watermelon + Lime Granita

- 1 small seedless watermelon, coarsely chopped (8 cups)
- 1/8 teaspoon pink salt
- Zest of 1 large lime
- 2 tablespoons freshly squeezed lime juice
- 1 tablespoon honey

First, make sure you have a level space in your freezer to accommodate the pan.

Fill an 8-cup (2-L) blender container with watermelon. Add the remaining ingredients and purée until smooth. Pour the mixture into a 9 × 13-inch (23 × 33-cm) baking dish or shallow vessel and place it in the freezer. Every hour or so, use a fork to scrape the sides and give the mixture a quick stir. After the fourth time, cover with plastic wrap and freeze until solid.

To serve, chill 8 glasses in the freezer for 10 minutes. This will keep the granita from melting.

Scrape the surface of the granita with a fork to produce fluffy shaved ice. Scoop it into the chilled glasses and serve.

Granita can be stored for up to a month in glass jars.

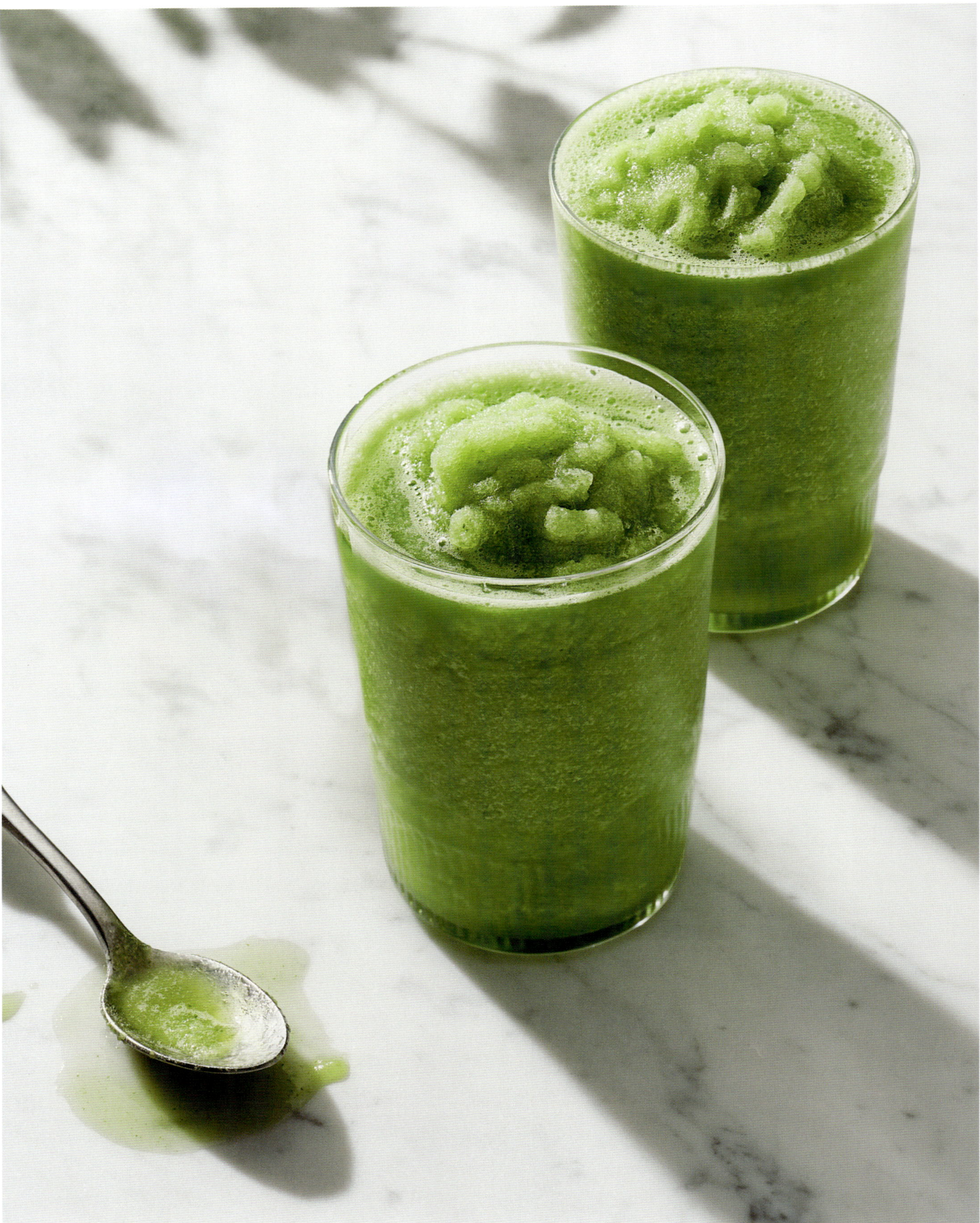

Hydrate and replenish your electrolytes in the summer heat with this refreshingly tart and tangy slushy!

SERVES 2

Summer Slushy with Lime + Mint

½ English cucumber, ends trimmed

¼ cup (4 g) lightly packed mint leaves

1½ cups (360 g) cold filtered water

Zest of 1 lime

¼ cup (60 g) freshly squeezed lime juice (see Note)

¼ cup (85 g) honey

Good pinch of pink salt

3 level cups (385 g) ice

Combine all ingredients, except ice, in a high-speed blender and process until broken down and combined. Add the ice and process until fully blended and slush-like. Serve immediately!

NOTE

It's not unusual for a lime to produce very little juice, so I suggest stocking 4 limes just in case. Use a Microplane to zest the lime and a citrus reamer to capture all the juice.

For the serious dark chocolate aficionado! Crispy edges give way to a gooey center and molten puddles of deep dark chocolate. They're best enjoyed fresh from the oven, so I recommend freezing any extra balls of dough to bake another time.

Emily and Heather who own Botanica Restaurant and Market in Los Angeles were kind enough to share the recipe for one of the cookies they sell in their adjacent market. This is my adapted version of their Dark Chocolate Almond Cookie.

Blackout Cookies with 100% Chocolate + Flake Salt

MAKES 14 COOKIES

- ⅓ cup (70 g) virgin coconut oil
- ½ cup (130 g) well-stirred almond butter
- 1⅓ cups (190 g) coconut sugar
- 2 large eggs, room temperature
- 1 tablespoon vanilla extract
- 1 teaspoon baking soda
- 1 teaspoon pink salt
- 1½ cups (155 g) super-fine blanched almond flour
- ¼ cup (30 g) Valrhona cocoa powder
- 3 oz (85 g) 100% unsweetened chocolate, coarsely chopped (see Note)
- Maldon flake salt, for sprinkling

In a medium bowl, combine coconut oil, almond butter, coconut sugar, eggs, and vanilla. Using an electric mixer, mix on high for 2 minutes, until smooth. Add the remaining ingredients, except flake salt, and blend on low speed with each addition until combined. (Overmixing this dough or mixing it by hand may cause the oils to separate.) Using a rubber spatula, fold the mixture a few times to ensure the chocolate is evenly distributed. Cover, then refrigerate for 4 hours or overnight.

Preheat oven to 350°F. Line a rimmed baking sheet with parchment paper.

Once the oven is preheated, use a large (size 20) cookie scoop to scoop the dough onto the prepared parchment paper, evenly spacing them a couple inches apart. Lightly flatten each ball by slipping a small piece of parchment paper over the dough and pressing gently with the flat bottom of a glass. Keep them chubby because they'll spread out while they bake. Sprinkle each one with flake salt.

Bake for 12–14 minutes. Let cookies cool for 10 minutes in the pan. Serve warm.

NOTES

I use Guittard 100% cacao baking bars. Look for a baking bar that contains only cacao beans. Bars with added cocoa butter do not hold their form and may scorch in this application.

Enjoy fresh-baked cookies on any whim by scooping dough into balls, wrapping them well, and storing in the fridge for a week or in the freezer for up to a month to bake later.

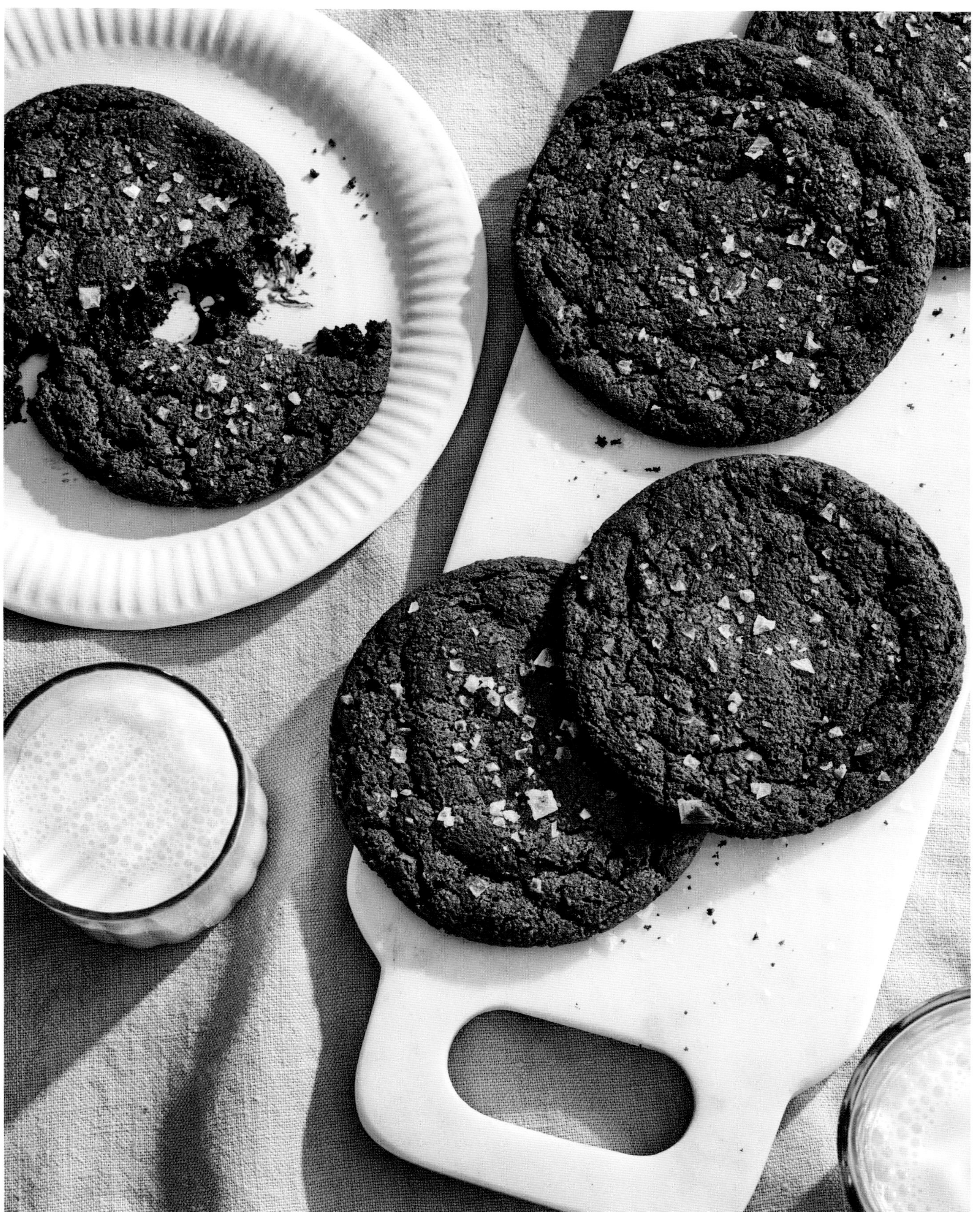

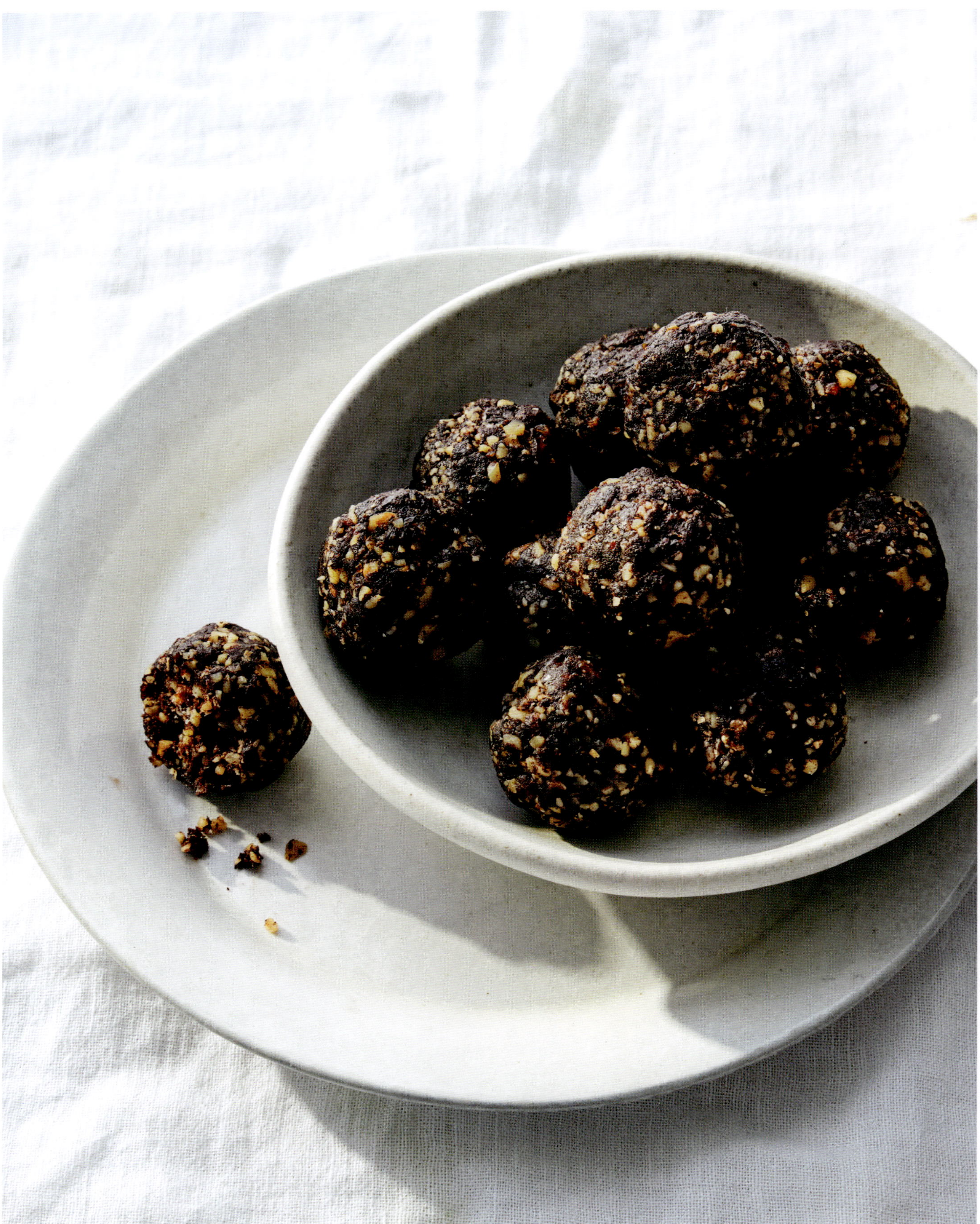

Reach for one of these rich, chocolatey walnut bites when less-than-healthy treats are beckoning! These energy-packed snacks last for a couple weeks when refrigerated and even longer when frozen. They're loaded with walnuts, a nutrient-dense source of alpha-linolenic acid (ALA), a plant-derived omega-3 fatty acid. Among tree nuts, walnuts boast the highest levels of ALA, making these morsels both delicious and healthful.

Walnut Fudge Brownie Balls

MAKES ABOUT 13 BALLS

1½ cups (160 g) toasted walnuts
10 plump Medjool dates, pitted
¼ cup (30 g) Valrhona cocoa powder
2 tablespoons pure maple syrup
1 tablespoon coconut flour (use a knife to level)
Scant 1 teaspoon pink salt
1 teaspoon vanilla extract

Combine all ingredients in a food processor and pulse until combined with visible walnut bits. Be careful not to overprocess it or the oils will separate and make the balls greasy.

Using a medium (size 40) cookie scoop, scoop the dough and roll into balls. Place them on a small baking sheet lined with parchment paper, keep uncovered, and freeze them for 1 hour to hold their shape. Transfer to a glass jar and store in the fridge for up to 2 weeks or in the freezer for up to a month. (They hold up best when frozen.)

Tender, rich, double-chocolatey muffins with melty bits. Use chocolate chips for the quickest option or add an extra layer of flavor by using the dark chocolate bar of your choosing. I like to use an orange- or mint-flavored bar—just look for one that contains essential oils.

MAKES 10 MUFFINS

Choc-a-Lot Muffins

- $2\frac{1}{2}$ cups (260 g) super-fine blanched almond flour
- $\frac{1}{4}$ cup (30 g) Valrhona cocoa powder
- 1 teaspoon baking soda
- $\frac{3}{4}$ teaspoon pink salt
- 3 large eggs, room temperature
- $\frac{3}{4}$ cup (235 g) pure maple syrup
- 5 oz (142 g) 70% dark chocolate or $\frac{3}{4}$ cup (135 g) chocolate chips (see Note)

Preheat oven to 350°F. Line a muffin tin with 10 paper liners.

The best method for measuring almond flour by the cup can be found on page 25.

In a medium mixing bowl, whisk together almond flour, cocoa, baking soda, and salt, breaking up any lumps. Add the remaining ingredients, except chocolate, and whisk until batter is smooth.

If using chocolate chips: Add them to the batter and set aside a handful if you wish to sprinkle some on top. Using a spoon, divide the batter among 10 cups of the prepared muffin tin and sprinkle reserved chocolate chips on top.

If using chocolate bars: Break the chocolate into 60 pieces (6 pieces per muffin). Using a spoon, fill each muffin cup by a third. Place 3 chocolate pieces on top of each cup of batter. Spoon the remaining batter over the chocolate pieces. Top each muffin with 3 more chocolate pieces and use your finger to gently press chocolate into the batter, just until the top of the chocolate is level with the batter. (Note: Cups will be full because almond flour doesn't rise as much as all-purpose flour.)

Bake on the center rack for 21 minutes. Let muffins cool in the pan for 10 minutes.

Leftover muffins can be stored at room temperature for up to 4 days or in the freezer (wrapped in plastic wrap) for up to a month.

NOTE

My favorite bars for these muffins are Theo's orange-flavored chocolate bar and Alter Eco's sea salt bar. When using chocolate chips, I use Guittard brand because they're soy-free. If you're avoiding cane sugar, Guittard has a coconut sugar-sweetened option.

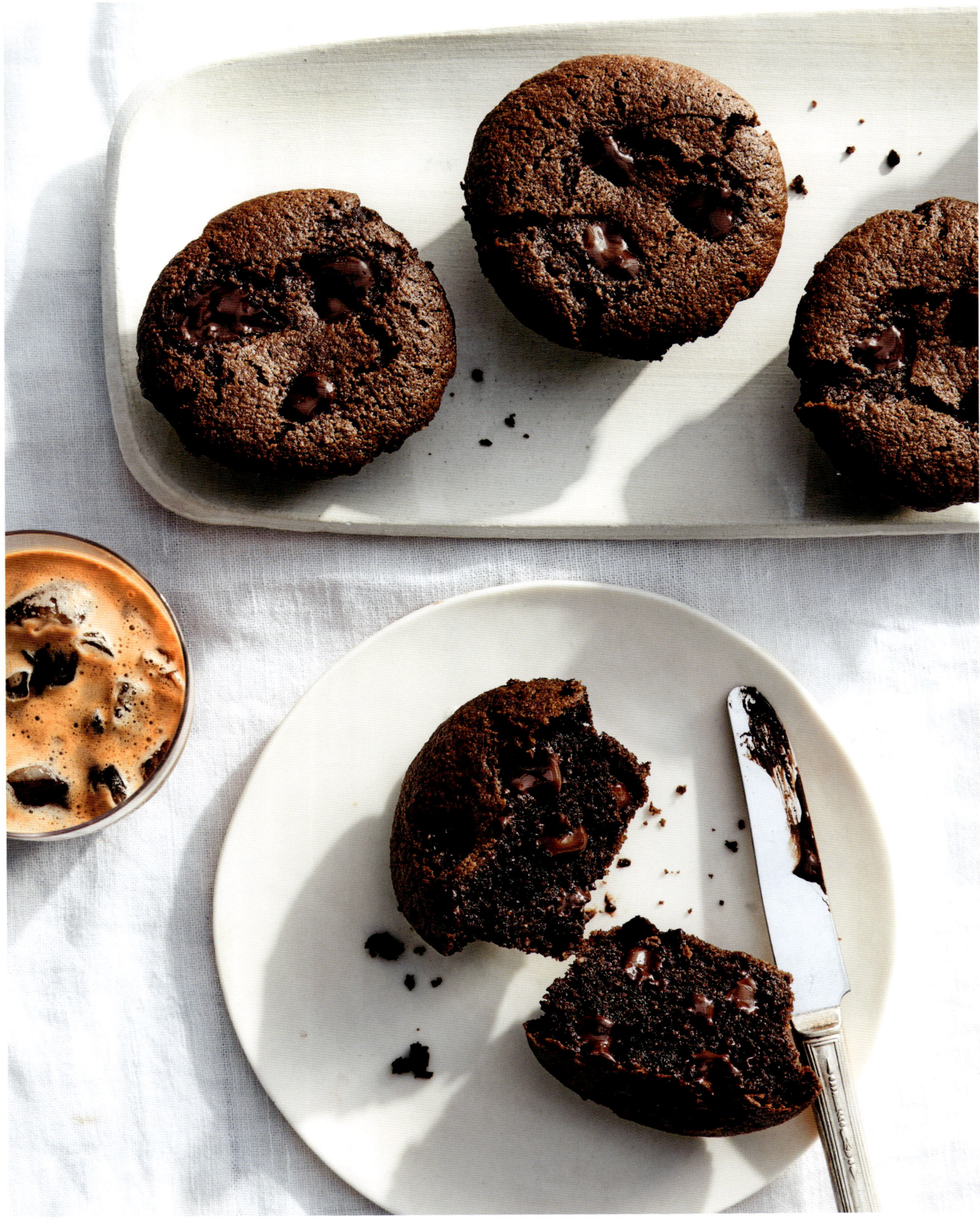

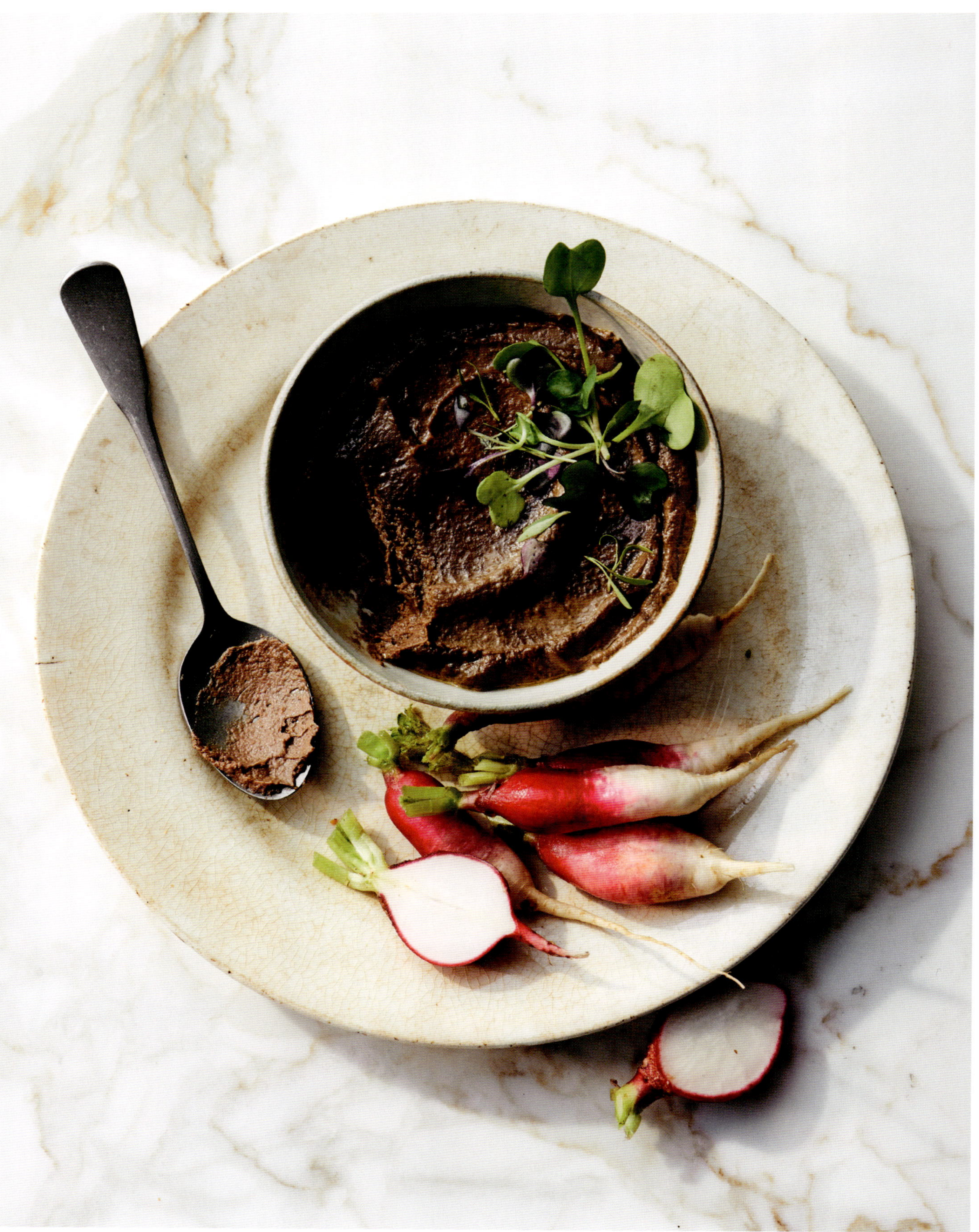

Iron deficiency can be challenging to detect and is increasingly common, partly due to the growing trend of reducing red meat consumption. Liver stands out as one of the most bioavailable foods, making it an excellent choice for boosting iron and B vitamin intake.

A toasted baguette would be ideal with this mousse, but I just enjoy it by the spoonful. If there's a gluten-free cracker you like, use it for dipping! Cornichons are a classic accompaniment, too.

Chicken Liver Mousse with Apple + Thyme

SERVES 4

- 1 lb (454 g) fresh, organic chicken livers, rinsed well
- 3/4 cup (153 g) ghee, such as 4th & Heart's original (divided)
- 2 medium shallots, thinly sliced
- 1 Granny Smith apple, peeled, cored, and finely chopped
- 3 tablespoons cream sherry (divided; see Note)
- 2 teaspoons chopped thyme leaves
- 1½ teaspoons pink salt
- Crackers, toast, or veggies, to serve

Pat the liver dry. Trim off any fat or connective tissue and cut the larger pieces in half to ensure even sizing and uniform cooking.

Melt ¼ cup (51 g) of ghee in a medium skillet over medium-low heat. Add shallots and apple and sauté for 10 minutes, until softened but not browned. Add liver, 2 tablespoons of cream sherry, and thyme. Increase the heat to medium and cook for another 6–8 minutes, stirring occasionally and flipping the larger pieces occasionally, until liver is cooked but still very pink inside. (Avoid overcooking, or it will become dry and mealy.)

Pour the mixture into a food processor. Add the remaining ½ cup (102 g) of ghee, 1 tablespoon cream sherry, and salt and process until smooth. Pour into ramekins or a vessel of your choice. Press a piece of plastic wrap directly onto the surface and refrigerate for 2 hours, until firm.

To serve, bring the mousse to room temperature for 15–30 minutes. Serve it with the accompaniments of your choice. It will keep in the fridge for up to a week or in the freezer for up to a month.

NOTE

Cream sherry is very different than cooking sherry and is an important component to this mousse. I recommend using Harveys Bristol Cream Sherry. It's widely available, lasts for years, and is also used in the Cream of Porcini Mushroom Soup recipe on page 91.

Fellow Swifties! This pink and orange board is an homage to Taylor Swift's 2016 Grammys look. Though I'm not a fan of cooked carrots, my husband and I were drawn to the vibrant hue of the carrot tahini from the mezze platter at Shed (Sonoma County's beloved but shuttered restaurant). I set out to replicate its color and texture, while enhancing the delicate flavor to mask any strong taste of cooked carrots. The result is a velvety light spread with a hint of cumin, a whiff of nuttiness, and a subtle sweetness.

Creamy Carrot Tahini

MAKES 1½ CUPS

- 1 lb (454 g) carrots, peeled, trimmed, and halved crosswise
- 1 garlic clove
- 2 tablespoons well-stirred tahini (see Note)
- 1 teaspoon red wine vinegar
- 2 teaspoons freshly squeezed lemon juice
- ½ teaspoon pink salt
- Scant ¼ teaspoon ground cumin
- ¼ teaspoon ground coriander
- Crackers or veggies, to serve

Place carrots in a steaming basket set over a pot of boiling water, cover, and steam for 20–25 minutes, until they can be easily pierced with a knife.

Transfer the carrots to a food processor and purée until smooth. Remove the lid from the processor to allow steam to escape and let it cool to room temperature.

Add the remaining ingredients and process until smooth. Transfer to a bowl and refrigerate until ready to use.

NOTE

For optimal flavor, be sure to use tahini made with toasted sesame seeds rather than raw.

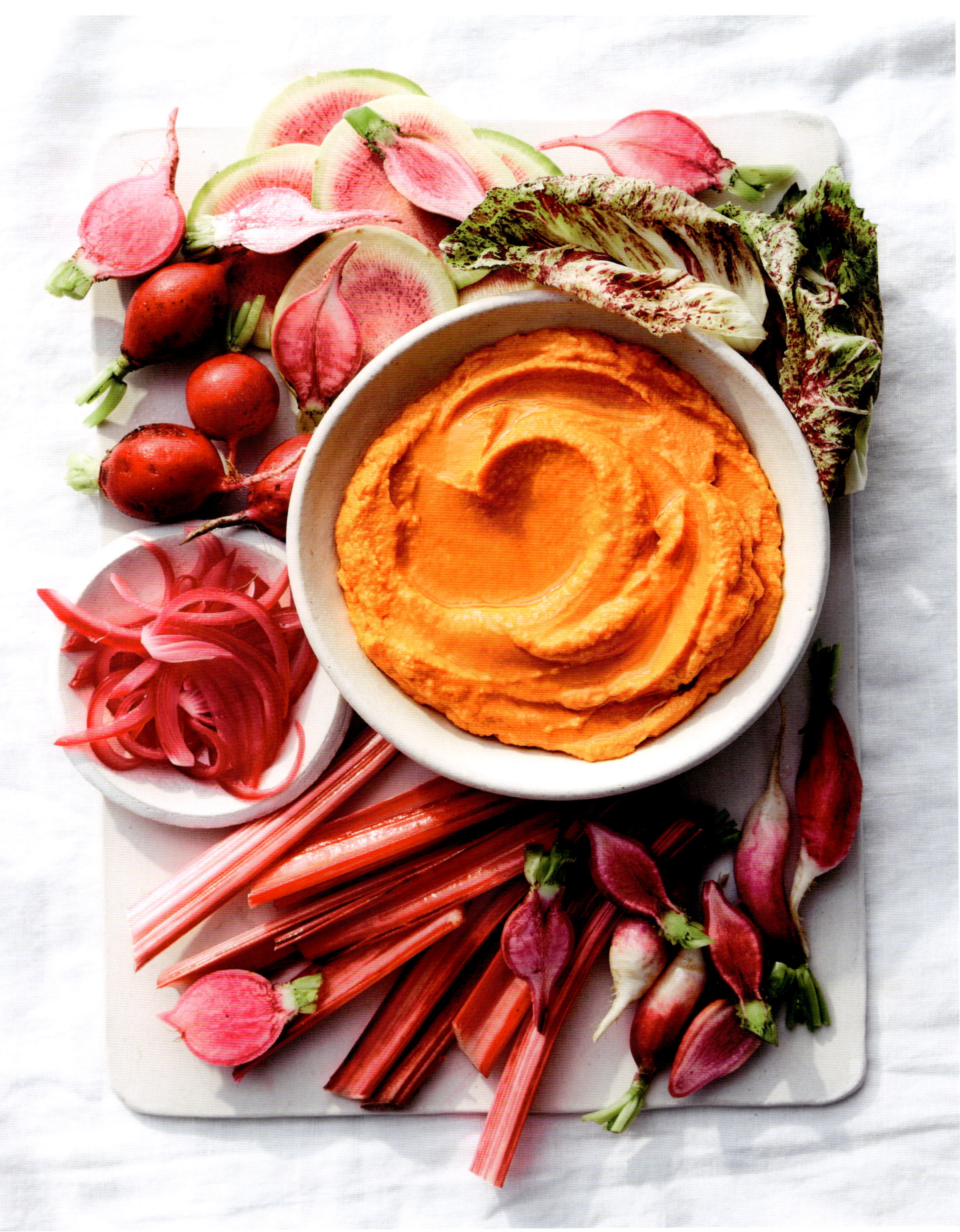

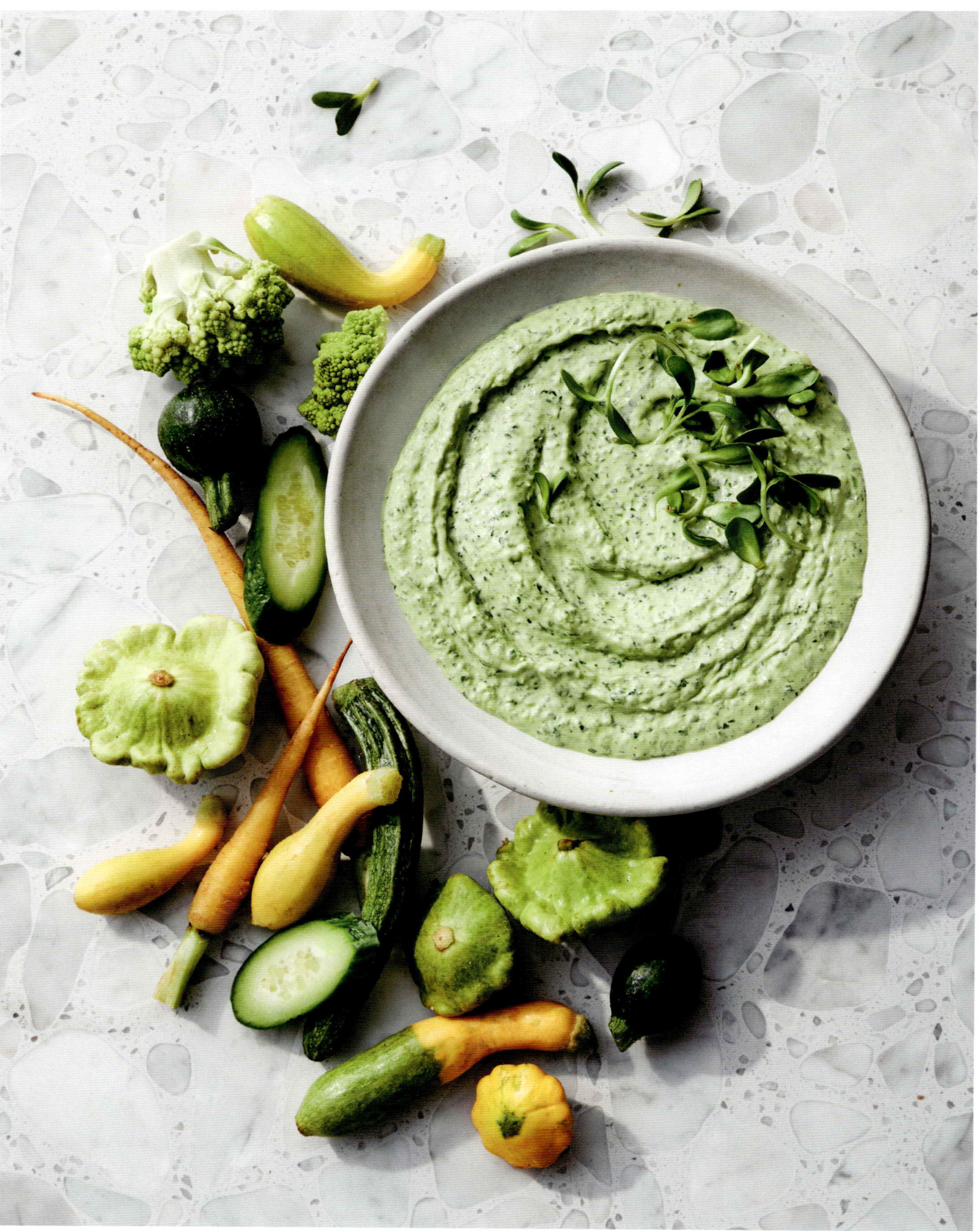

Considering parsley's status as a nutritional powerhouse, I wanted to find a way to incorporate more of it into my diet beyond the occasional garnish. This punchy dip packs a serious amount of parsley while not being overly assertive. I keep it thick for dipping, but thin it slightly to drizzle over roasted vegetables, and thin it even further for a salad dressing.

Make the dressing a few hours in advance so the garlic can mellow and the flavors can develop. Carrots are my favorite veg to pair with this dip!

Zesty Herbed Tahini Dip

MAKES 2 CUPS

- Large bunch of flat-leaf parsley (3.5–4.5 oz/100–125 g), trimmed
- 3 garlic cloves
- 1 teaspoon pink salt
- ½ cup (120 g) filtered water
- ⅓ cup (80 g) freshly squeezed lemon juice
- 1 cup (240 g) well-stirred tahini (see Note)
- Crackers or veggies, to serve

Submerge parsley, including stems, in a large bowl of water or, ideally, a salad spinner. Swish to loosen any dirt from the leaves. Drain, then spin or pat dry.

Add garlic to a food processor and pulse until minced. Add parsley (including stems) and the remaining ingredients. Process until smooth. Refrigerate until ready to use.

NOTE

For optimal flavor, be sure to use tahini made with toasted sesame seeds rather than raw.

Tonnato is an Italian classic that could be likened to a tuna aioli. A few minutes on the grill add a light smokiness, while the vegetables become sweeter, and their bite softens. This is a unique and flavorsome starter to have in your repertoire. My favorite is the 4.94-ounce (140-g) can of Tonnino tuna.

Creamy, Salty + Tangy Tonnato Sauce with Grilled Veg

SERVES 4

Tonnato sauce

- 1 garlic clove
- 2 oil-packed anchovy fillets
- 1 tablespoon drained capers (if salted, rinse first)
- Zest of 1 lemon
- 1 tablespoon freshly squeezed lemon juice
- ½ teaspoon pink salt
- 2 tablespoons extra-virgin olive oil
- ¾ cup (172 g) mayonnaise
- 1 (5-oz/140-g) can oil-packed tuna, drained

Grilled vegetables

- Bunch of asparagus spears
- 8 radishes, halved
- 1 radicchio, cut into wedges
- 1 red onion, cut into wedges with core attached
- 4 Belgian endives, halved lengthwise
- Extra-virgin olive oil, for drizzling
- Pink salt

Tonnato sauce Make the tonnato sauce at least a few hours or up to a day in advance to allow the flavors to develop.

Add each sauce ingredient to a mini food processor in the order listed, pulsing a couple times after each addition. Once everything has been added, process until smooth and creamy. Transfer to a bowl, then cover and refrigerate.

Grilled vegetables Preheat a grill pan or outdoor grill.

Lightly drizzle oil over the vegetables, sprinkle with salt, and toss to coat. Place vegetables on the grill and grill until tender-crisp. The red onions can take some extra time, depending on the thickness of the wedges.

To serve, arrange the grilled vegetables on a platter and serve at room temperature with a bowl of the tonnato sauce.

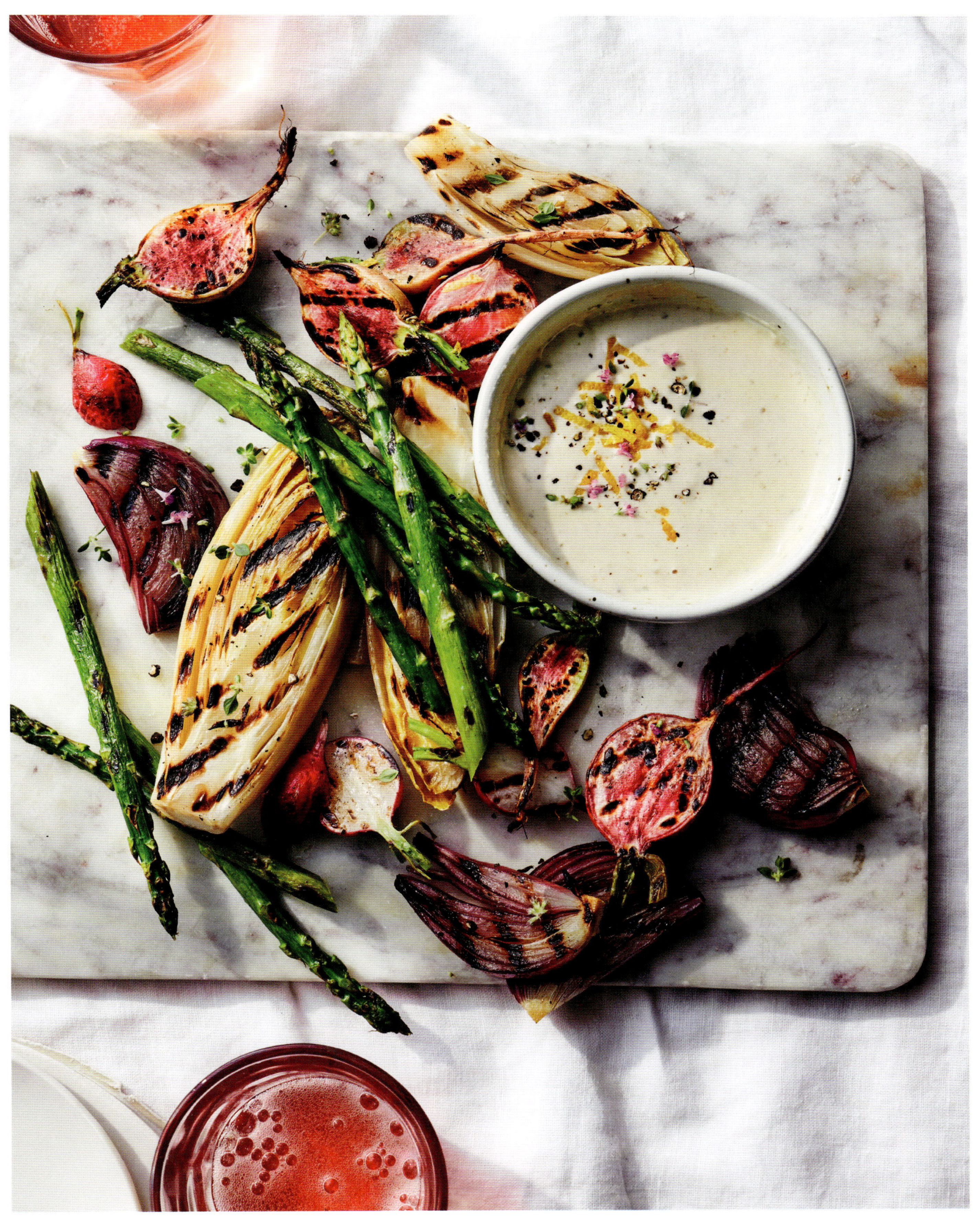

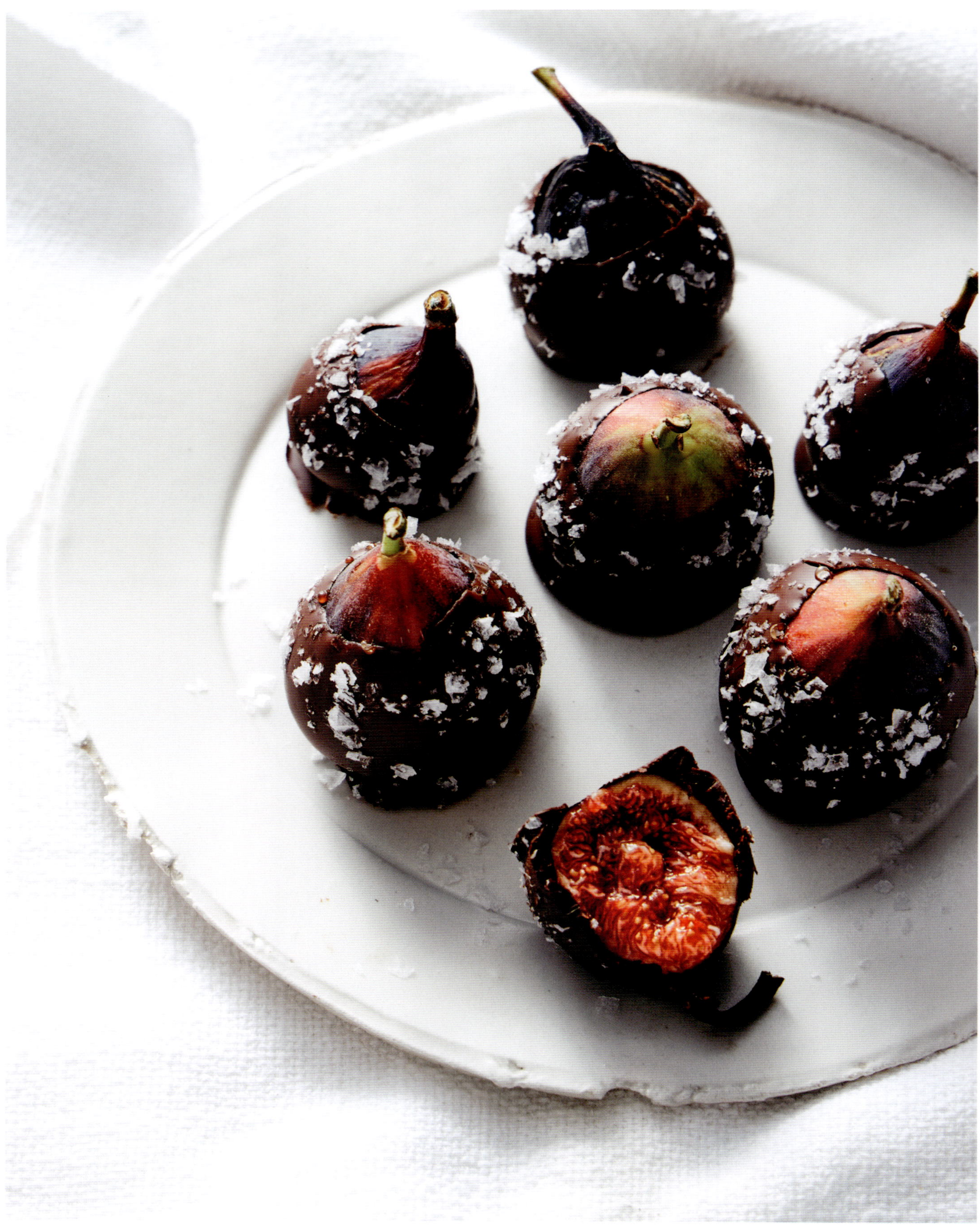

This recipe (if you can call it that) is an ode to the beauty of simple food. Ripe, juicy, and subtly fragrant Mission figs take a dip in rich, velvety dark chocolate and are finished with a salty sprinkle of Maldon. Serve these gems at your next dinner party. Fig season is ruefully short, so enjoy them while you can!

MAKES 12 PIECES

Fresh Figs in Dark Chocolate

8 oz (228 g) up-to-72% dark chocolate (see Note)

12 black Mission figs, ripe but not mushy

Maldon flake salt

Line a rimmed baking sheet with parchment paper. Chop the chocolate for easier melting. In a small microwave-safe bowl, heat chocolate in 30-second intervals until melted, stirring each time.

Holding each fig by the stem, dip it in the melted chocolate, then shake off any excess chocolate into the bowl. Sprinkle lightly with salt and place on the prepared baking sheet.

Refrigerate for 5 minutes to firm up. (Set a timer, because if you leave them in the fridge too long, they'll develop condensation.) They are best enjoyed the same day, at room temperature.

NOTE

Chocolate chips are not ideal for this recipe, as most brands contain stabilizers and can be matte and brittle once melted and cooled. I recommend using Trader Joe's Pound Plus dark chocolate bar, made by Callebaut—it's an affordable and high-quality option.

A cleaned-up classic! Make sure your bananas are plenty ripe because there's very little added sweetener here. Measuring the bananas out after they've been mashed ensures the right moisture balance.

MAKES 12 MUFFINS

Banana + Toasted Walnut Muffins

- 2 cups (220 g) super-fine blanched almond flour
- 3 tablespoons coconut flour (use a knife to level)
- 1½ teaspoons baking soda
- 1 teaspoon ground cinnamon
- ½ teaspoon pink salt
- 3–4 overripe bananas, mashed (1¼ cups/306 g)
- 3 large eggs, room temperature
- ⅓ cup (105 g) pure maple syrup
- 2 tablespoons extra-virgin olive oil
- 1 teaspoon vanilla extract
- 1½ cups (180 g) finely chopped walnuts (divided)
- Maldon flake salt, for sprinkling

Preheat oven to 350°F. Line a muffin tin with 12 paper liners.

The best method for measuring almond flour by the cup can be found on page 25.

In a medium mixing bowl, combine almond flour, coconut flour, baking soda, cinnamon, and pink salt. Whisk to combine and break up any lumps. Add the remaining ingredients, except for walnuts and flake salt, and whisk until combined. Add ¾ cup (90 g) of the walnuts and whisk to distribute. Using a spoon, divide the batter among the muffin cups. (Note: Cups will be full because almond flour doesn't rise as much as all-purpose flour.)

Sprinkle the remaining ¾ cup (90 g) of walnuts over the tops of muffins, covering as much of the batter as possible. Finish with a light sprinkle of flake salt. Bake on the center rack for 25 minutes. Allow them to cool in the pan for 10 minutes.

Muffins can be covered and stored at room temperature for 2 days or wrapped in plastic and stored in the freezer for up to a month.

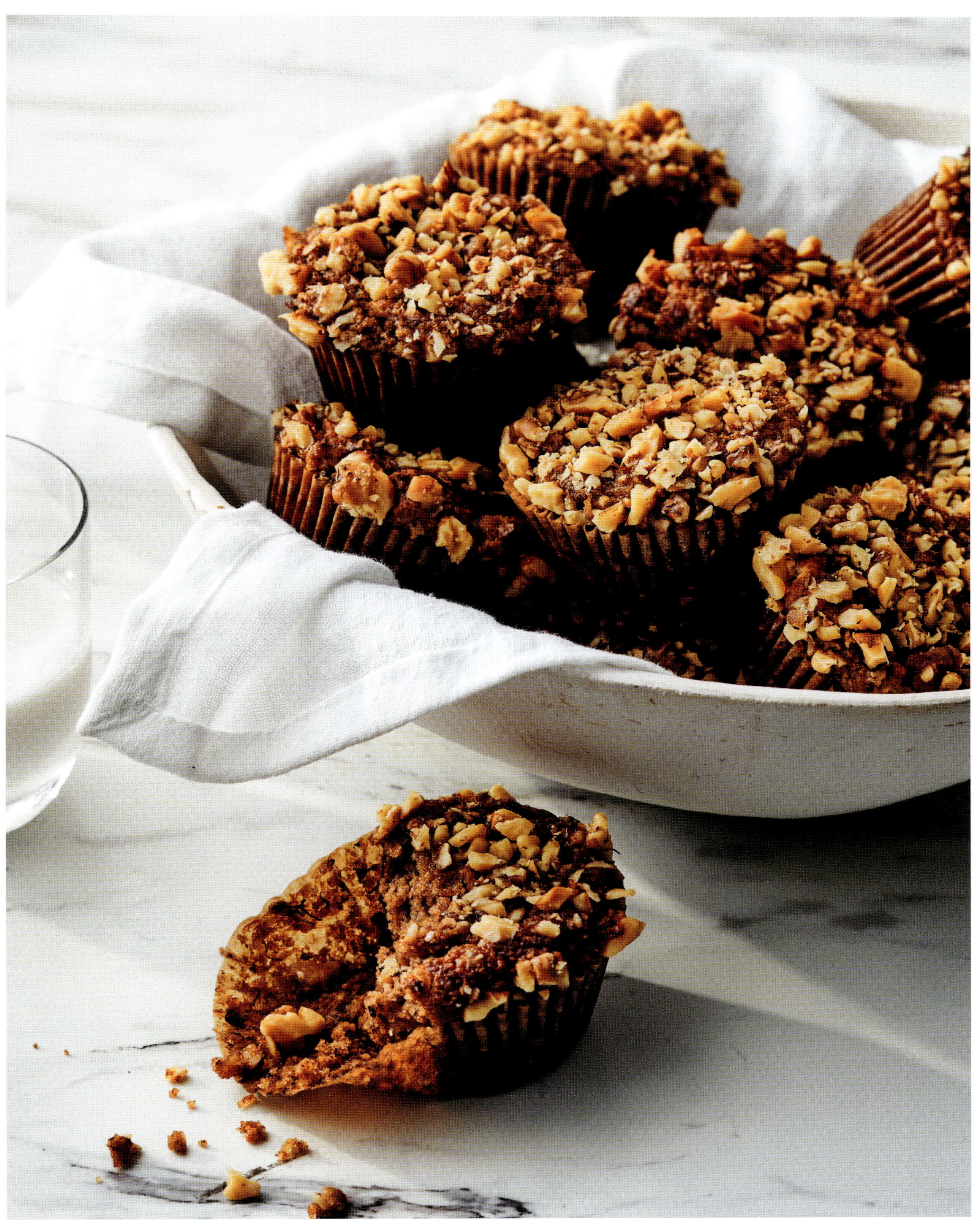

SIDE SALADS

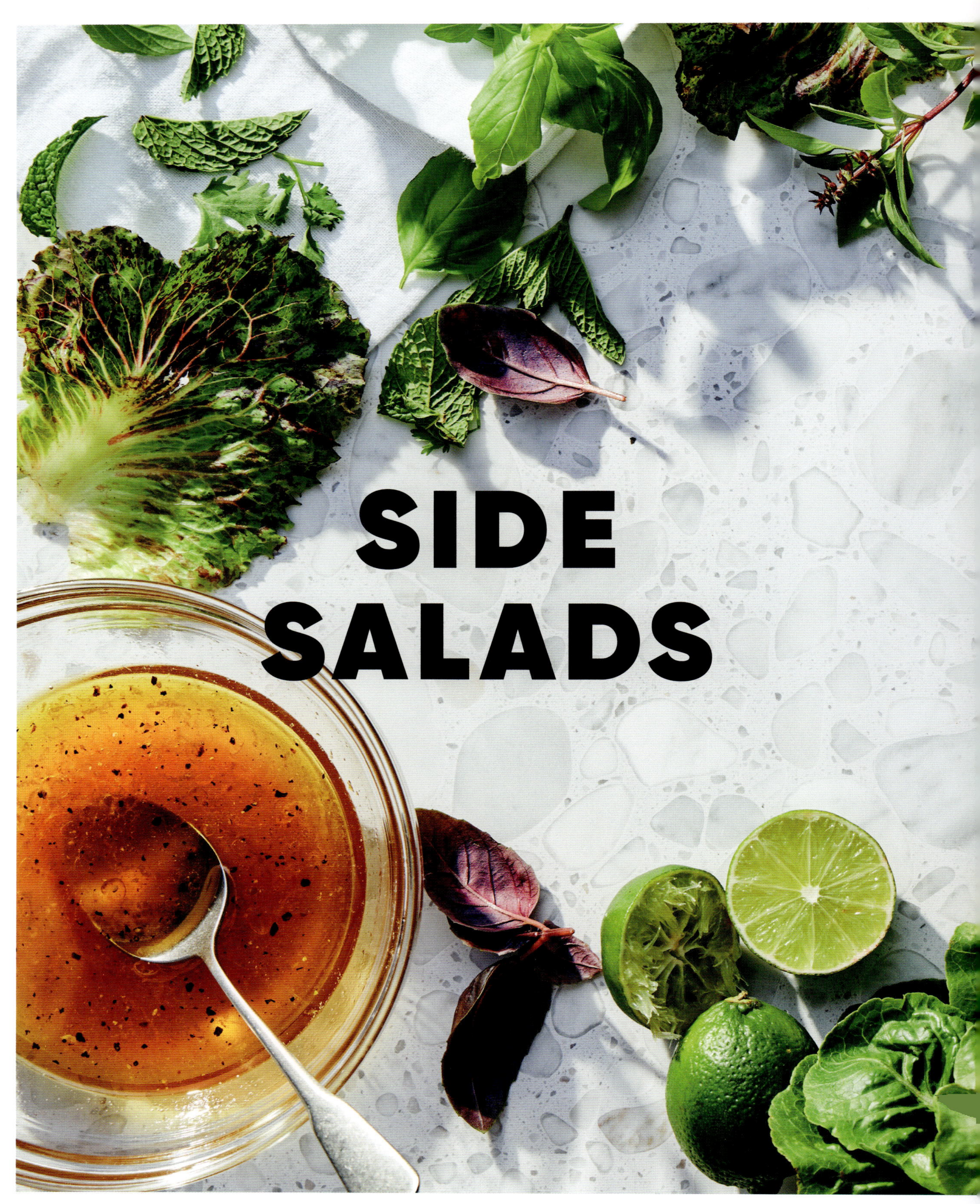

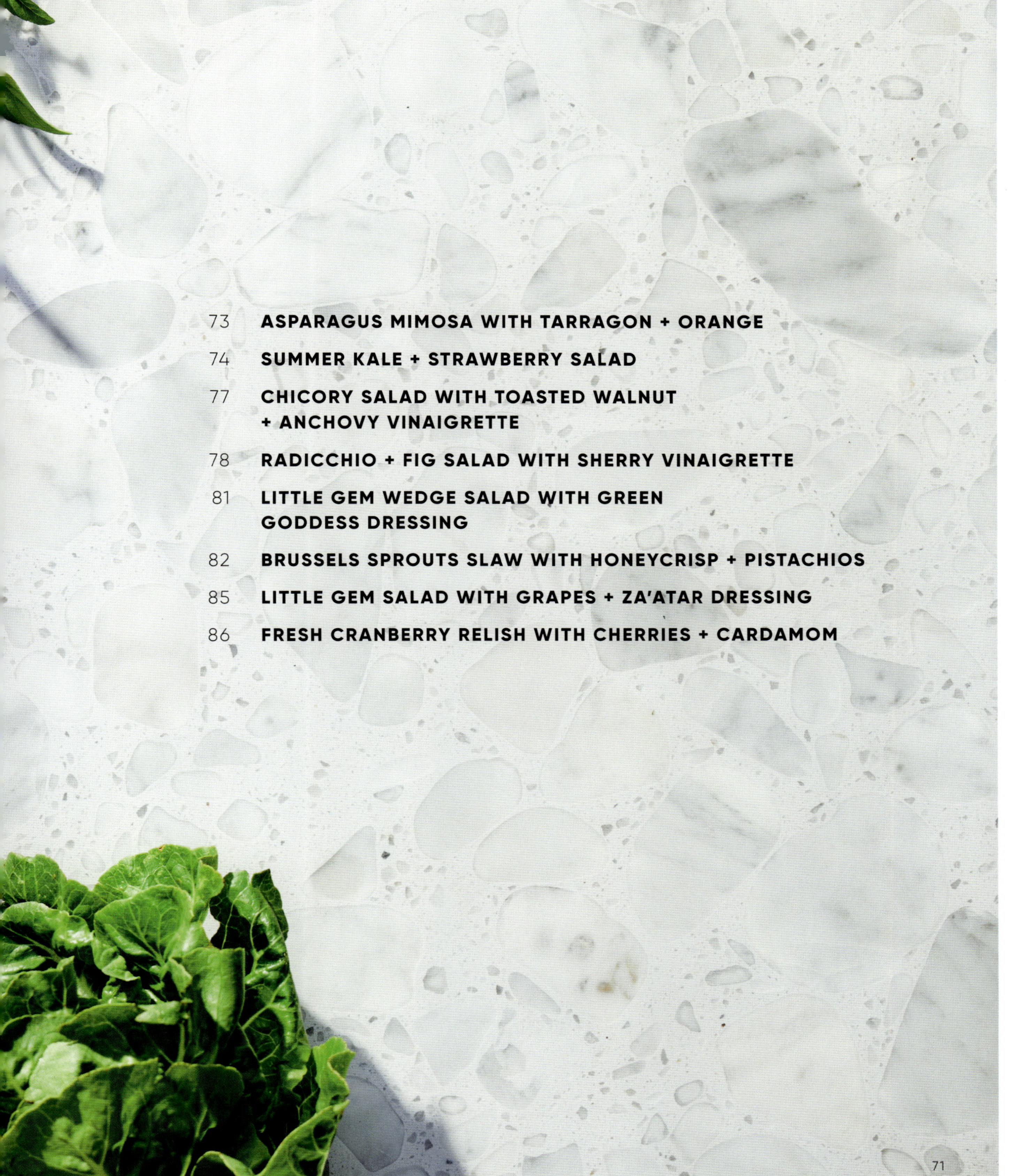

73 **ASPARAGUS MIMOSA WITH TARRAGON + ORANGE**

74 **SUMMER KALE + STRAWBERRY SALAD**

77 **CHICORY SALAD WITH TOASTED WALNUT + ANCHOVY VINAIGRETTE**

78 **RADICCHIO + FIG SALAD WITH SHERRY VINAIGRETTE**

81 **LITTLE GEM WEDGE SALAD WITH GREEN GODDESS DRESSING**

82 **BRUSSELS SPROUTS SLAW WITH HONEYCRISP + PISTACHIOS**

85 **LITTLE GEM SALAD WITH GRAPES + ZA'ATAR DRESSING**

86 **FRESH CRANBERRY RELISH WITH CHERRIES + CARDAMOM**

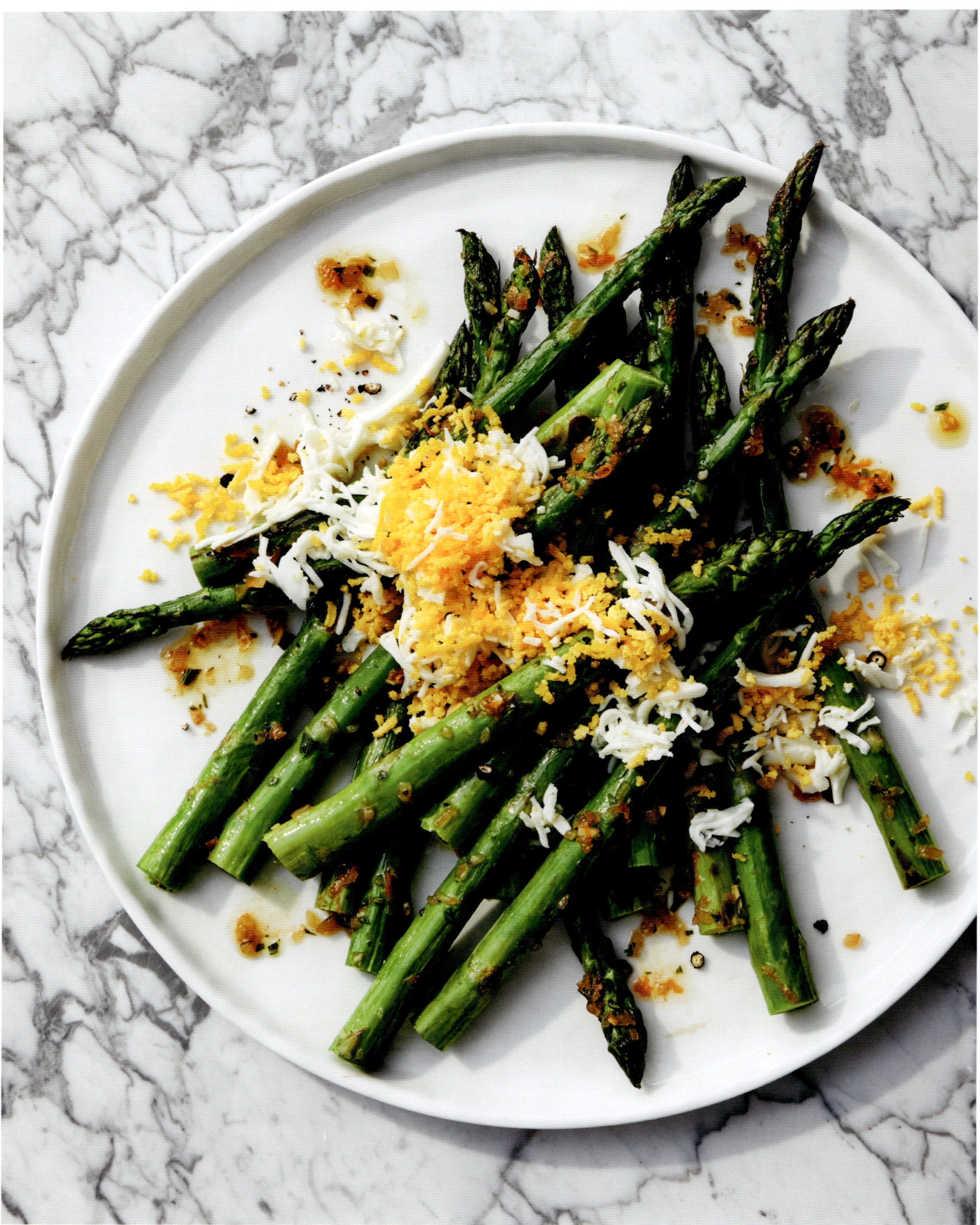

This updated French classic screams brunch! It gets its name from the fluffy grated egg yolks that resemble bright yellow mimosa flowers. Traditionally, it's made with a lemon-based vinaigrette, but I'm mixing it up with tarragon and orange. Look for Spanish sherry vinegar labeled *vinagre de Jerez* for the most complex flavor.

Make the vinaigrette several hours or a day ahead so the flavors have a chance to mingle. It's best served at room temperature.

Asparagus Mimosa with Tarragon + Orange

SERVES 4

Dressing

- 1 small shallot, finely chopped
- 1 garlic clove, finely chopped
- 1 tablespoon + 1 teaspoon vinagre de Jerez sherry vinegar
- 1 teaspoon honey
- 1 oil-packed anchovy fillet, chopped
- ½ teaspoon pink salt
- Zest and juice of 1 large navel orange
- 1 tablespoon finely chopped tarragon, plus extra for sprinkling
- ¼ cup (50 g) extra-virgin olive oil

Asparagus

- 2 lbs (907 g) asparagus, preferably large diameter, trimmed
- Extra-virgin olive oil, for drizzling
- Pinch of pink salt
- 2 hard-boiled eggs, chilled
- Maldon flake salt and freshly cracked black pepper, to taste

Dressing In a small saucepan, combine all dressing ingredients, except orange zest, tarragon, and oil—use a citrus reamer to get all the orange juice. Simmer over medium-low heat for 8 minutes, until the mixture has reduced by half and thickened. Remove from the heat, then whisk in the zest, tarragon, and oil, until combined. Transfer to a small bowl and refrigerate until ready to use.

Asparagus Position an oven rack 6 inches (15 cm) from the broil element. (In my oven, that's the second notch from the top.) Preheat the oven to broil. Line a rimmed baking sheet with parchment paper.

Place asparagus on the prepared baking sheet. Lightly drizzle with oil, sprinkle with pink salt, and toss to coat. Arrange them in a single layer, working in two batches if necessary.

Broil for 3–4 minutes, until tender. Using tongs, transfer asparagus to a plate to prevent them from overcooking.

Peel eggs, then grate them on a box grater into a small bowl.

To serve, arrange asparagus on a platter. Drizzle with a small amount of the dressing and toss gently to coat. Drizzle with the remaining dressing. Spoon grated eggs over the top, as pictured. Sprinkle with tarragon leaves, finish with flake salt and pepper, and enjoy at room temperature.

I wanted this salad dressing to be sweet and summery like lemonade. And because strawberries and freshly cracked black pepper play so well together, there's a good bit of pepper here to add balance and a little edge. Don't worry if there's extra; it holds up beautifully in the fridge!

SERVES 4–6

Summer Kale + Strawberry Salad

Dressing

Zest of 2 lemons

⅓ cup (80 g) freshly squeezed lemon juice

⅓ cup (67 g) extra-virgin olive oil

¼ cup (80 g) pure maple syrup

¼ teaspoon pink salt

½ teaspoon freshly cracked black pepper

Salad

Bunch of curly kale, stemmed and torn into bite-sized pieces (see Note)

½ cup (50 g) unsweetened finely shredded coconut

12 oz (340 g) strawberries, stemmed and quartered

½ cup (60 g) unsalted dry-roasted almonds, roughly chopped, or toasted slivered almonds (see Note)

Dressing Combine all dressing ingredients in a small bowl and whisk. Cover and refrigerate until ready to use.

Salad Place kale in a large bowl. Add a quarter of the dressing and toss to combine. Using your hands, give the leaves 2–3 aggressive squeezes. (This breaks down the fibers and allows the dressing to absorb.) You'll notice the kale becomes darker, glossier, and reduced in volume. Add the remaining salad ingredients and enough dressing to thoroughly coat it all. Give it another toss to combine and serve immediately or refrigerate to enjoy later.

NOTES

Bunches of curly kale can vary in size, so use your best judgment to know how much you'll need.

For maximum crunch, add the almonds right before serving.

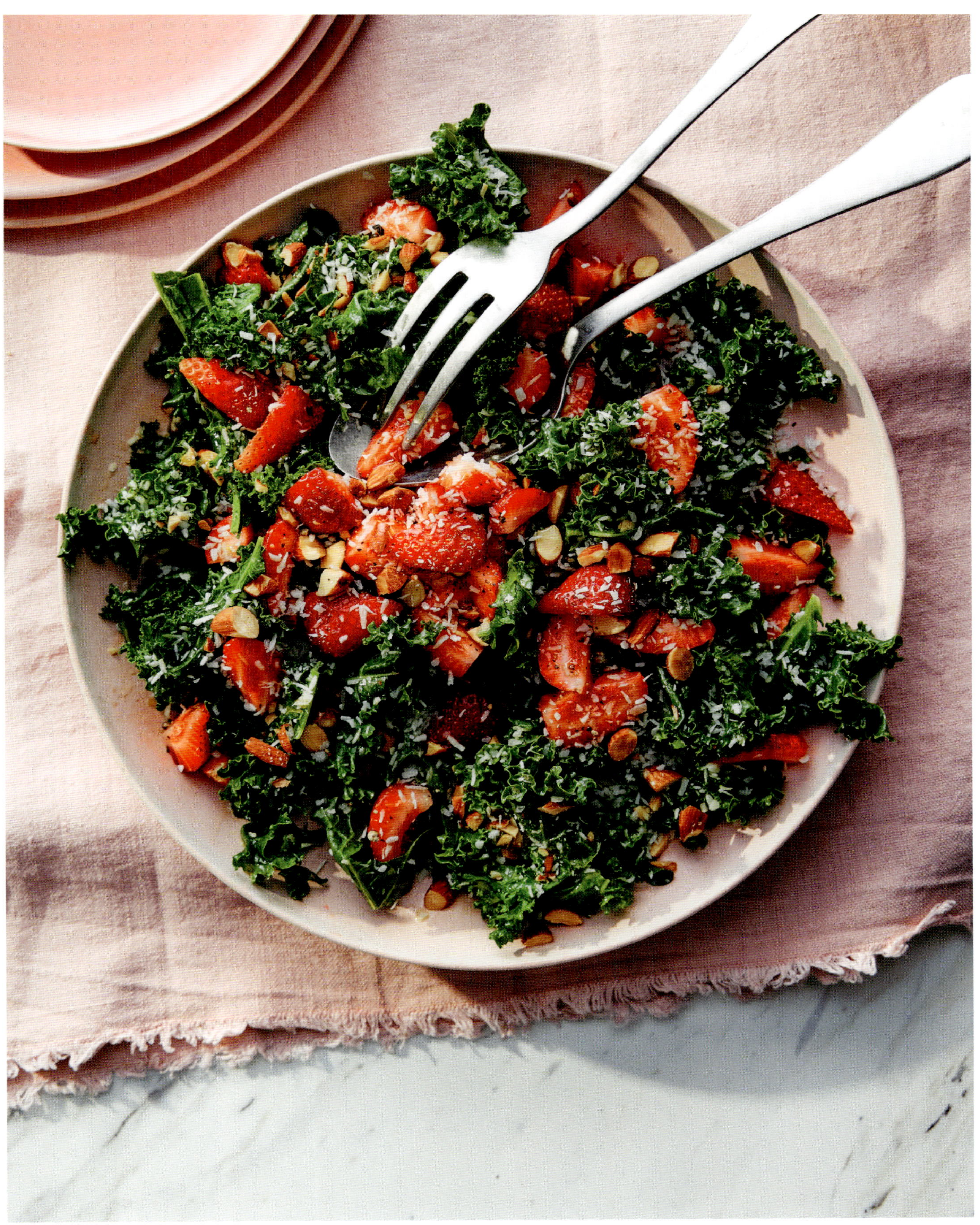

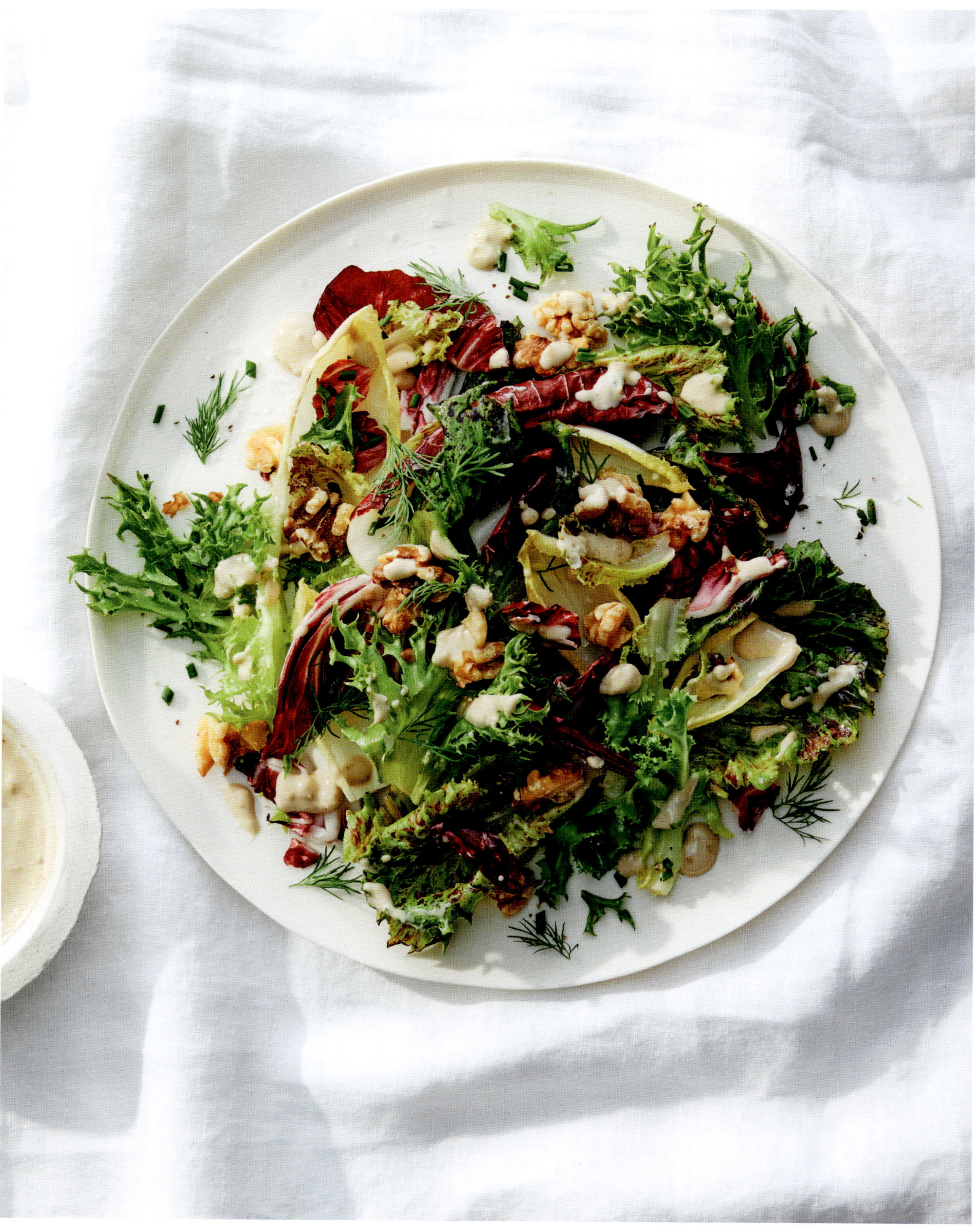

Radicchio sort of begs for Parmigiano. And while there's no way to replicate the king of cheeses, the aim here is to approximate that vibe. Radicchio and the other chicories have a lovely crunch and a subtle bitter edge that stands up well to a bold dressing. Toast your nuts within an inch of their life to maximize their flavor and crunch—just make sure to watch them like a hawk so they don't burn.

Chicory Salad with Toasted Walnut + Anchovy Vinaigrette

SERVES 4

Dressing

3 garlic cloves

4 oil-packed anchovy fillets

¼ cup (28 g) toasted walnuts

¼ cup (50 g) extra-virgin olive oil

2 tablespoons freshly squeezed lemon juice

1 teaspoon pink salt

1 teaspoon vinagre de Jerez sherry vinegar

1 teaspoon Dijon mustard

2 teaspoons honey

¼ teaspoon freshly cracked black pepper

Salad

1 small head of radicchio, torn into pieces

8 oz (227 g) mixed chicories, such as Belgian endive and frisée, leaves separated and torn into bite-sized pieces

1 cup (100 g) toasted walnuts, roughly chopped

¼ cup (10 g) chopped chives

Handful of dill, torn into small pieces

Freshly cracked black pepper

Dressing Using a mini food processor, pulse the garlic first to mince. Add the remaining dressing ingredients, pulsing with each addition until creamy and combined. Transfer to a small bowl and refrigerate until ready to use.

Salad In a large serving bowl, combine radicchio, chicories, walnuts, and chives. Drizzle with a generous amount of dressing and toss to coat.

Scatter dill over the top, season with pepper, and serve.

Elevate a simple roast chicken with this harmonious blend of bitter radicchio, sweet luscious figs, and toasty walnuts. My husband calls this an "adult salad" because of radicchio's divisive bitterness. But when coated in a sweet sherry vinaigrette, it's all brought back into balance. Fig season is short, so snag some when you can!

Radicchio + Fig Salad with Sherry Vinaigrette

SERVES 4

Dressing

- ½ teaspoon fennel seeds
- ¼ cup (50 g) extra-virgin olive oil
- 2 tablespoons vinagre de Jerez sherry vinegar
- 2 tablespoons honey
- ¼ teaspoon pink salt
- 4 grinds of freshly cracked black pepper

Salad

- 1 small shallot, thinly sliced crosswise
- 1 small head of radicchio, core removed and torn into bite-sized pieces
- 8 ripe figs, quartered
- 2 tablespoons finely chopped chives
- 1 cup (115 g) chopped well-toasted walnuts
- Maldon flake salt

Dressing Toast fennel seeds in a small skillet for 3–5 minutes over medium-low heat, until fragrant and lightly golden.

Whisk together all dressing ingredients in a small bowl. Refrigerate until ready to use. Making the dressing a few hours in advance allows the flavors to develop.

Salad Separate shallot rings. Soak them in a small bowl of water for 5 minutes to soften the bite. Drain, then pat dry.

In a medium bowl, combine shallots, radicchio, and the dressing and toss until well coated. Divide it among 4 plates. Layer the remaining ingredients, adding walnuts last so they retain their crunch. If there's any remaining dressing, drizzle it over each salad. Sprinkle with flake salt and serve.

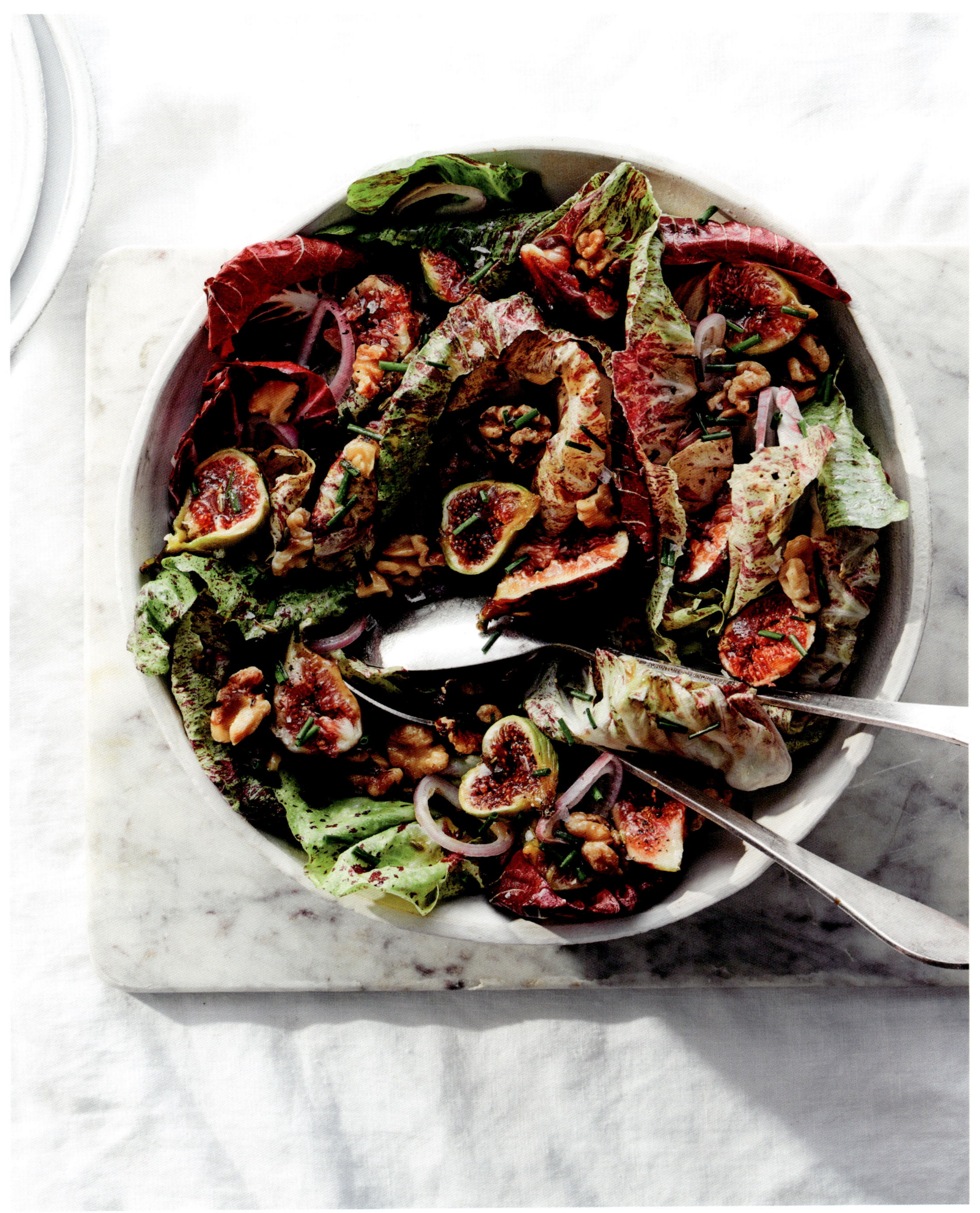

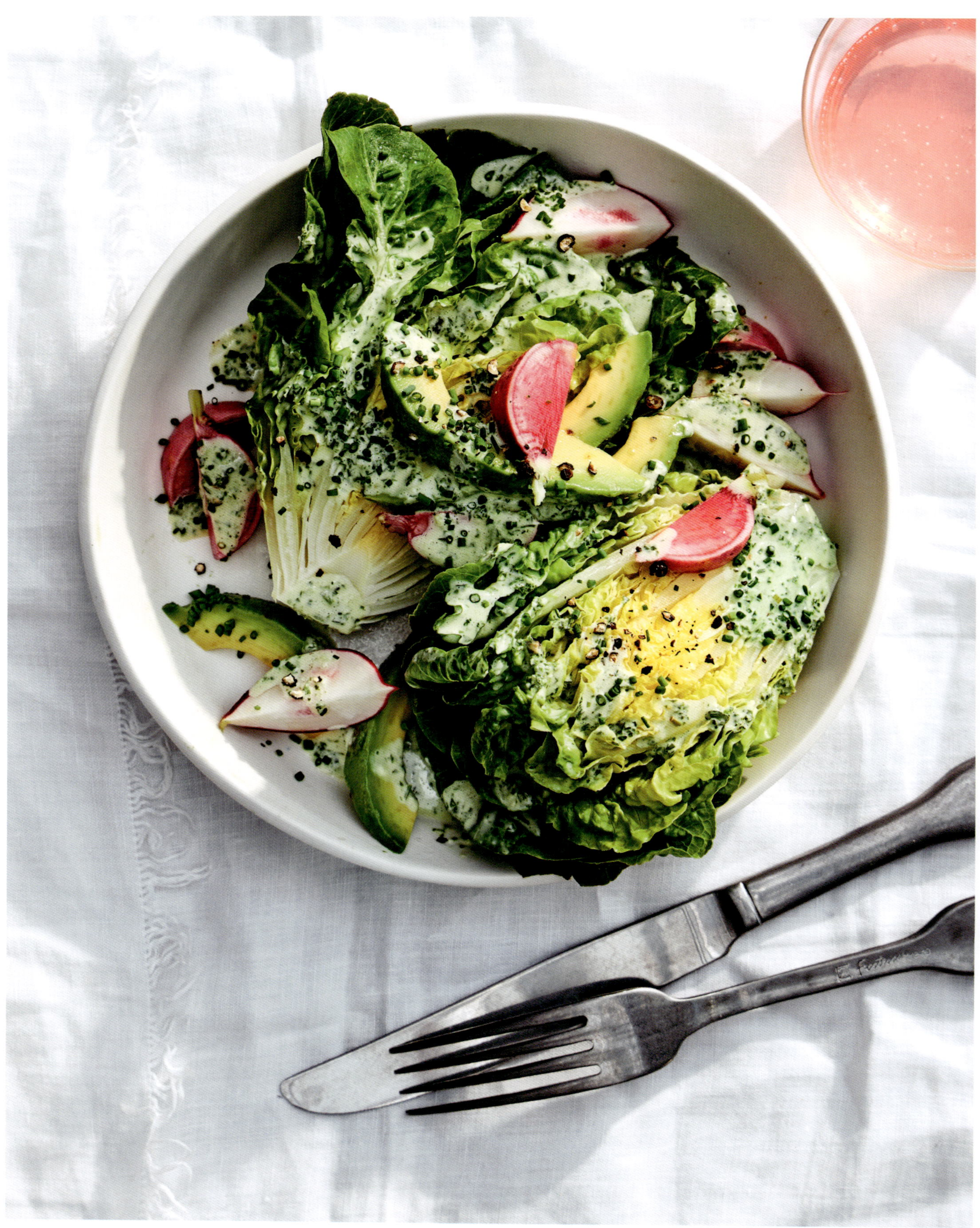

A newfangled wedge salad bursting with the savory herbaceousness of green goddess dressing! Little Gem lettuce can be tricky to source—if you can't find them, romaine hearts are the perfect stand-in. Make the dressing a few hours in advance so the flavors can develop.

Little Gem Wedge Salad with Green Goddess Dressing

SERVES 4

Dressing

4 garlic cloves

4 oil-packed anchovy fillets

3 tablespoons freshly squeezed lemon juice

1 tablespoon Champagne vinegar

1 cup (27 g) packed flat-leaf parsley, including tender stems

1 cup (25 g) packed basil leaves

1 (3/4-oz/21-g) package fresh tarragon, leaves only

1 teaspoon pink salt

1/4 cup (50 g) extra-virgin olive oil

1 cup (235 g) mayonnaise

Salad

4 heads of Little Gem lettuce or 2 romaine hearts, halved lengthwise

3 radishes, quartered

1 ripe avocado, thinly sliced

Chopped chives, for garnish

Freshly cracked black pepper, to taste

Dressing Using a food processor, pulse the garlic first to mince. Add the remaining dressing ingredients, except the mayo, and process until broken down. Add mayo and blend until creamy and combined. Transfer to a bowl and refrigerate until ready to use.

Salad Divide lettuce wedges among 4 plates. Add radishes and avocado slices to each, then drizzle with dressing. Sprinkle with chives and a few grinds of pepper. Serve.

This irresistibly crisp and bright slaw is scrumptious in any season, and it packs a nutritional punch! Brussels sprouts are rich in fiber, antioxidants, and plant-based omega-3s. They are also a great source of B vitamins necessary for cellular energy production and contain a good hit of vitamin A for eye health.

Brussels Sprouts Slaw with Honeycrisp + Pistachios

SERVES 4

Dressing

1 small shallot, finely chopped

1 garlic clove, finely chopped

½ teaspoon pink salt

¼ cup (50 g) extra-virgin olive oil

2 tablespoons honey

1 tablespoon apple cider vinegar

1 tablespoon Dijon mustard

2 grinds of freshly cracked black pepper

Slaw

1 lb (454 g) Brussels sprouts, trimmed

1 Honeycrisp apple

⅓ cup (46 g) shelled and salted pistachios

Dressing Whisk all dressing ingredients together in a small bowl until combined. Refrigerate until ready to use. Making the dressing a few hours in advance gives the shallot time to mellow and allows the flavors to meld.

Slaw Prepare the Brussels sprouts by removing any unsightly leaves. Shred them in a food processor fitted with the slicing attachment. (Alternatively, thinly slice them by hand.) Transfer Brussels sprouts to a large mixing bowl, add the dressing, and toss to coat. It's best dressed an hour or so in advance of serving.

To serve, core and slice apple. Add to the salad and toss to combine. Divide among 4 plates and sprinkle pistachios on top.

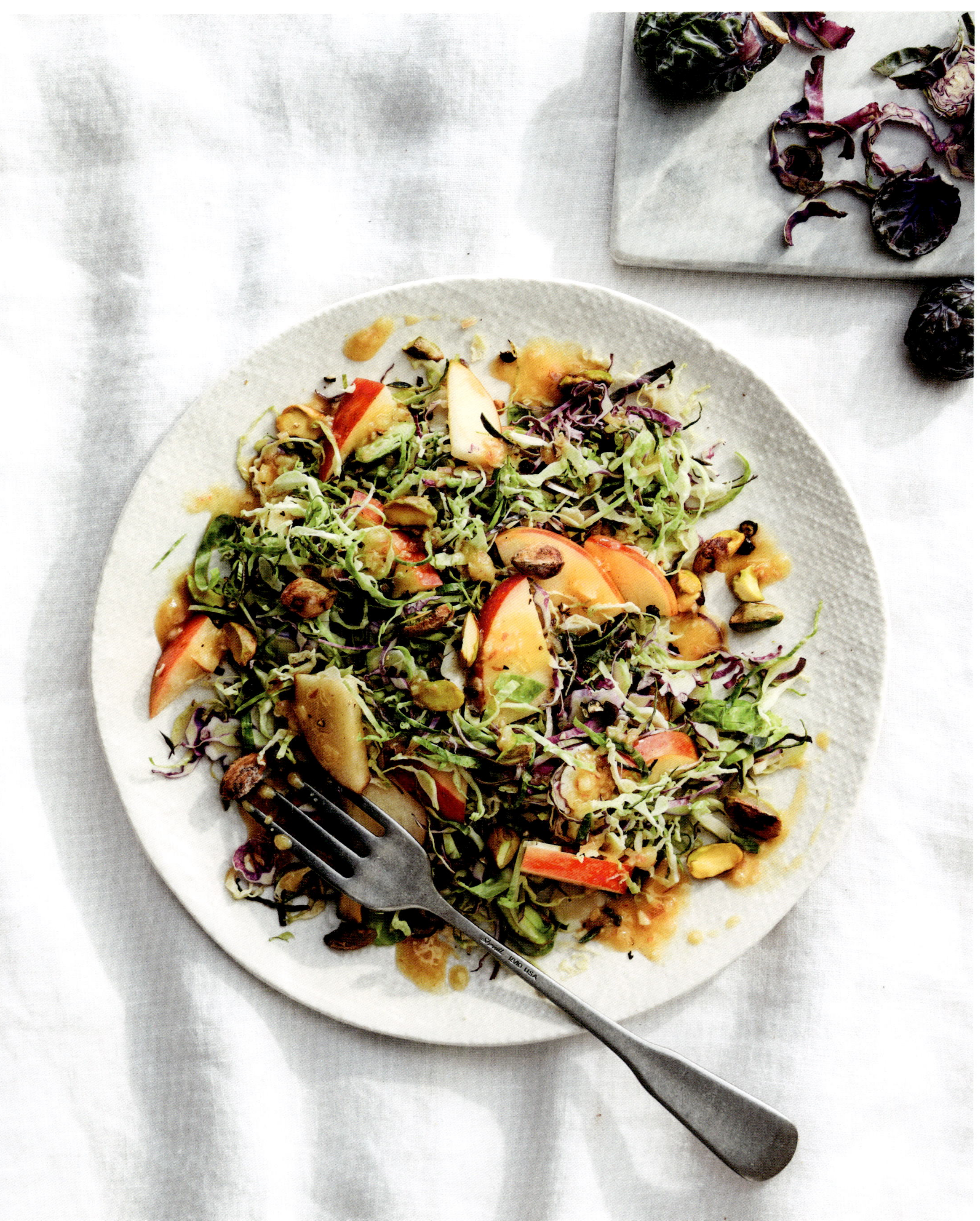

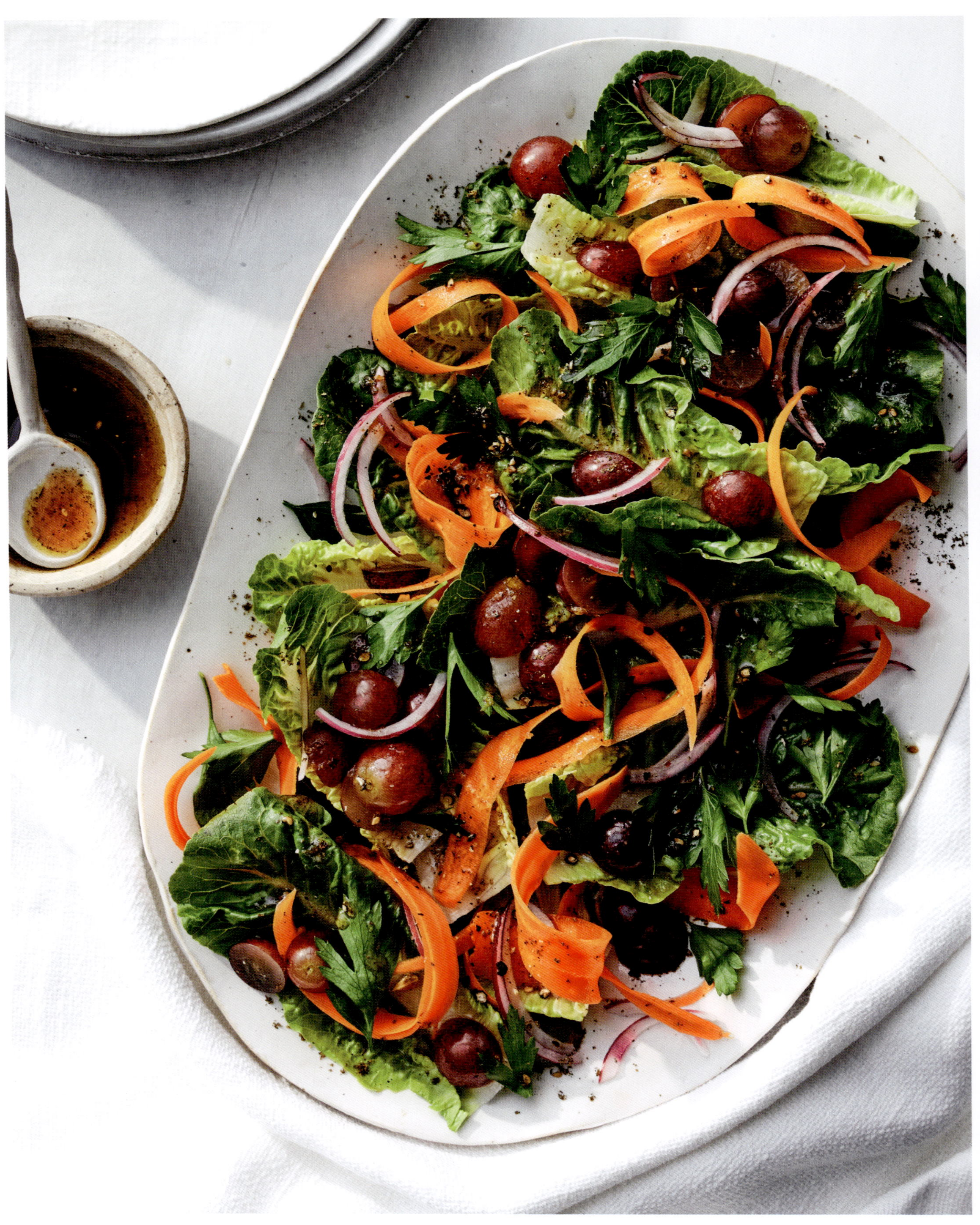

The dressing adds just the right amount of zip to this refreshingly crisp and juicy salad. It's packed with so much flavor that I'm tempted to drizzle it on anything that gets in the way.

Za'atar is a savory Middle Eastern spice blend traditionally made with hyssop, which is considered to have extensive health benefits. (Some less traditional versions substitute thyme as an alternative.) You'll also find it featured in the Za'atar Roast Chicken on page 135.

Little Gem Salad with Grapes + Za'atar Dressing

SERVES 4

Dressing

½ cup (100 g) extra-virgin olive oil

1 tablespoon za'atar (see Note)

Zest of 1 lemon

2 tablespoons freshly squeezed lemon juice

1 tablespoon honey

1 teaspoon pink salt

Salad

4 heads of Little Gem lettuce or 2 romaine hearts, leaves separated (see Note)

¼ small red onion, thinly sliced

1 carrot, shaved into ribbons with a vegetable peeler

Large handful of flat-leaf parsley with tender stems, roughly chopped

1½ cups (250 g) red seedless grapes, halved

Dressing Whisk together all dressing ingredients in a small bowl. Refrigerate until ready to use. Make it in advance so flavors can develop.

Salad Place all salad ingredients in a large bowl, add a generous amount of dressing, and toss to coat.

NOTES

My preferred brand of za'atar—The Spice Way's traditional Lebanese za'atar with hyssop—is available online. Avoid brands that substitute thyme and oregano for the hyssop.

If you can't find Little Gem lettuce, use romaine hearts (just the crisp inside leaves), separated and quartered.

Native to North America, cranberries are as American as apple pie. By the time October rolls around each year, I'm on cranberry watch because we only get three short months with these crimson beauties. They're loaded with antioxidants, and in a sea of heavy Thanksgiving dishes, this light, crisp relish brings balance into the mix. It's bursting with flavor and offers a fresh alternative to the usual cranberry concoctions.

Fresh Cranberry Relish with Cherries + Cardamom

SERVES 6

1 (12-oz/340-g) bag fresh cranberries
3/4 cup (100 g) dried tart cherries, chopped
1/2 cup (157 g) pure maple syrup
1/2 teaspoon ground cardamom
1/4 teaspoon ground cinnamon
Scant 1/4 teaspoon pink salt

Make this a day ahead so the cherries can hydrate in the juices and flavors have a chance to meld.

Discard any rotten or mushy cranberries. Rinse, then pat dry with a paper towel so they don't make the relish too juicy.

Combine all ingredients in a food processor and pulse until all cranberries are coarsely chopped. Transfer to a bowl and refrigerate until ready to use. It holds up in the fridge for up to 5 days.

NOTE

You don't have to reserve this relish for turkey—it's the perfect complement to roast chicken and can be enjoyed all season long. For a quick salad, toss baby romaine lightly in olive oil and sprinkle with flake salt. Add shredded rotisserie chicken and thinly shaved red onion (use a mandoline for best results), then top it all with a generous scoop of cranberry relish.

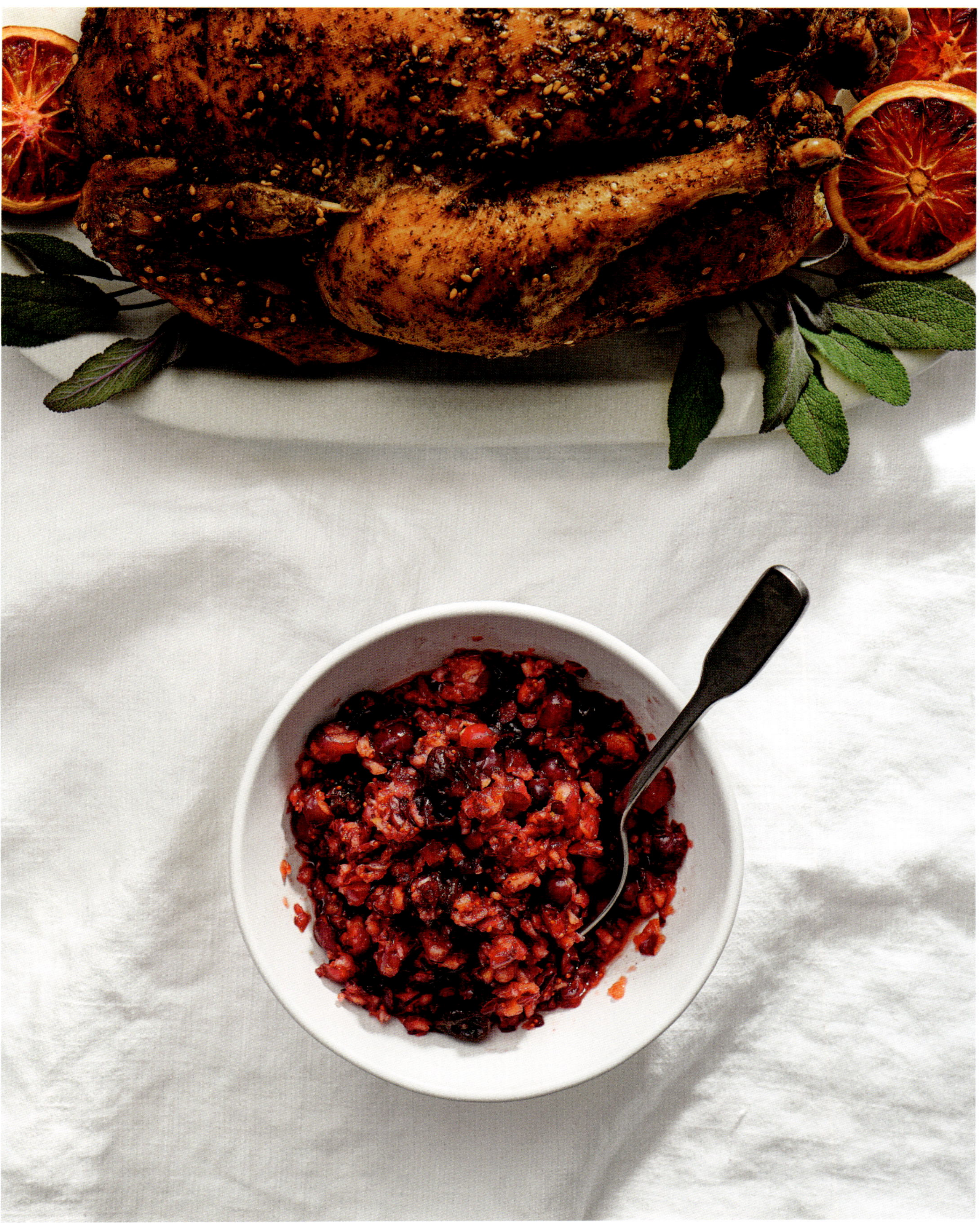

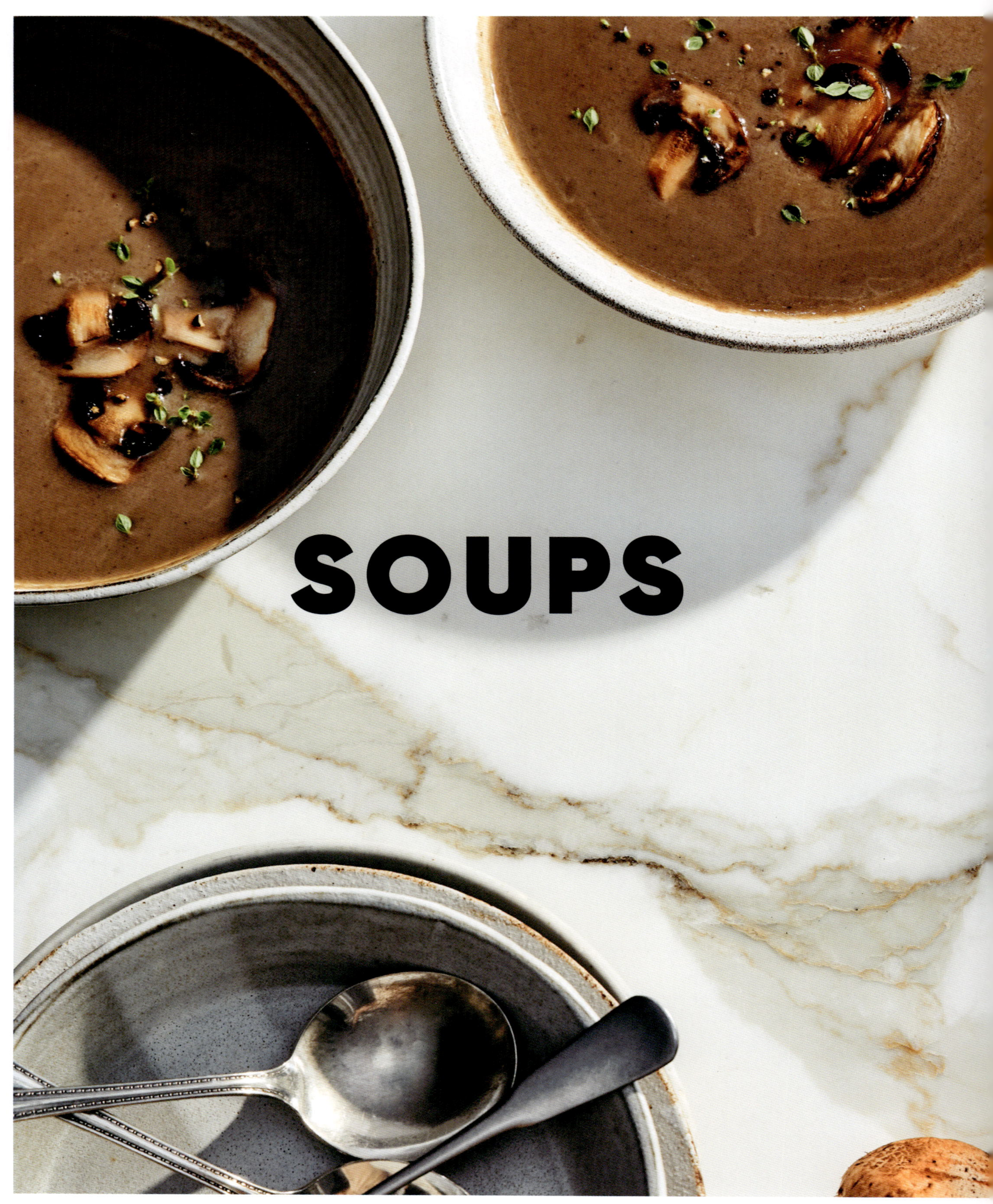

SOUPS

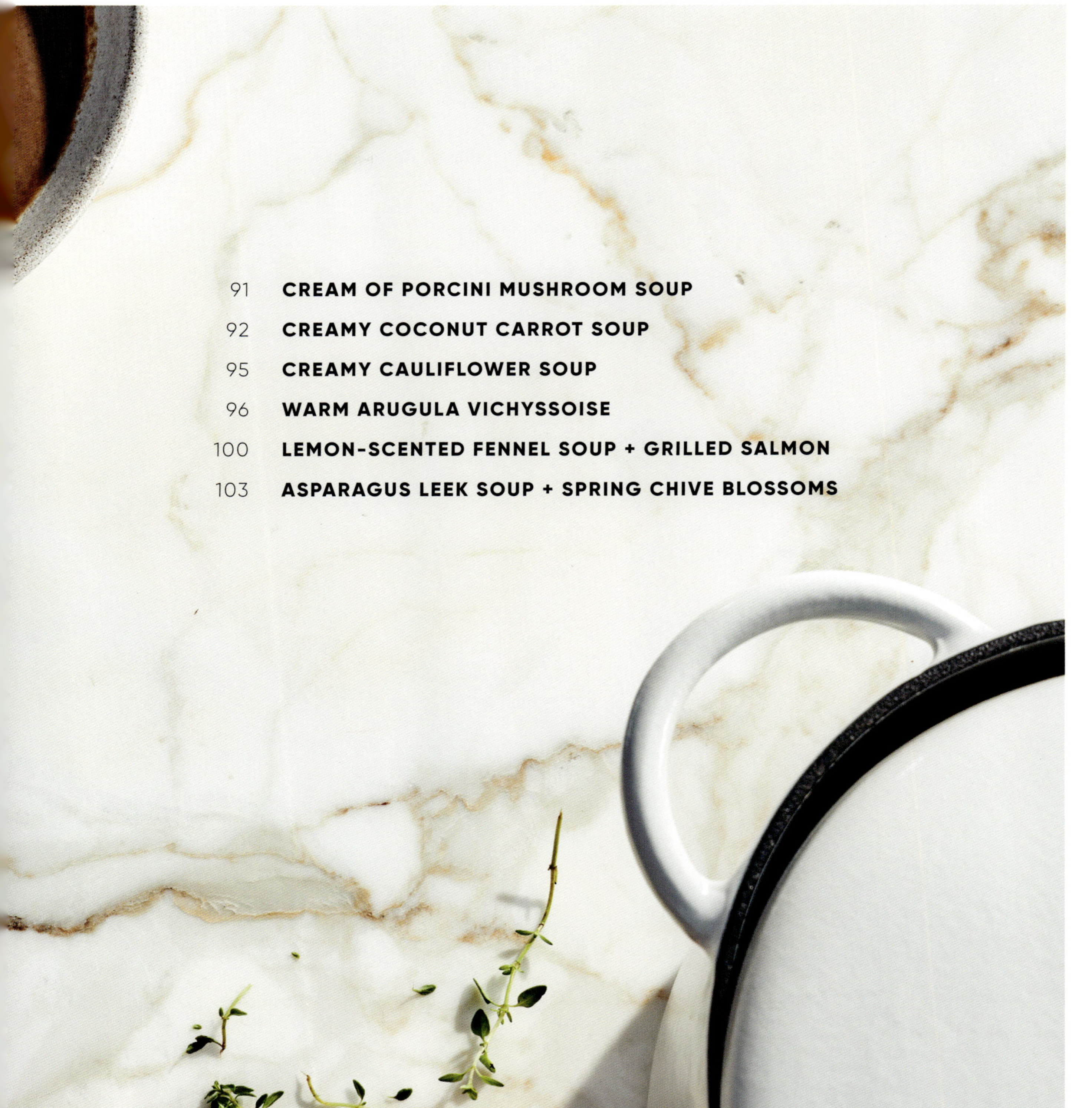

91 CREAM OF PORCINI MUSHROOM SOUP

92 CREAMY COCONUT CARROT SOUP

95 CREAMY CAULIFLOWER SOUP

96 WARM ARUGULA VICHYSSOISE

100 LEMON-SCENTED FENNEL SOUP + GRILLED SALMON

103 ASPARAGUS LEEK SOUP + SPRING CHIVE BLOSSOMS

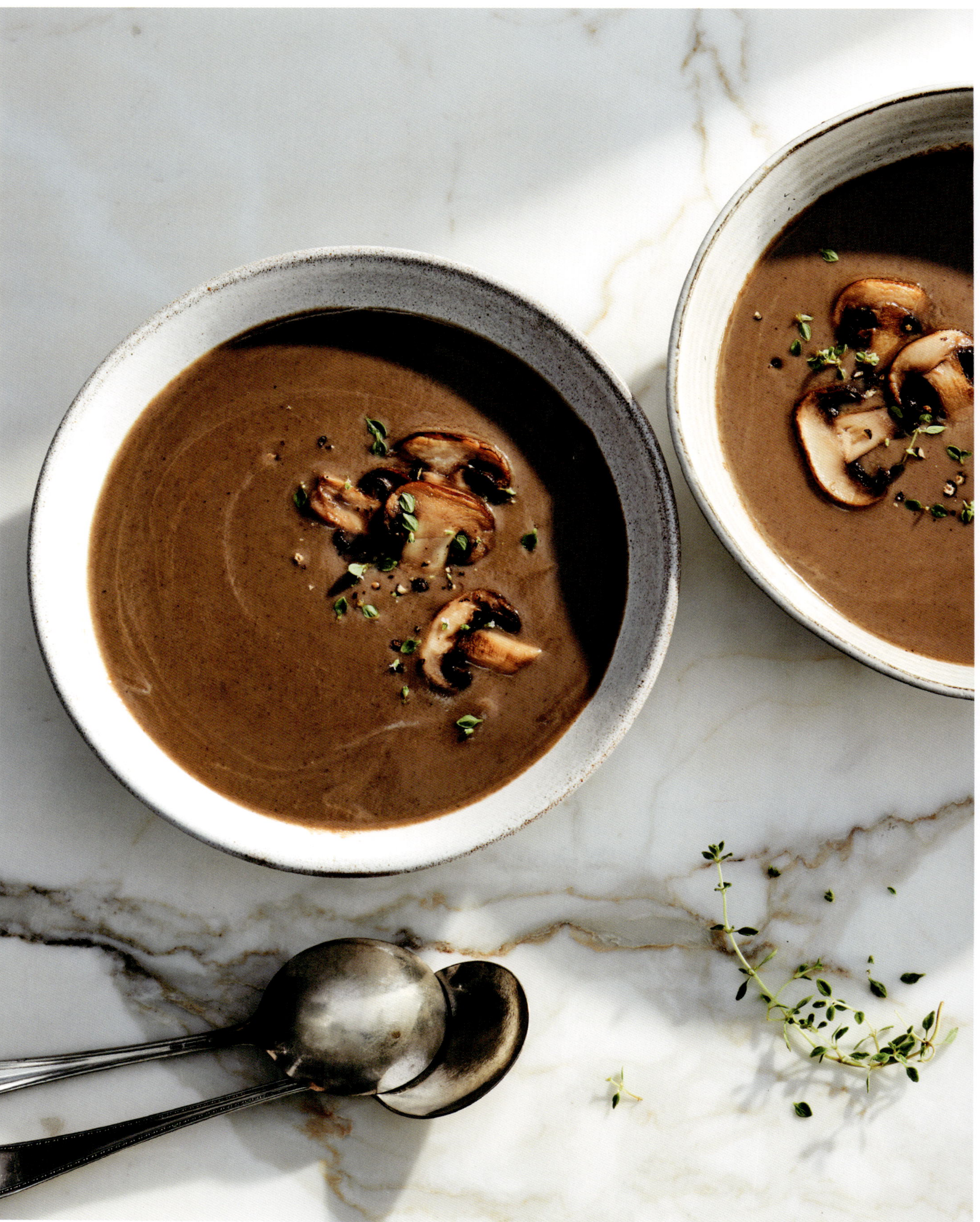

Indulge in this rich and savory soup while enjoying a long list of health benefits. Cremini mushrooms (sometimes also called baby portobellos) are an excellent source of B vitamins and packed with phytonutrients that help boost immune function, tame inflammation, prevent arthritis, and protect against heart disease. This earthy combination of cremini and porcini mushrooms is further elevated by the heady scent of cream sherry.

Cream of Porcini Mushroom Soup

SERVES 6

- 24 oz (680 g) cremini mushrooms
- 8 cups (1.89 L) chicken stock (divided)
- 1 oz (28 g) dried porcini mushrooms
- Extra-virgin olive oil, for the pan
- 1 large yellow onion, finely chopped
- 2 large leeks, white and light green parts only, thinly sliced
- 6 garlic cloves, finely chopped
- 2 tablespoons thyme leaves, plus extra thyme sprigs for garnish
- 2 teaspoons pink salt
- Black pepper, to taste
- ¼ cup (60 g) cream sherry (see Note)
- 1 (13.5-oz/400-ml) can full-fat, additive-free coconut milk

Rinse cremini mushrooms quickly under cold running water to prevent waterlogging, then let them drain on paper towels. Slightly trim the stems, then thinly slice.

Pour 1 cup of the stock in a small microwave-safe bowl and heat until very hot. Add dried porcini and set aside to soak until hydrated. Give them a quick stir and allow to sit undisturbed.

Meanwhile, add a splash of olive oil, onion, and cremini mushrooms to a large stockpot and sauté over medium-high heat until the mushroom liquid has evaporated and mushrooms are browned.

Add leeks, garlic, thyme, salt, and pepper. Sauté for another 2 minutes, until fragrant.

Remove porcini from the soaking liquid and chop, then add them to the pot. Pour the soaking liquid into the pot, taking care to not add in any of the grit that has settled to the bottom. Add the remaining 7 cups of stock and bring to a boil over high heat. Reduce heat to medium, then simmer for 20 minutes, uncovered, until it is slightly reduced and flavors are concentrated. Turn off the heat.

Using an immersion blender, blend until creamy or to your desired consistency. (Alternatively, use a regular blender for a creamier consistency.) Stir in cream sherry and coconut milk and blend to combine.

Ladle into bowls, then garnish each bowl with a sprig of thyme, if desired.

NOTE

I recommend using Harveys Bristol Cream Sherry. It's easy to find, has a long shelf life, and is also featured in the Chicken Liver Mousse recipe (page 59).

Though redolent of fall, you'll want this one in your year-round rotation! Creamy, complex, and loaded with nutritious veg, it is truly greater than the sum of its parts. I've also provided a vegan option in the Note.

SERVES 6

Creamy Coconut Carrot Soup

- Extra-virgin olive oil, for the pan
- 2 yellow onions, chopped
- 1 lb (454 g) carrots, peeled and sliced into coins
- 6 large celery stalks, plus tender celery leaves, chopped
- 6 garlic cloves, roughly chopped
- 2 teaspoons pink salt
- 1 teaspoon pumpkin pie spice
- ⅛ teaspoon cayenne (optional; see Note)
- 4 cups (946 ml) chicken stock (see Note)
- 1 (13.5-oz/400-ml) can full-fat, additive-free coconut milk
- Sliced scallions or chives, for garnish (optional)

Heat a splash of oil in a stockpot over medium-high heat. Add onions and sauté for 15 minutes, until lightly golden around the edges. Add carrots and celery and stir. Add the remaining ingredients (except the coconut milk), cover, and bring to a boil. Reduce heat to low and simmer for 30 minutes, until the vegetables are very tender. Turn off the heat.

Stir in the coconut milk, then carefully transfer the soup to a blender. Purée until smooth. (Alternatively, use an immersion blender, but it won't be as smooth.) Season to taste with salt.

Ladle the soup into bowls, then garnish with scallions or chives, if desired.

NOTES

If you're avoiding nightshades, omit the cayenne.

For a vegan option, replace the chicken stock with 3 cups (720 g) filtered water plus a second (13.5-oz/400-ml) can of coconut milk. Add the water when directed to add the chicken stock. Reserve the additional can of coconut milk until the end, adding it at the same time as the first can of coconut milk.

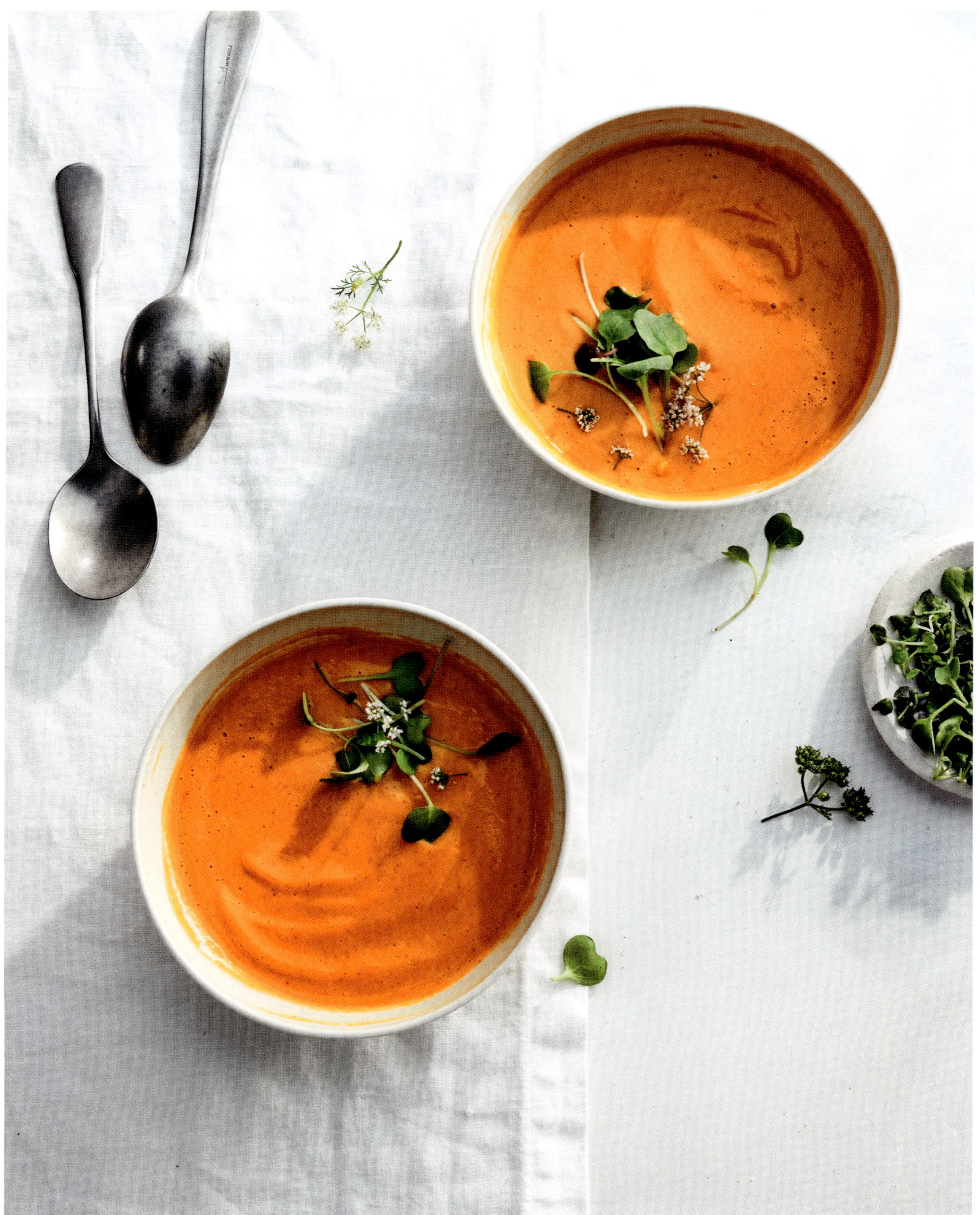

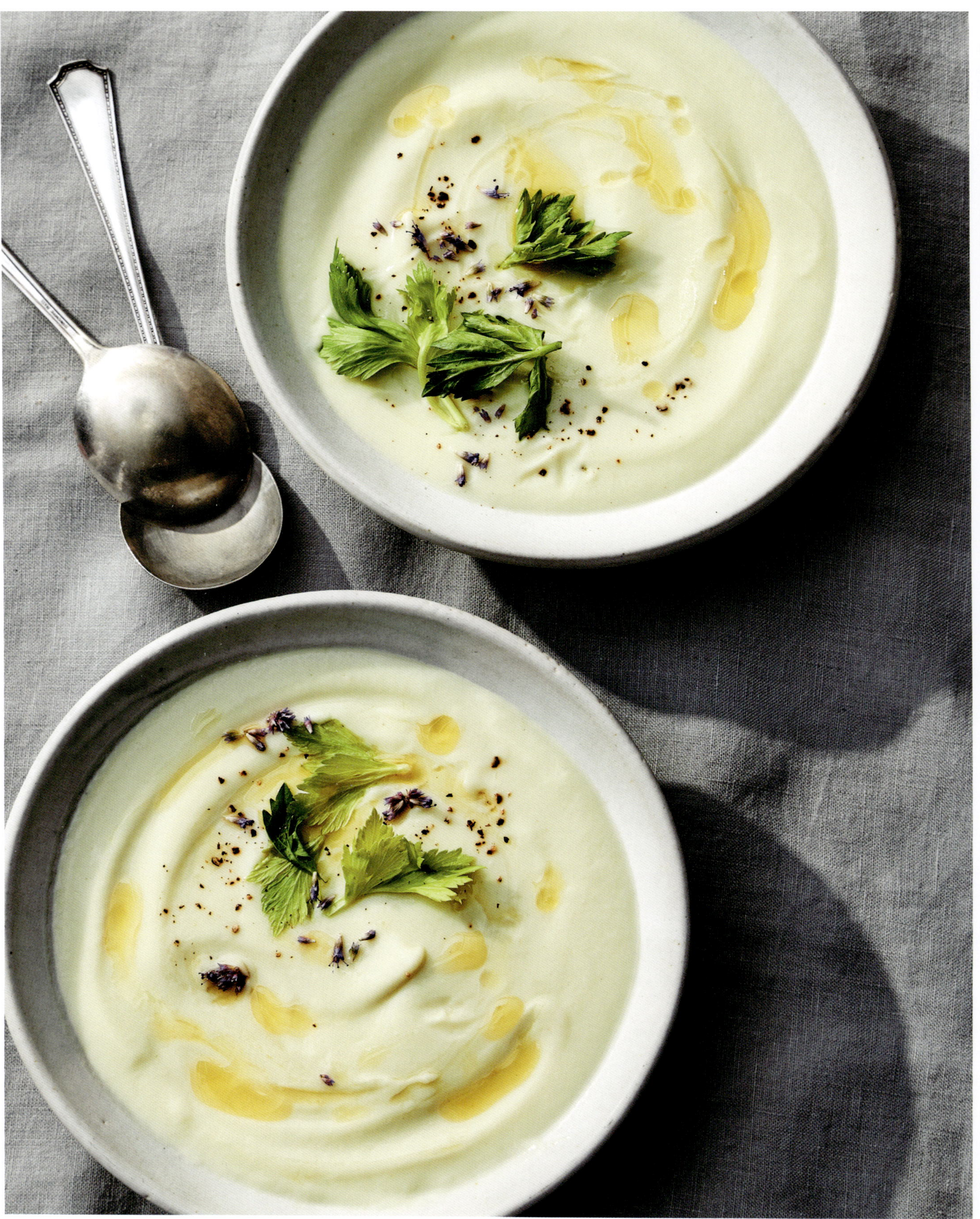

If you're on the fence about cauliflower, this silky soup is unexpectedly subtle and might just win you over. It's the perfect thing to help bring balance during the winter months when holiday goodies leave us feeling less than optimal. Cozy up to a warm, comforting bowl of this seasonal soup, and pair it with Roast Chicken (page 135) or a mild flaky white fish for a complete meal.

Creamy Cauliflower Soup

SERVES 4

- 2 small shallots, roughly chopped
- 3 garlic cloves, roughly chopped
- 4 large celery stalks, chopped
- 1 large head of cauliflower, finely chopped
- 2 cups (480 g) filtered water
- 1½ teaspoons pink salt
- ¼ teaspoon white pepper
- 1 (13.5-oz/400-ml) can full-fat, additive-free coconut milk
- Celery leaves, for garnish
- Extra-virgin olive oil, for drizzling

Combine all ingredients, except coconut milk, celery leaves, and oil, in a large saucepan over high heat. Cover, and when it reaches a boil, reduce the heat to medium-low and simmer for 15 minutes, until vegetables are very tender. Turn off the heat, then stir in coconut milk.

Carefully transfer the soup to a blender and blend until smooth. (Alternatively, use an immersion blender, but it won't be as smooth.) Season to taste with salt.

Ladle the soup into bowls, then garnish with celery leaves and finish with a drizzle of olive oil.

Your daily greens disguised as potato soup! This warm and creamy arugula vichyssoise was broadly adapted from Giada De Laurentiis's fantastic recipe. I've omitted the two forms of dairy (Parmesan and mascarpone) contained in the original recipe, and I've replaced the Yukon Gold potatoes with Hannah sweet potatoes, which are white-fleshed and less sweet than other sweet potatoes. I limit the sweet potatoes to one pound, allowing the other ingredients to take center stage and balance their subtle sweetness. To make it a complete meal, I top each bowl with a halved jammy egg.

Warm Arugula Vichyssoise

SERVES 4

- ¼ cup (50 g) extra-virgin olive oil (divided)
- 2 large leeks, white and light green parts only, thinly sliced
- 4 garlic cloves, roughly chopped
- 1½ teaspoons pink salt
- 1 lb (454 g) Hannah sweet potatoes, peeled and diced
- 4 cups (946 ml) chicken stock
- ¼ teaspoon red pepper flakes (optional; see Note)
- 1 (5-oz/142-g) bag baby arugula
- 1 teaspoon lemon zest
- 2 tablespoons freshly squeezed lemon juice
- 4 soft-boiled eggs, for garnish (optional)
- Maldon flake salt, for sprinkling

Heat 2 tablespoons of oil in a large saucepan over medium-high heat. Add leeks, garlic, and salt and sauté for 5 minutes, until the leeks are soft but not brown.

Add sweet potatoes, stock, and red pepper flakes. Stir, then bring to a boil. Cover, reduce the heat, and gently simmer for 20 minutes, until potatoes are very tender. Turn off the heat, then add arugula. Stir for 1 minute, until wilted.

Add the remaining 2 tablespoons of oil, lemon zest, and juice. Carefully transfer the soup to a blender and blend until smooth. (Alternatively, use an immersion blender, but it won't be as smooth.)

Ladle into bowls and top with soft-boiled eggs, if desired, and flake salt.

NOTE

If you are avoiding nightshades, omit the red pepper flakes.

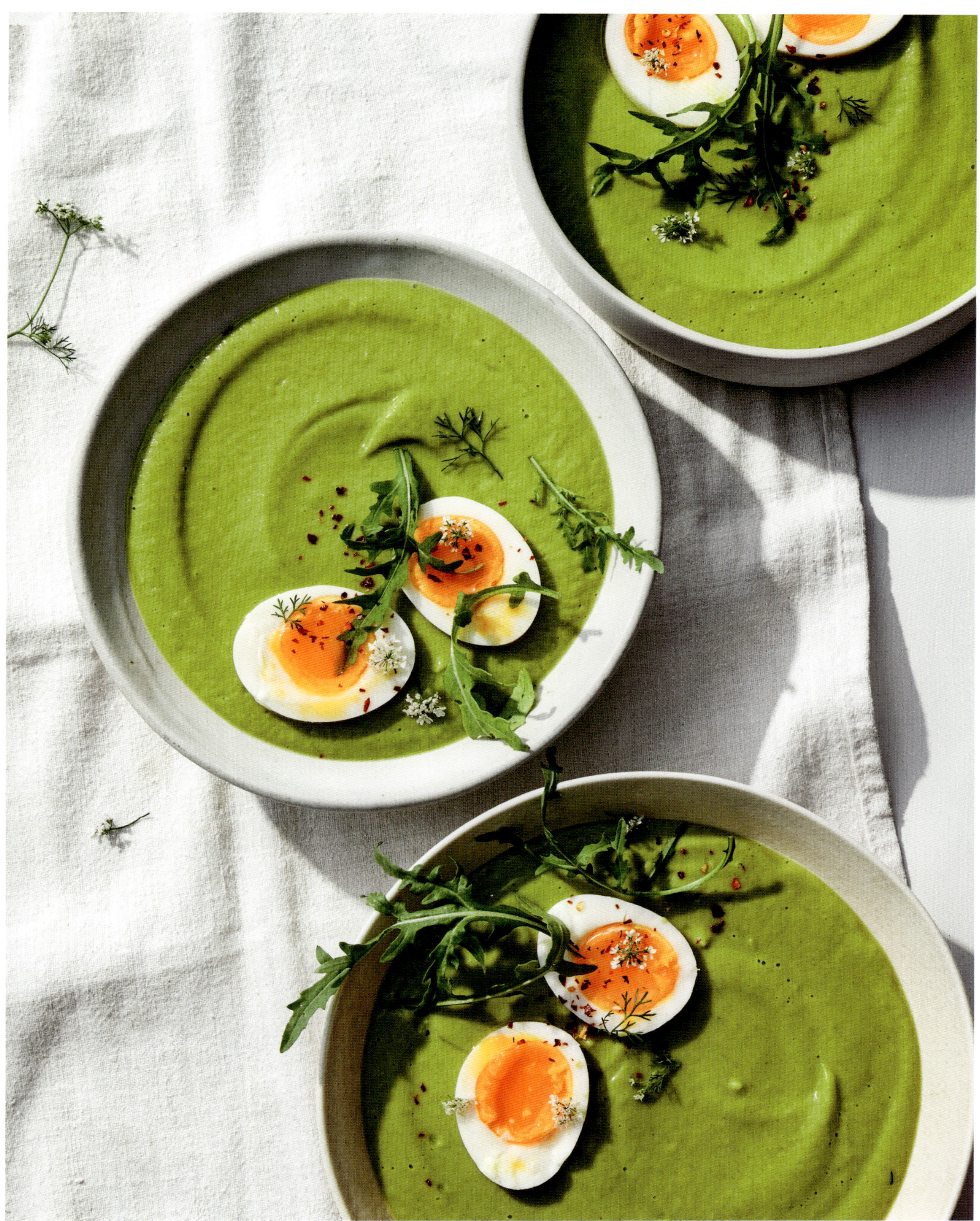

Once crowned with a buttery bite of salmon, this light and luxurious soup is what dinners alfresco are made of.

Lemon-Scented Fennel Soup + Grilled Salmon

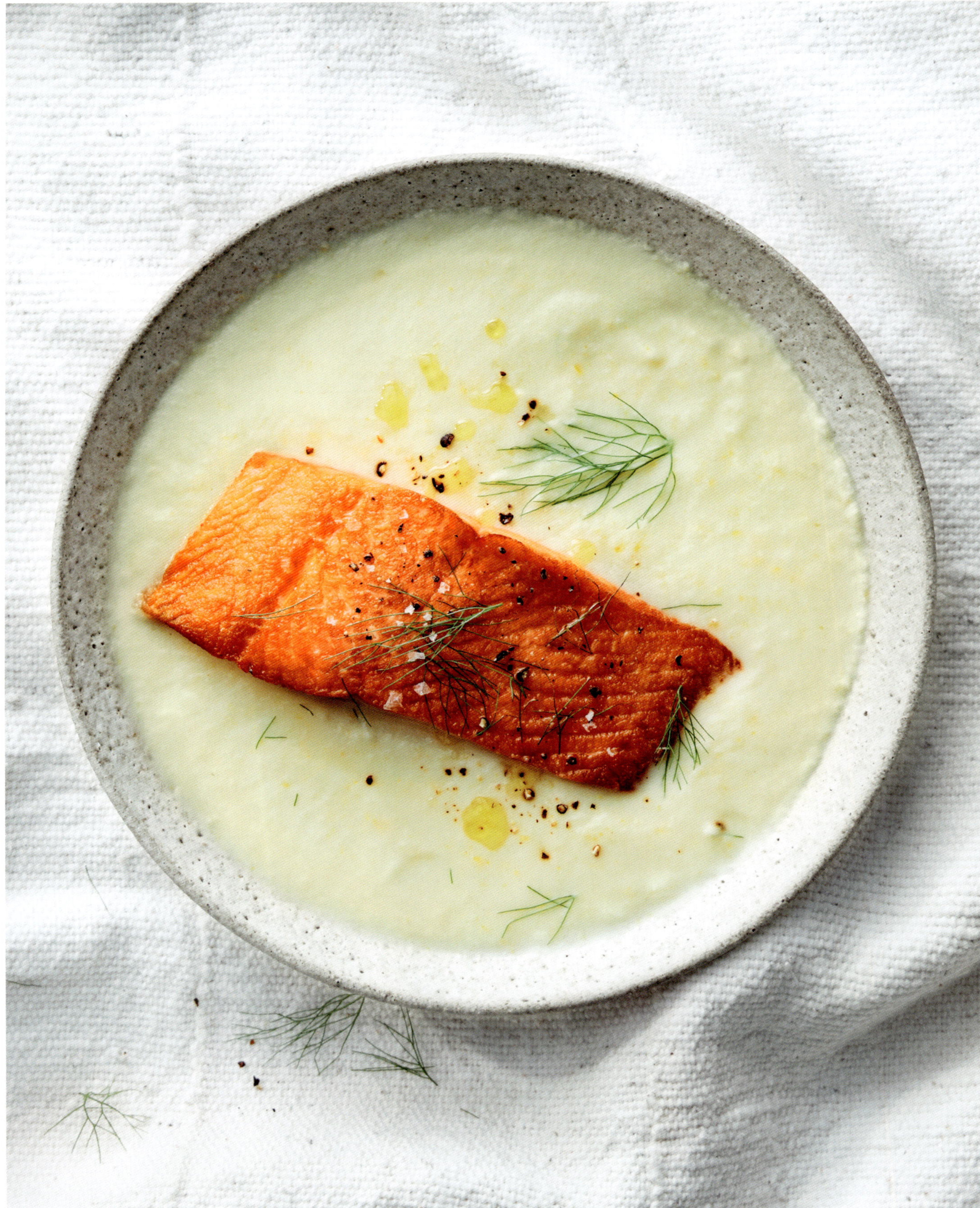

This light and luxurious fennel soup is a study in subtlety and restraint. And once crowned with a buttery bite of salmon, it's what summer dinners alfresco are made of. For pairing, opt for a mild salmon such as king or Atlantic, as a delicate flavor complements the soup better than fuller-flavored varieties like sockeye. A generous amount of lemon zest lends a sublime floral note to the finish.

Lemon-Scented Fennel Soup + Grilled Salmon

SERVES 4

Salmon

4 (6-oz/170-g) fresh salmon fillets

Extra-virgin olive oil, for coating

Pink salt, for sprinkling

Soup

3 medium-large fennel bulbs

¼ cup (50 g) extra-virgin olive oil (see Note)

2 teaspoons pink salt

5 cups (1.15 L) filtered water

Zest of 3 lemons (see Note)

Maldon flake salt, for finishing

Salmon Bring salmon to room temperature by removing it from the fridge and setting aside for 30 minutes. This ensures even doneness.

Soup To prepare fennel, remove cores, thinly slice, and reserve fronds for garnish. In large saucepan, combine oil, pink salt, and fennel slices and stir to coat. Cover and cook over medium heat, stirring occasionally, for 10 minutes, until the fennel is softened. Reduce the heat, if necessary, to prevent the fennel from browning.

Add the water, cover, and bring to a boil. Reduce heat to low and simmer gently for 20 minutes, until fennel is very tender. Uncover, then allow it to cool for 10 minutes.

Carefully transfer the soup to a blender and blend until smooth. Stir in lemon zest and blend again until it's incorporated. (We add the zest last to preserve its vibrant flavor.) Keep soup warm.

Assembly Preheat outdoor grill over medium-high heat.

Pat dry salmon. Coat each one with oil and sprinkle generously with pink salt. Grill, skin-side down, until golden, crisp, and nearly cooked through. Flip over and cook for another 1–2 minutes, until an instant-read thermometer inserted in the thickest part of the fillet registers 125°F. (Alternatively, arrange salmon skin-side down in a cool, dry [no oil] nonstick skillet—you may need to do this in batches. Cook undisturbed on medium heat for 8–10 minutes, until the skin is golden and crispy. Briefly press down with a spatula to ensure the fillet is making full contact with the pan. Flip them over and cook for another 1–2 minutes.)

To serve, ladle soup into 4 wide, shallow bowls. Top each with a grilled salmon fillet and garnish with hand-torn fennel fronds. Sprinkle with flake salt and serve warm.

NOTES

Since olive oil plays a starring role, select a high-quality option that is well balanced, avoiding those that are overly fruity or grassy.

You may be tempted to add a squeeze of lemon juice, but don't. Save your naked lemons for another use such as lemonade.

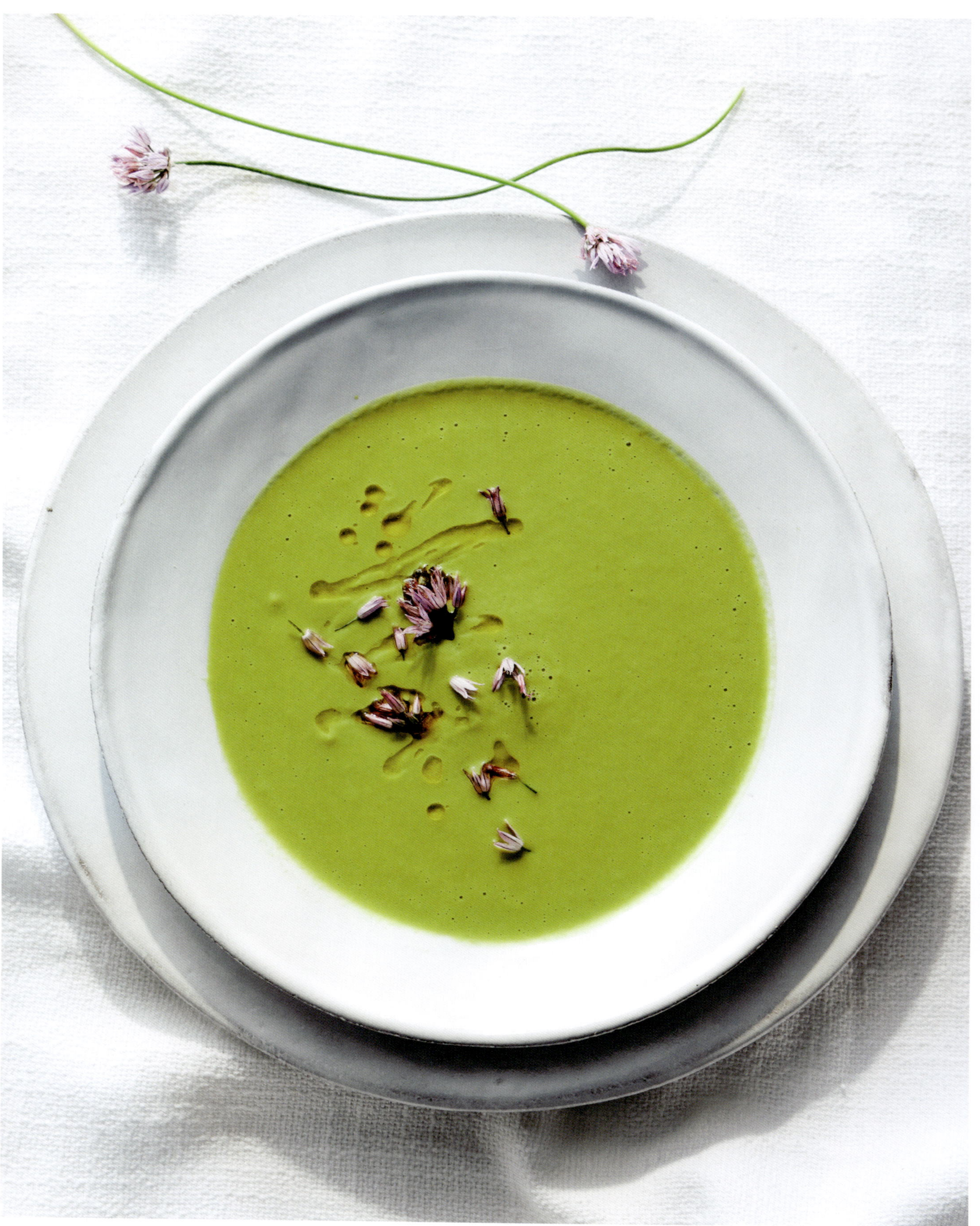

I love making this light and colorful soup in early spring, when asparagus and leeks begin to make an appearance at the local farmers' market—but it's become a year-round staple for us, too. Chive blossoms have a short window of availability, but adding them as a garnish, when possible, provides both a dainty purple pop of color and a hint of garlic flavor!

Asparagus Leek Soup + Spring Chive Blossoms

SERVES 4–6

- Extra-virgin olive oil, for the pan
- 2 leeks, white and light green parts only, thinly sliced
- 2 lbs (907 g) asparagus, trimmed and quartered into segments
- 2 garlic cloves, roughly chopped
- 1½ teaspoons pink salt, plus extra to taste
- ⅛ teaspoon cayenne (optional; see Note)
- 4 cups (946 ml) chicken stock
- ½ cup (120 g) canned full-fat, additive-free coconut milk
- 1 tablespoon freshly squeezed lime juice, plus extra to taste
- Chopped chives and chive blossoms, for garnish (optional)

Heat a splash of oil in a large saucepan over medium heat. Add leeks and asparagus and sauté for 4–5 minutes, until asparagus turns bright green. Add the garlic, salt, and cayenne, then pour in stock. Cover, increase heat to high, and bring to a boil. Reduce the heat to low and gently simmer for 8–10 minutes, until asparagus is tender. Turn off the heat.

Stir in coconut milk. Carefully transfer the soup to a blender and blend until smooth. (Alternatively, use an immersion blender, but it won't be as smooth.) Add lime juice and give it one last whirl. Season to taste with more salt or lime juice.

To serve, ladle soup into bowls and garnish with chopped chives and chive blossoms, if desired.

NOTE

If you're avoiding nightshades, omit the cayenne.

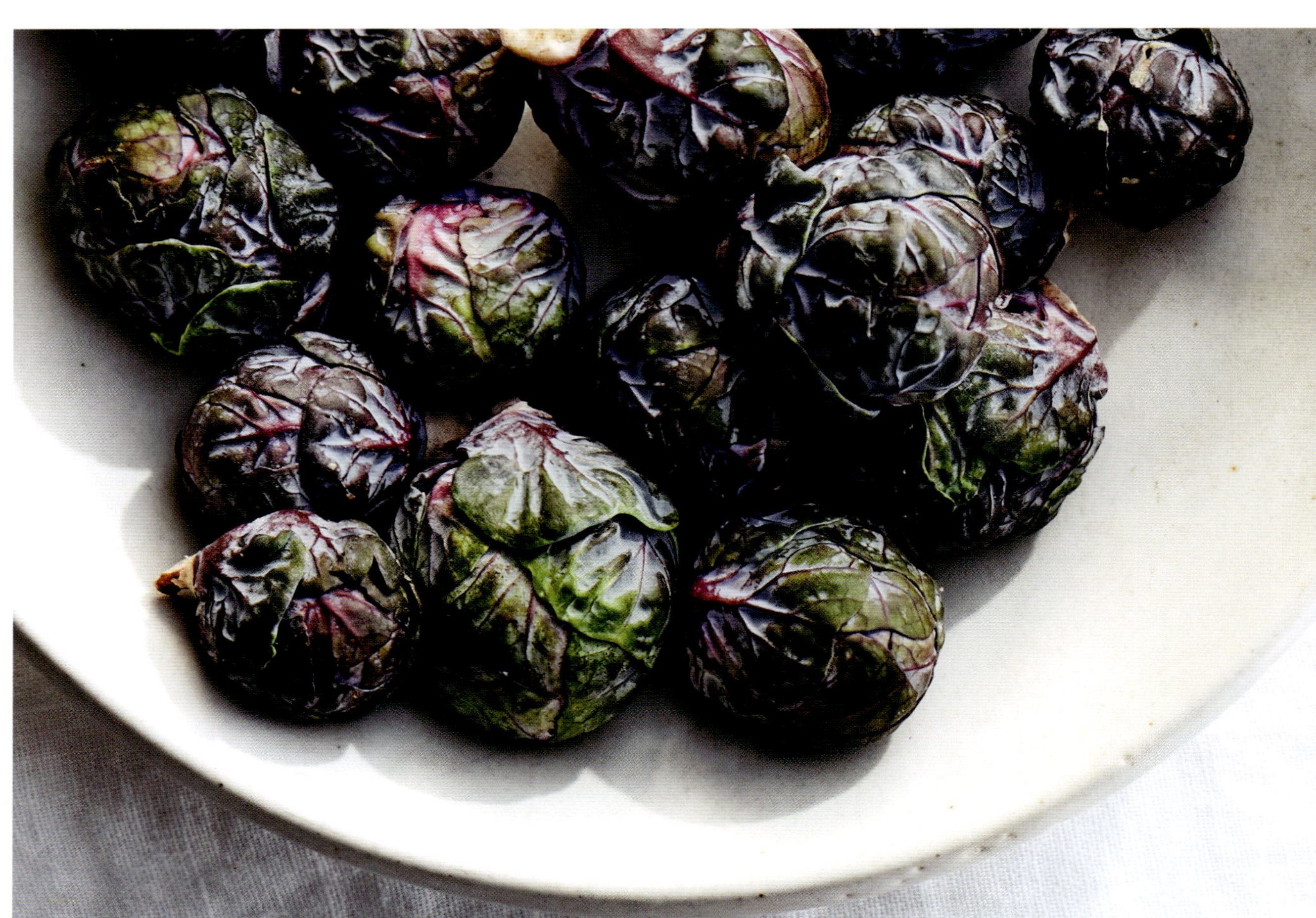

VEGETABLES

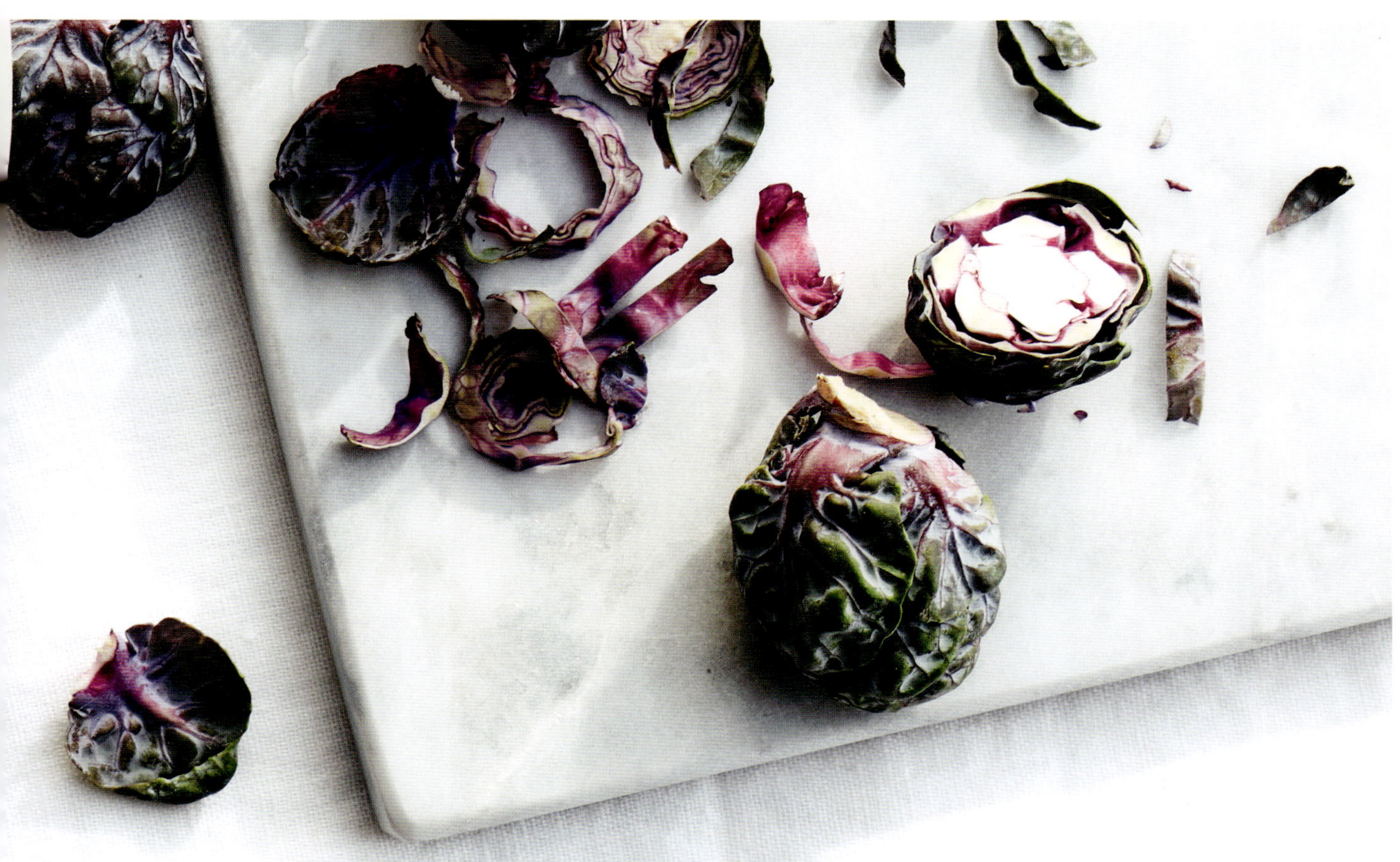

107 **CHARRED BROCCOLI + LEMON TAHINI SAUCE**

108 **TAHINI-CHARRED CAULIFLOWER WITH DATES + MINT**

111 **HARICOTS VERTS WITH HAZELNUTS + ORANGE**

112 **GARLIC MASHED CAULIFLOWER**

114 **RUSTIC FENNEL + CELERY ROOT MASH**

115 **RUTABAGA MASH WITH SAGE + CRISPY SHALLOTS**

117 **CHARRED ASPARAGUS + LEMON-PISTACHIO GREMOLATA**

120 **ROASTED BRUSSELS SPROUTS + BLOOD ORANGES WITH SWEET WHITE BALSAMIC**

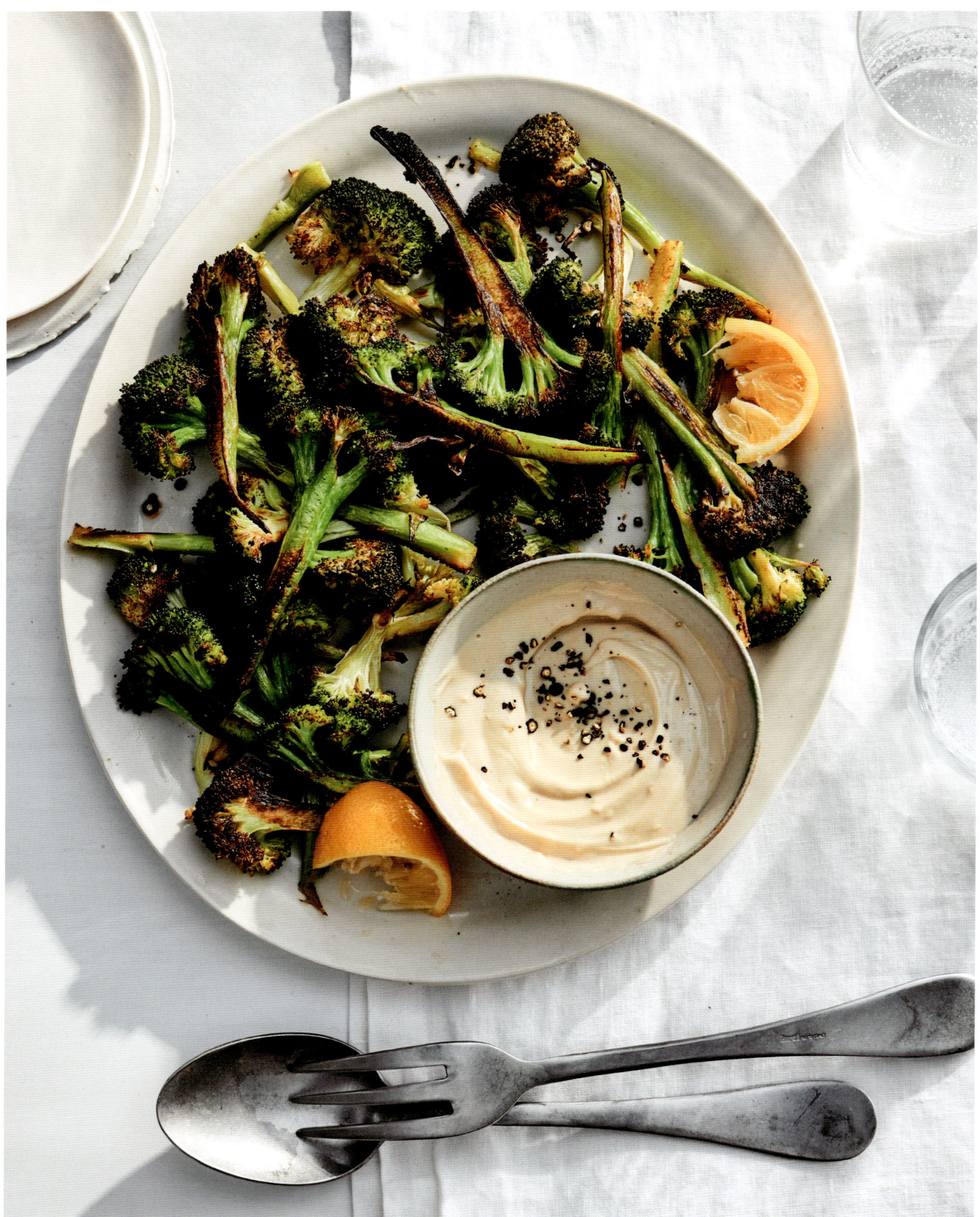

What if you could up your broccoli game? Try broiling it dry before tossing it in oil—it's a total game changer. Broiling is quicker than roasting and delivers perfectly charred, tender-crisp broccoli without the mush. It's an easy way to rediscover your love for this versatile veggie!

Charred Broccoli + Lemon Tahini Sauce

SERVES 4

Lemon tahini sauce

3 tablespoons freshly squeezed lemon juice

2 garlic cloves, finely chopped

1 tablespoon pure maple syrup

½ teaspoon pink salt

½ cup (120 g) well-stirred tahini (see Note)

⅓ cup (80 g) filtered water

Broccoli

1 (2-lb/908-g) head of broccoli, sliced into florets (see Note)

Maldon flake salt, for sprinkling

Extra-virgin olive oil, for drizzling

Lemon tahini sauce Whisk together all sauce ingredients in a small bowl, until combined and thickened. Refrigerate until ready to use.

Broccoli Position an oven rack about 3½ inches (9 cm) from the broil element. Preheat oven to broil. Line a rimmed baking sheet with parchment paper.

Spread out broccoli on the prepared baking sheet and broil for about 7 minutes, rotating once midway, until stalks have some char and florets are slightly frizzled and crispy. Keep a watchful eye while broiling.

Using tongs, quickly transfer broccoli to a plate, then sprinkle with flake salt and drizzle with oil. Toss until evenly coated. (You'll notice the vibrancy returns once you add oil.) Drizzle with the tahini sauce and enjoy while hot.

NOTES

Choose a tahini made with *toasted* sesame rather than raw, and prepare the sauce a few hours in advance, if possible, so the flavors can develop.

Cut the broccoli into slender pieces, otherwise they'll char before they cook all the way through. The cook time is just a guideline, as every oven is different. After doing this once, you'll have your perfect formula going forward.

Cauliflower florets oven-fried in nutty tahini get a squeeze of lemon, a sprinkle of fresh herbs, and a sweet pop of caramel from the Medjool dates. This is a perennial fave!

Tahini-Charred Cauliflower with Dates + Mint

SERVES 4

Sauce

1/3 cup (80 g) well-stirred tahini

1 large garlic clove, grated

1/4 teaspoon Aleppo pepper (optional; see Note)

3/4 teaspoon pink salt

Cauliflower

1 large head of cauliflower, cut into small florets

1 lemon

Handful of mint leaves, torn in half

Handful of dill, torn into smaller bits

4 Medjool dates, pitted and chopped (see Note)

Maldon flake salt, for sprinkling

Sauce Combine all sauce ingredients in a small bowl and mix well.

This can be made in advance so the flavors have a chance to mingle, but don't refrigerate because it needs to be pourable.

Cauliflower Position a rack in the top third of your oven. Preheat oven to 500°F. Line a rimmed baking sheet with parchment paper.

Place cauliflower florets in a large mixing bowl, then drizzle with tahini sauce. Using a rubber spatula, toss for 3 minutes, scraping from the bottom and turning the bowl, until it's all well coated. Place florets on the prepared baking sheet, spreading them out with as much space as possible.

Bake for 20 minutes, until charred and tender but not mushy. Remove from the oven and let the cauliflower cool for 5 minutes. Transfer it to a platter.

Using a Microplane, grate a dusting of lemon zest over cauliflower. Cut lemon in half, then add a light squeeze of juice. Top with mint, dill, and dates. Sprinkle with flake salt. Serve warm or at room temperature.

NOTES

If you are avoiding nightshades, omit the Aleppo pepper.

Choose the drier, firmer dates from the package to use here, as they are less likely to stick together once chopped.

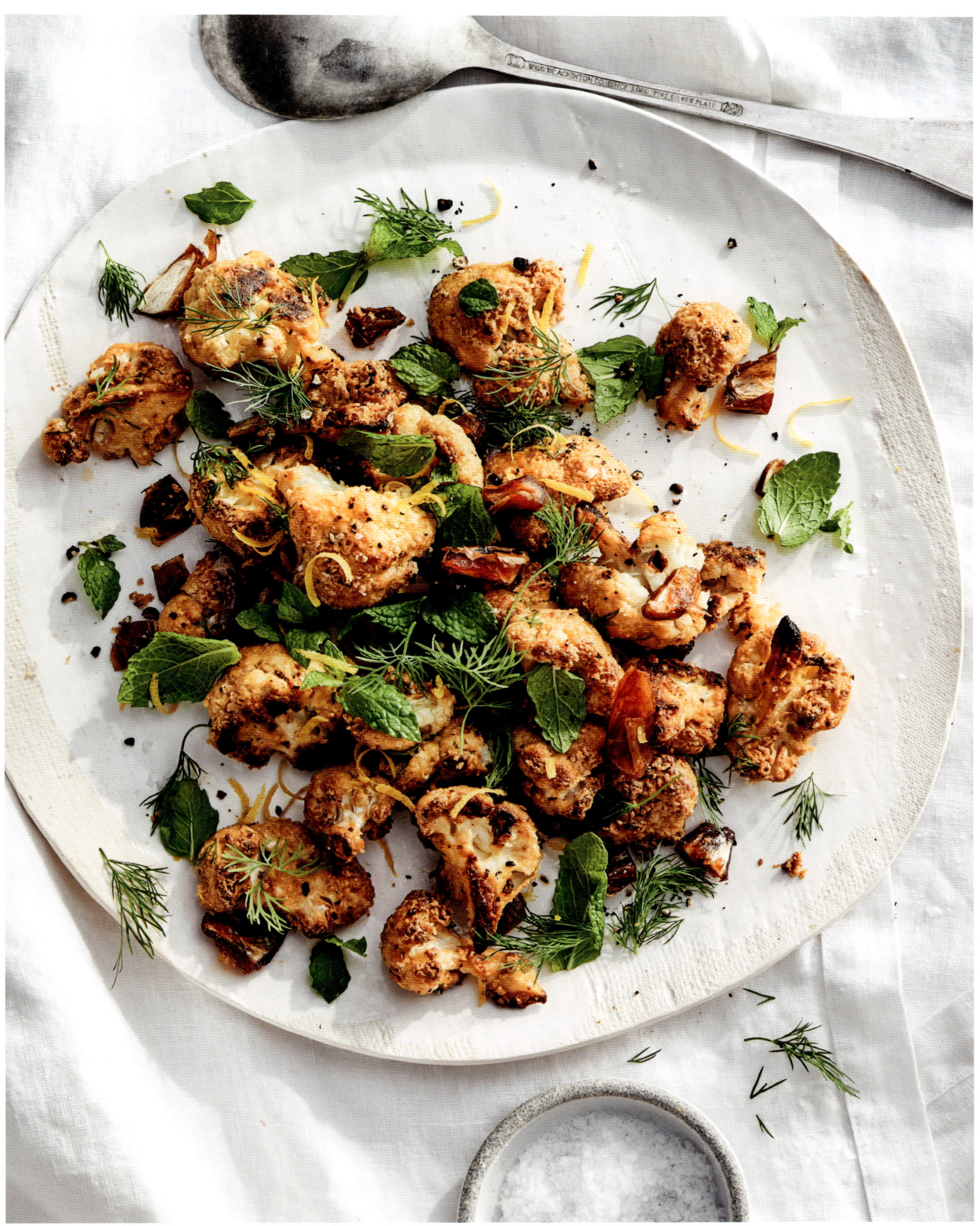
BLACKINTON CO. SINCE
FINE SILVER PLATE

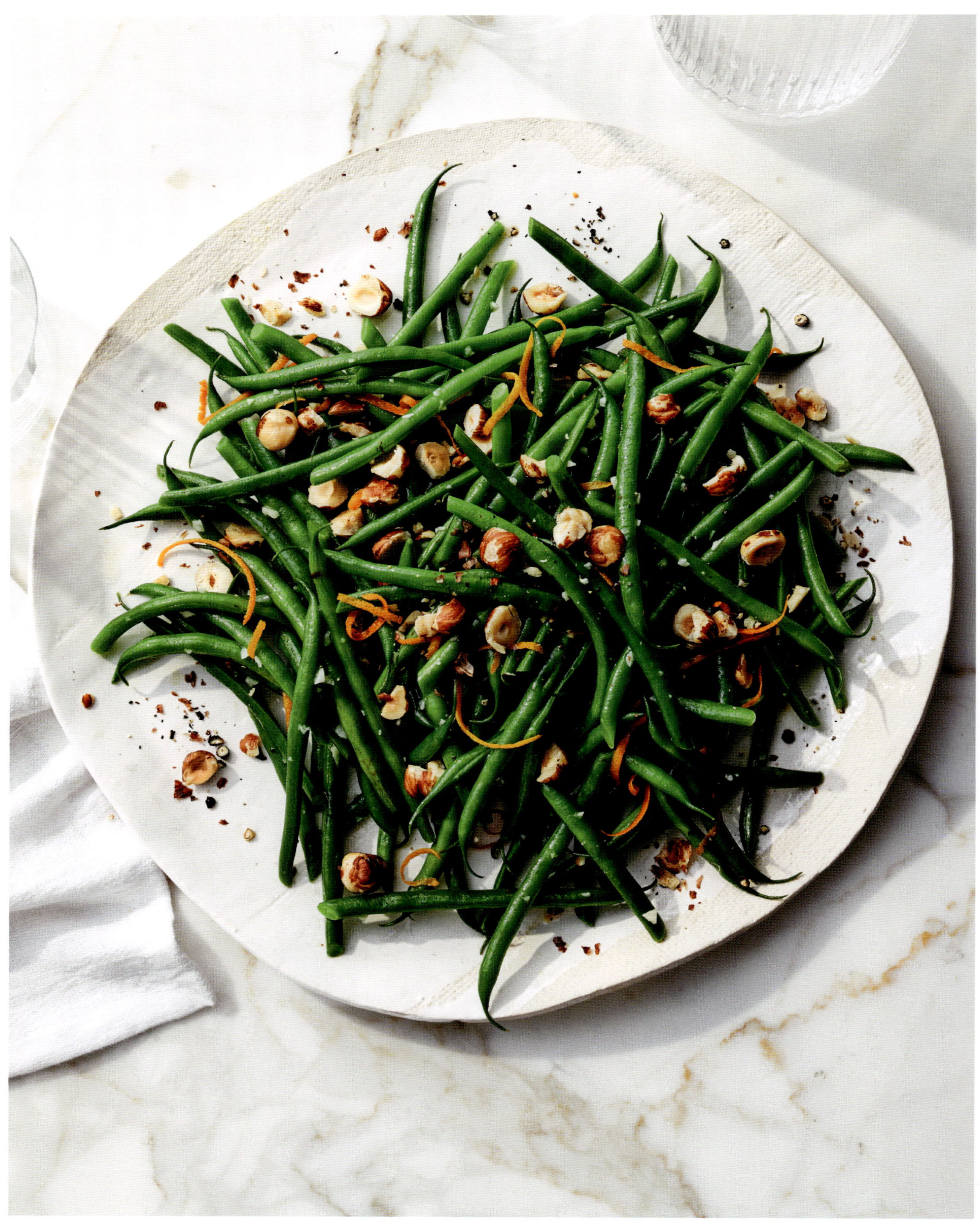

This recipe was inspired by Ottolenghi's French Beans and Mangetout. They're suitable for all occasions and bring a welcome pop of freshness to the table. They can be prepared a day ahead and served at room temperature. Wait until the last minute to sprinkle the toasted hazelnuts so they retain their crunch!

Haricots Verts with Hazelnuts + Orange

SERVES 6

- 1½ lbs (680 g) French beans, stalk ends trimmed
- 1 large navel orange
- 1 tablespoon minced garlic
- ½ teaspoon pink salt
- 3 grinds of freshly cracked black pepper
- ¼ cup (50 g) extra-virgin olive oil
- Maldon flake salt, for finishing
- ⅔ cup (85 g) well-toasted hazelnuts, roughly chopped

Bring a large saucepan of water to a boil. Add French beans and cook for 5 minutes. Using tongs, transfer them to a large bowl of ice water to stop the cooking. Cool completely, then transfer them to a clean kitchen towel (or paper towels) to dry. Dry the bowl and set it aside for later when tossing the beans in dressing.

Use a citrus zester (not a Microplane; see Note) to remove zest from orange in long strips. Set aside. Cut orange in half, then juice it into a small saucepan, using a citrus reamer to get all the juice. Simmer over medium heat until it has reduced to 2 tablespoons. Turn off the heat. Add garlic, pink salt, pepper, and oil to the pan, then whisk to combine.

Transfer the dry beans to the bowl. Add the dressing and orange strips and toss to coat. Refrigerate until ready to serve.

To serve, bring the beans to room temperature, then arrange them on a platter. Sprinkle generously with flake salt and top with hazelnuts at the last minute to retain their crunch.

NOTE

A citrus zester, sometimes called a lemon zester, looks like a small handle with five round holes on one end.

This creamy cauliflower mash is a righteous stand-in for mashed potatoes. Simmering the cauliflower in coconut milk—instead of boiling in water and pouring it away—preserves its nutrients. Serve it alongside Roast Chicken (page 135), Savory French Onion Beef (page 139), or Bison Meatloaf (page 140). It reheats well, so you can make it in advance if that's more convenient.

SERVES 6–8

Garlic Mashed Cauliflower

2 large heads of cauliflower, finely chopped

1 (13.5-oz/400-ml) can full-fat, additive-free coconut milk

3 large garlic cloves, roughly chopped

2 teaspoons pink salt, plus extra to taste

Maldon flake salt, for sprinkling

Chopped chives, for garnish

In a stockpot, combine cauliflower, coconut milk, garlic, and pink salt. Cover and bring to a boil. Reduce heat to medium-low and gently simmer for 20 minutes, until cauliflower is very tender. Remove from the heat, uncover, and allow it to sit for 10 minutes so the excess moisture can evaporate.

Transfer the mixture to a food processor and process until smooth. (Alternatively, you can use an immersion blender for a denser, silkier purée.) Season to taste with more pink salt.

Transfer to a serving bowl, then sprinkle with flake salt and chives.

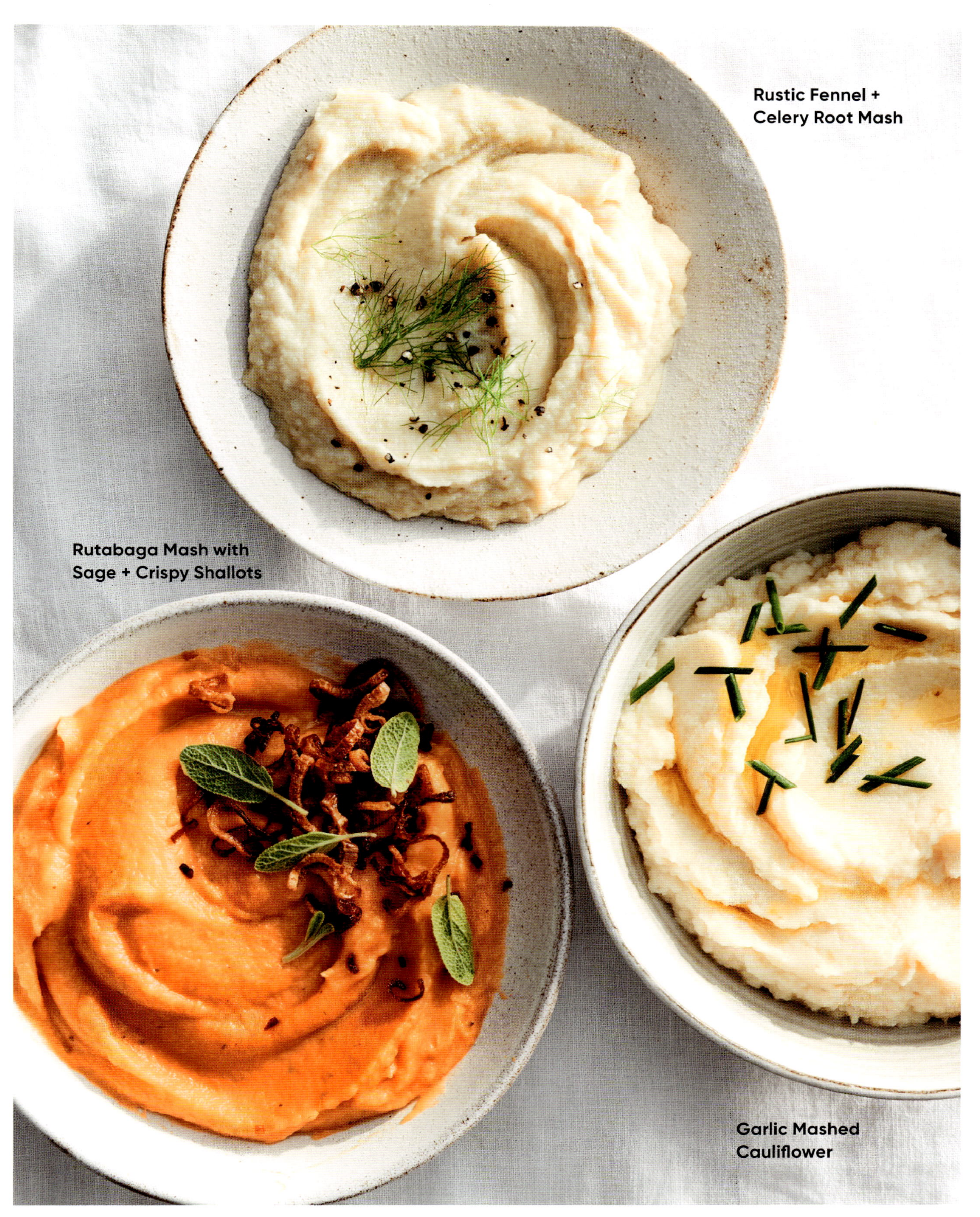
Rustic Fennel +
Celery Root Mash
Rutabaga Mash with
Sage + Crispy Shallots
Garlic Mashed
Cauliflower

Celeriac (a.k.a. celery root) is the star of the show in this complex and silky purée—and it's a roast chicken's perfect companion! It isn't exactly winning any beauty contests, but this underappreciated root vegetable is a nutritional powerhouse. It contains huge amounts of dietary fiber, which helps maintain a healthy digestive system, and it's also a good source of B vitamins, which play a major role in macronutrient synthesis. The vegetables are simmered in coconut milk instead of boiled in water to retain all the nutrients instead of draining them away.

SERVES 6

Rustic Fennel + Celery Root Mash

2 lbs (907 g) celery root

1 fennel bulb

1 tablespoon virgin coconut oil, for the pan

2 shallots, chopped

2 garlic cloves, chopped

1½ teaspoons pink salt, plus extra to taste

⅛ teaspoon white pepper

1 cup (240 g) canned full-fat, additive-free coconut milk

Fennel fronds, for garnish

Freshly cracked black pepper, for garnish

Peel celery root, then cut into ½-inch (12-mm) dice (otherwise, it takes ages to cook).

For the fennel, remove stalks and core, and reserve fronds for garnish. Roughly chop fennel bulb.

Heat coconut oil in a stockpot over medium heat. Add celery root, fennel, shallots, garlic, salt, and white pepper. Sauté for 4–5 minutes, until the vegetables begin to soften.

Pour in coconut milk, then cover. Bring to a boil, then reduce heat to low and simmer for 35–40 minutes, stirring occasionally, until vegetables are cooked through and very soft. Turn off the heat.

Pour mixture into a food processor and process until smooth. Season to taste with pink salt. Transfer to a serving bowl, then garnish with fennel fronds and black pepper.

It's time to become acquainted with this oft-forgotten root vegetable! Rutabagas feel old-fashioned to me—in the best way. I grew up on my mom's rutabaga and mashed potato combo, never to have them again until eyeballing them recently with renewed interest. This nutritious member of the Brassicaceae family (which includes broccoli, cauliflower, and kale) is a robustly flavored cross between cabbage and turnips. Rutabagas have a reputation for being on the bitter side, but I've added shallots and apple to round out the flavor. This light and silky purée is the perfect foil for Roast Chicken (page 135).

Rutabaga Mash with Sage + Crispy Shallots

SERVES 4

Crispy shallots

1 shallot

2 tablespoons olive oil

Pink salt, for sprinkling

Rutabaga mash

2 lbs (907 g) rutabaga

1 large shallot, roughly chopped

1 Honeycrisp apple, peeled, cored, and roughly chopped

1 garlic clove, roughly chopped

1 tablespoon finely chopped sage

1½ teaspoons pink salt, plus extra to taste

1 (13.5-oz/400-ml) can full-fat, additive-free coconut milk

¼ teaspoon freshly ground nutmeg

Freshly cracked black pepper, to taste

Crispy shallots Thinly slice shallot lengthwise into matchsticks or crosswise into thin rings.

Combine oil and shallots in a small (cold) skillet. Sauté over medium heat, stirring occasionally, for 10 minutes, or until golden. Using a slotted spoon, quickly transfer shallots onto a paper towel-lined plate. Immediately sprinkle with salt while they're hot. They will crisp up once cool.

Rutabaga mash To peel rutabaga, start by slicing off the top and bottom. Next, slice it in half so it's easier to manage. Cut away the thick skin and any especially tough spots because they can be bitter. Cut into ½-inch (12-mm) cubes.

In a large saucepan, combine rutabaga, shallot, apple, garlic, sage, and salt. (Wait to add the nutmeg.) Pour in coconut milk and stir. Cover, then bring to a boil over high heat. Reduce the heat to medium-low and simmer for 35 minutes, or until rutabaga are tender enough to be easily pierced with a fork. Remove from the heat.

Using an immersion blender, blend until smooth. (Alternatively, you can use a food processor instead of an immersion blender to produce a slightly lighter, fluffier mash.) Add nutmeg and blend until combined. Season to taste with salt.

Transfer mash to a serving bowl, then top with crispy shallots and season with pepper.

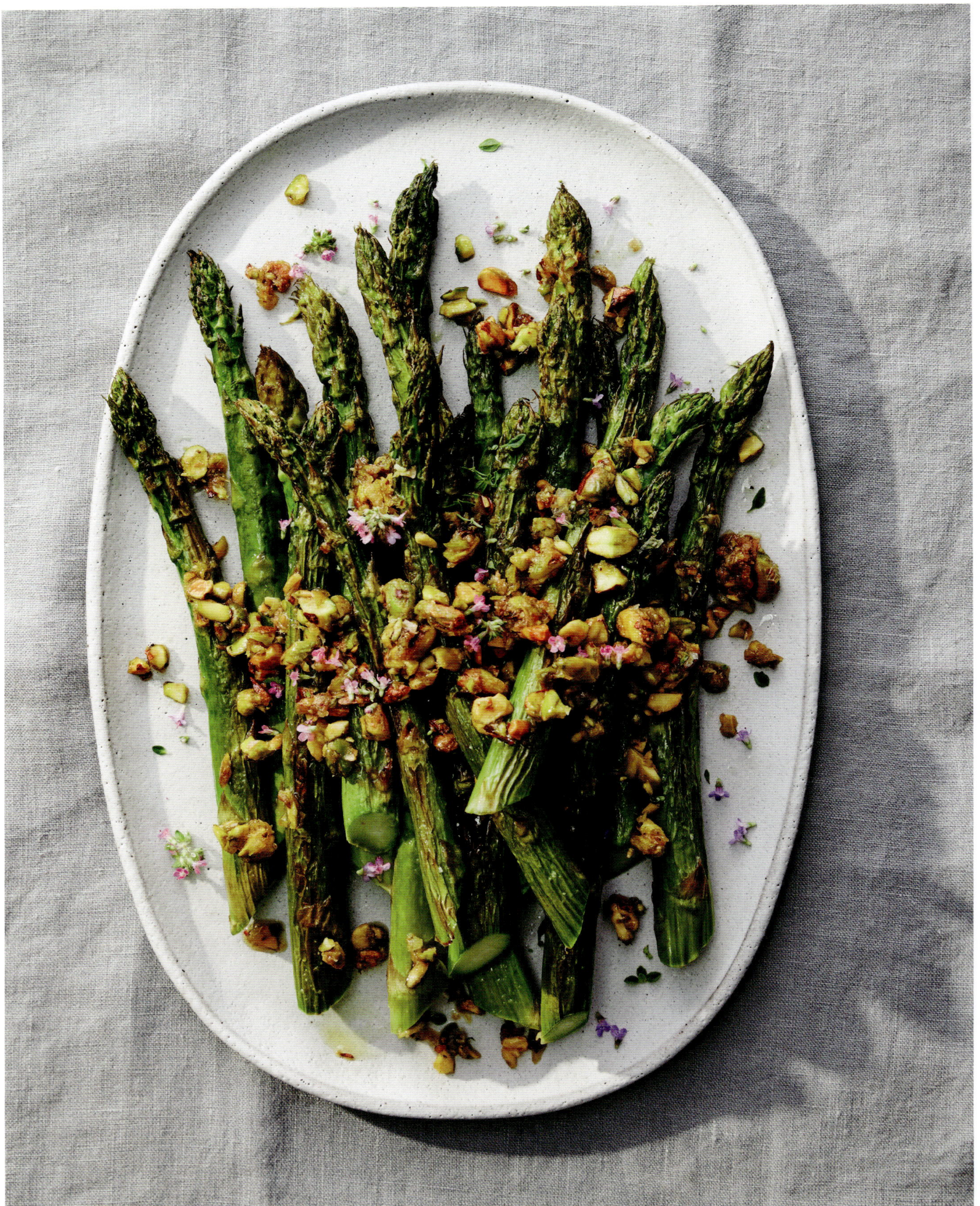

Fresh asparagus are lightly charred under the broiler, sprinkled with a vibrant gremolata, and finished with an earthy flutter of fresh thyme leaves—a sumptuous way to increase your asparagus consumption!

Asparagus is a rich source of glutathione, packed with vitamins and minerals, and great for digestive health.

Charred Asparagus + Lemon-Pistachio Gremolata

SERVES 4–6

Gremolata

1 oil-packed anchovy fillet, blotted to remove any excess oil

Zest of 2 lemons

1 garlic clove, grated on a Microplane

Heaping ½ cup (75 g) toasted, salted, shelled pistachios (see Note)

Asparagus

2 lbs (907 g) asparagus, preferably large diameter, trimmed

Extra-virgin olive oil, for drizzling

2 teaspoons thyme leaves

Maldon flake salt

Gremolata In a mini food processor, combine anchovy, lemon zest, garlic, and pistachios. Pulse until nuts are broken down and the mixture is coarse. Transfer the gremolata to a small bowl.

Asparagus Position an oven rack 6 inches (15 cm) from the broil element. (In my oven, that's the second notch from the top.) Preheat the oven to broil. Line a rimmed baking sheet with parchment paper.

Place asparagus on the prepared baking sheet. Lightly drizzle with oil and toss to coat. Arrange them in a single layer, working in two batches if necessary.

Broil for 4–5 minutes, until tender and slightly charred. Using tongs, transfer asparagus to a serving platter.

To serve, spoon gremolata over asparagus, then sprinkle with thyme and flake salt. Serve immediately.

NOTE

You can opt for shelled pistachios or shell them yourself, but be sure they are salted and toasted.

In season from November to March, blood oranges are a treasure waiting to be discovered. The crimson flesh and sweet raspberry notes are the perfect symphony of flavor to brighten your winter days.

Roasted Brussels Sprouts + Blood Oranges with Sweet White Balsamic

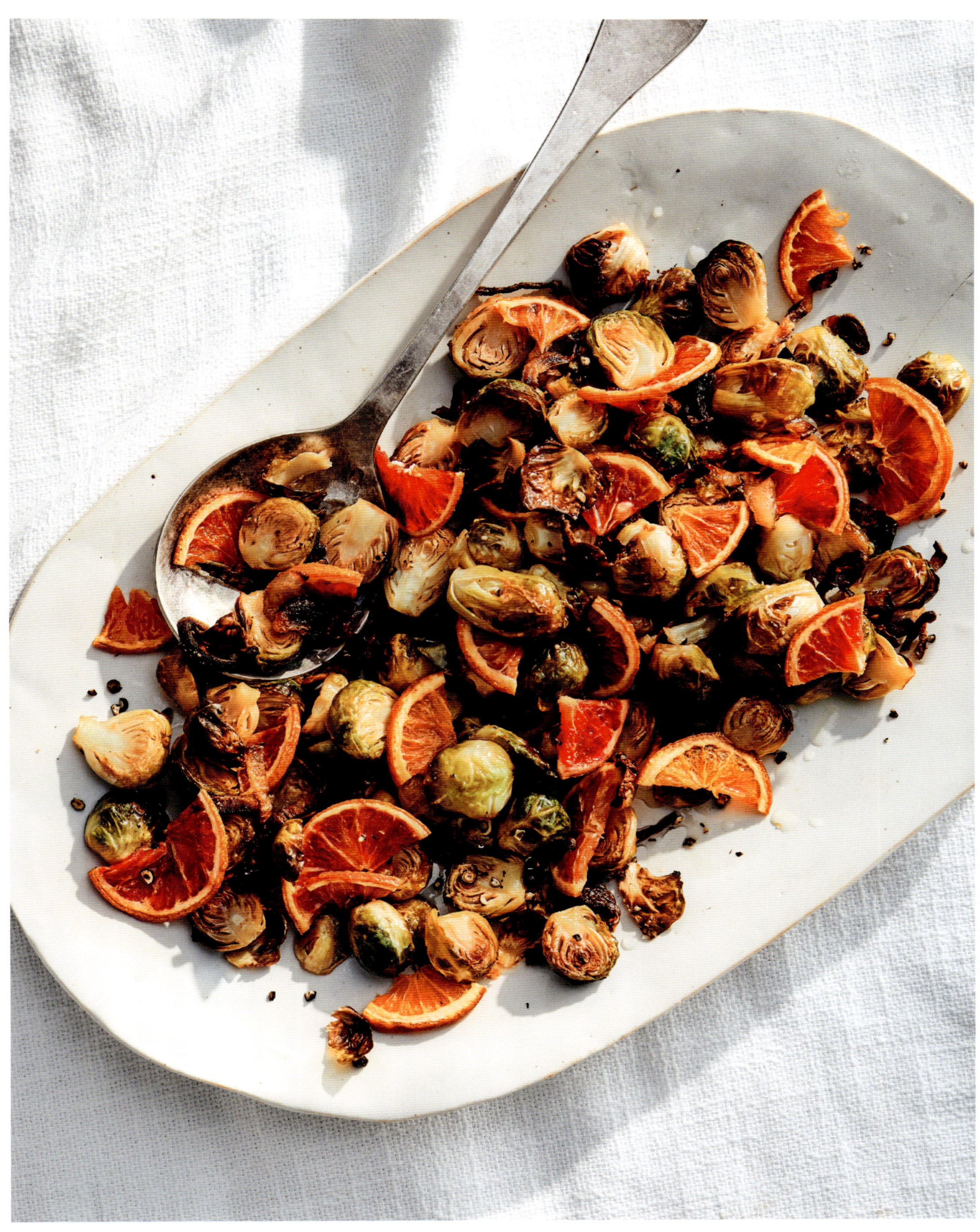

Marmalade lovers, this is your vibe! Blood oranges are typically in season November–March and are worth hunting down for their crimson-colored flesh and sweet hints of raspberry. If they're not available, small, thin-skinned oranges such as Valencia can be substituted. Navel oranges are not suitable because of their thick, bitter rinds. This dish is best when served slightly warm or at room temperature.

Roasted Brussels Sprouts + Blood Oranges with Sweet White Balsamic

SERVES 6

- 2 blood oranges
- Extra-virgin olive oil
- 1½ lbs (680 g) Brussels sprouts, trimmed
- 3 shallots, thinly sliced into rings
- Pink salt and freshly cracked black pepper, to taste
- 2 tablespoons sweet white balsamic vinegar (see Note)

Preheat oven to 325°F. Set a wire baking rack over a rimmed baking sheet lined with parchment paper.

Cut the oranges crosswise, into ¼-inch (6-mm) thick slices. Discard end pieces, which are all rind.

In a medium mixing bowl, combine orange slices and a splash of oil and use your hands to mix until coated. Space them out on the prepared baking rack in a single layer. Bake on the center rack for 25 minutes. Using tongs, flip the slices over and bake for another 15 minutes, until they're slightly charred around the edges and beginning to dry out. Set aside. Increase the oven temperature to 425°F.

Meanwhile, peel away any discolored outer leaves from the Brussels sprouts. Cut them in half and add them to the mixing bowl you used for the oranges.

Transfer the rack of orange slices somewhere to cool. Line the baking sheet with parchment paper.

Add a splash of oil and a good sprinkle of salt to the bowl of Brussels sprouts and toss with your hands until coated. Spread them out over the prepared baking sheet, leaving a quarter of the pan free for the shallots.

In the same mixing bowl, combine shallots, oil, and a sprinkle of salt. Toss to coat, separating the rings as much as possible. Spread them out on the baking sheet next to the Brussels sprouts.

Bake on the center rack for 16–25 minutes, until sprouts are lightly charred and tender. If needed, remove Brussels sprouts when they are ready and return the shallots to the oven for a few more minutes, until they start to become golden and crispy. Set them aside to cool.

Cut the orange slices into quarters. Use a paper towel to wipe any excess oil from the mixing bowl, then add the Brussels sprouts, shallots, and oranges back into the bowl. Drizzle with vinegar and gently toss to combine. Season to taste with salt and black pepper. Transfer to a serving bowl or platter.

NOTE

Look for a *sweet* white balsamic, such as Seggiano, Carandini, or Prelibato (Italian brands sometimes call it white dressing). While I generally like O brand white balsamic vinegar, it's not sweet enough for this dish.

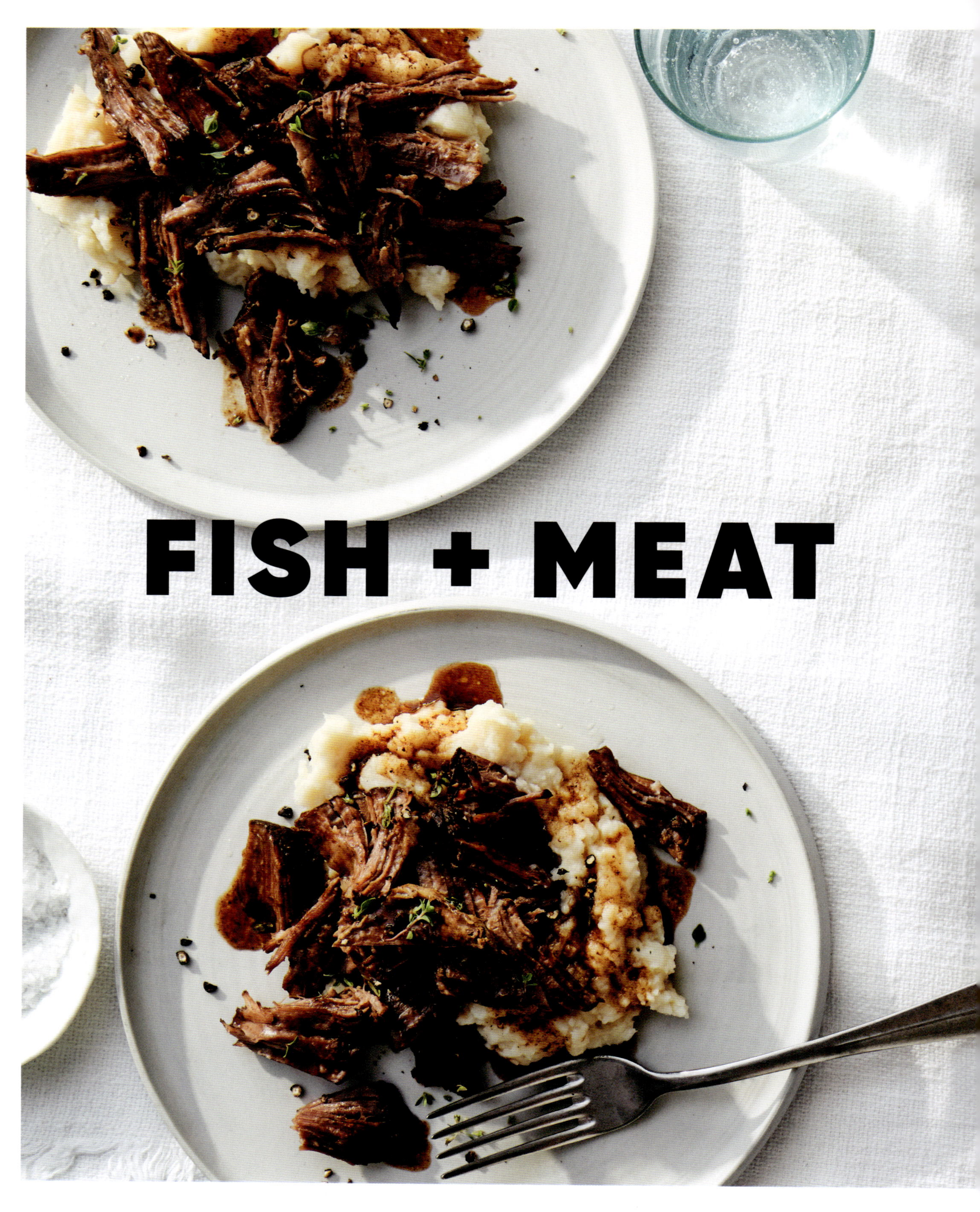

FISH + MEAT

125 WILD SALMON CAKES + LEMON AIOLI

126 WILD SALMON WITH BLACKBERRY GASTRIQUE + THYME

130 GINGER-MARINATED BLACK COD + ROASTED BABY BOK CHOY

132 EVERYTHING SEASONING ENCRUSTED HALIBUT + HORSERADISH AIOLI

135 ROAST CHICKEN: A UTILITARIAN APPROACH

136 GRILLED FLANK STEAK

139 SAVORY FRENCH ONION BEEF

140 BISON MEATLOAF + JUS

143 PAN-SEARED LAMB LOLLIPOPS WITH ROSEMARY, MAPLE + DIJON

144 LETTUCE WRAPPED LAMB BURGERS + LEMON AIOLI

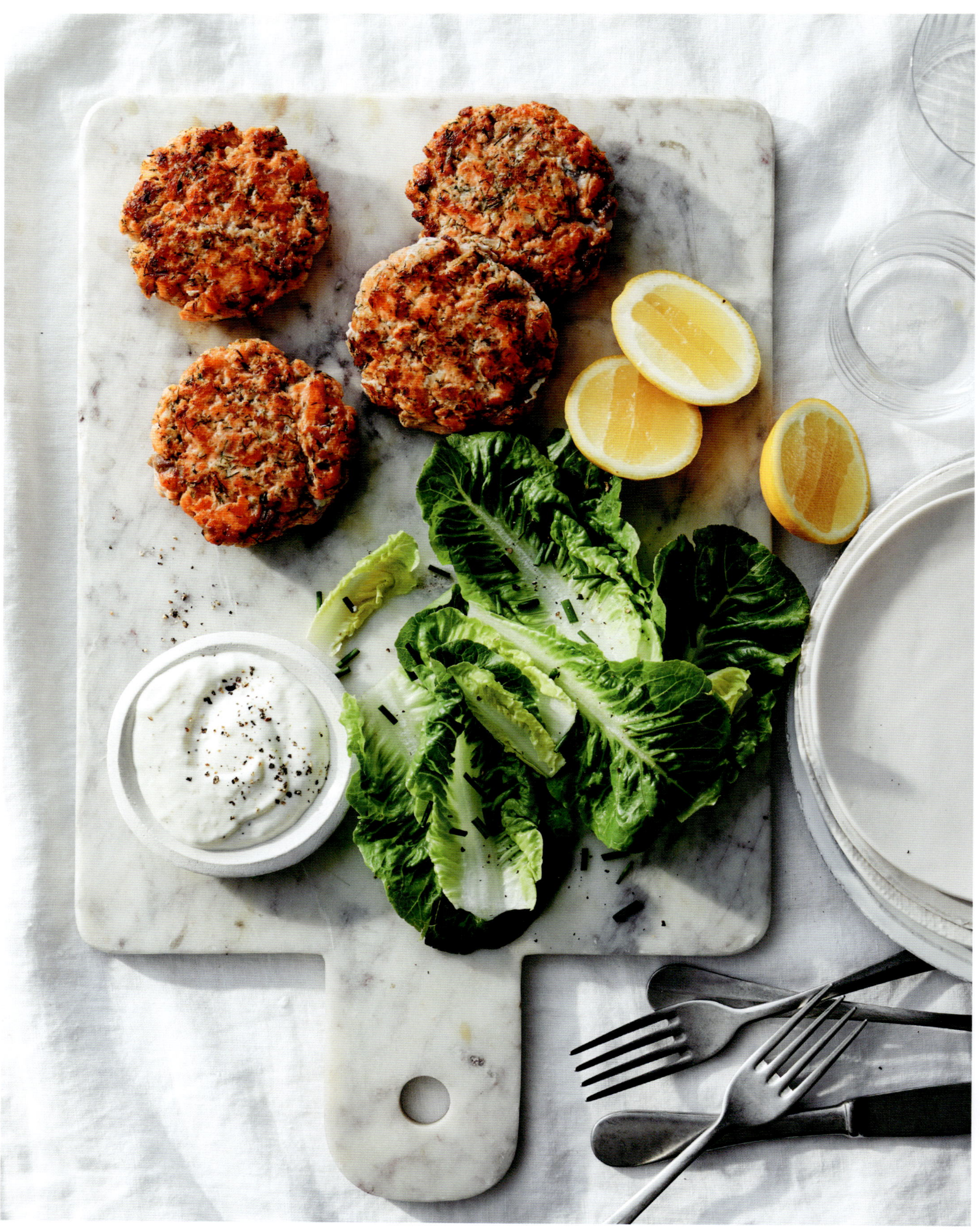

I created this recipe to work more wild salmon into my diet during the off-season when fresh wild salmon is unavailable. Wild salmon is such an excellent protein source and is loaded with all those good omega-3s. Sockeye is the most available form of frozen wild salmon, but it has a denser texture and more assertive flavor than my preferred king and coho. So, I've upped the freshness factor with citrus and herbs to enjoy these salmon cakes on repeat during the winter months.

SERVES 4

Wild Salmon Cakes + Lemon Aioli

Salmon cakes

- 2 lbs (908 g) frozen wild salmon, thawed
- 2 large garlic cloves
- ½ cup (12 g) finely chopped dill
- ½ cup (60 g) minced shallot
- 1 tablespoon extra-virgin olive oil, plus more for the pan
- Zest of 1 lemon
- 2 tablespoons freshly squeezed lemon juice
- 2 teaspoons Dijon mustard
- 1 teaspoon pink salt

Aioli

- 2 garlic cloves, grated
- ⅛ teaspoon pink salt
- ½ cup (117 g) mayonnaise
- Zest of 1 lemon
- 1 tablespoon freshly squeezed lemon juice

Salmon cakes Remove the skin from salmon (I find this easiest to do while salmon is still half-frozen), then pat it dry and roughly chop.

Add garlic cloves to a food processor and pulse until minced. Add the remaining ingredients, except salmon, and pulse once or twice until combined. Add salmon and pulse until salmon is chopped but before it becomes a paste. (Otherwise, the salmon cakes will have a mealy texture.) Transfer the mixture to a bowl, then refrigerate for at least 1 hour.

Aioli Combine all aioli ingredients in a small bowl and mix well. Refrigerate for at least 1 hour so the flavors can develop.

Assembly Form salmon mixture into 4 patties.

Heat a generous splash of oil in a nonstick skillet over medium-high heat. Add salmon cakes and pan-fry for 3–4 minutes on each side, until cooked through.

Serve with aioli.

Wild salmon season just happens to coincide with blackberry season, and they're a summer-centric match made in heaven. Make the sweet and tangy gastrique sauce in advance if you'd like—it gives the flavors more time to get to know each other. I like to serve this salmon with grilled or roasted asparagus.

Wild Salmon with Blackberry Gastrique + Thyme

SERVES 4

- 4 (6-oz/170-g) fresh wild-caught salmon fillets
- 18 oz (510 g) blackberries (divided)
- 1 tablespoon extra-virgin olive oil, plus extra for coating
- 1 medium shallot, finely minced
- ¼ cup (60 g) red wine vinegar
- ¼ cup (60 g) pomegranate juice
- 2 tablespoons pure maple syrup
- ¼ teaspoon pink salt
- Thyme leaves, for sprinkling
- Maldon flake salt and freshly cracked black pepper, to taste

Bring salmon to room temperature by removing it from the fridge and setting aside for 30 minutes. This ensures even doneness.

In a mini food processor, purée 1½ cups (12 oz/340 g) of berries. Reserve the remaining berries to use as garnish. Pour purée through a fine-mesh sieve into a small bowl, using a rubber spatula to push as much liquid through as possible. Discard seeds.

Heat oil in a small saucepan over medium heat. Add shallots and sauté for 4 minutes, until lightly golden. Add the blackberry purée, vinegar, pomegranate juice, maple syrup, and salt. Cook for about 8 minutes over medium heat until thickened, reduced by half, and bubbling profusely. If needed, turn the heat up a bit until it does. Stir often and keep a close eye on it. Transfer sauce to a bowl, then set it aside to cool or refrigerate until ready to use.

Preheat outdoor grill over medium-high heat.

Pat dry salmon. Coat each fillet with oil and sprinkle generously with pink salt. Grill, skin-side down, until golden, crisp, and nearly cooked through. Flip over and cook for another 1–2 minutes, until an instant-read thermometer inserted in the thickest part of the fillet registers 125°F. (Alternatively, arrange salmon skin-side down in a cool, dry [no oil] nonstick skillet—you may need to do this in batches. Cook undisturbed on medium heat for 8–10 minutes, until the skin is golden and crispy. Briefly press down with a spatula to ensure the fillet is making full contact with the pan. Flip them over and cook for another 1–2 minutes.)

To serve, plate salmon and spoon sauce over each one. Add a few berries and a generous sprinkle of thyme leaves. Season to taste with flake salt and pepper.

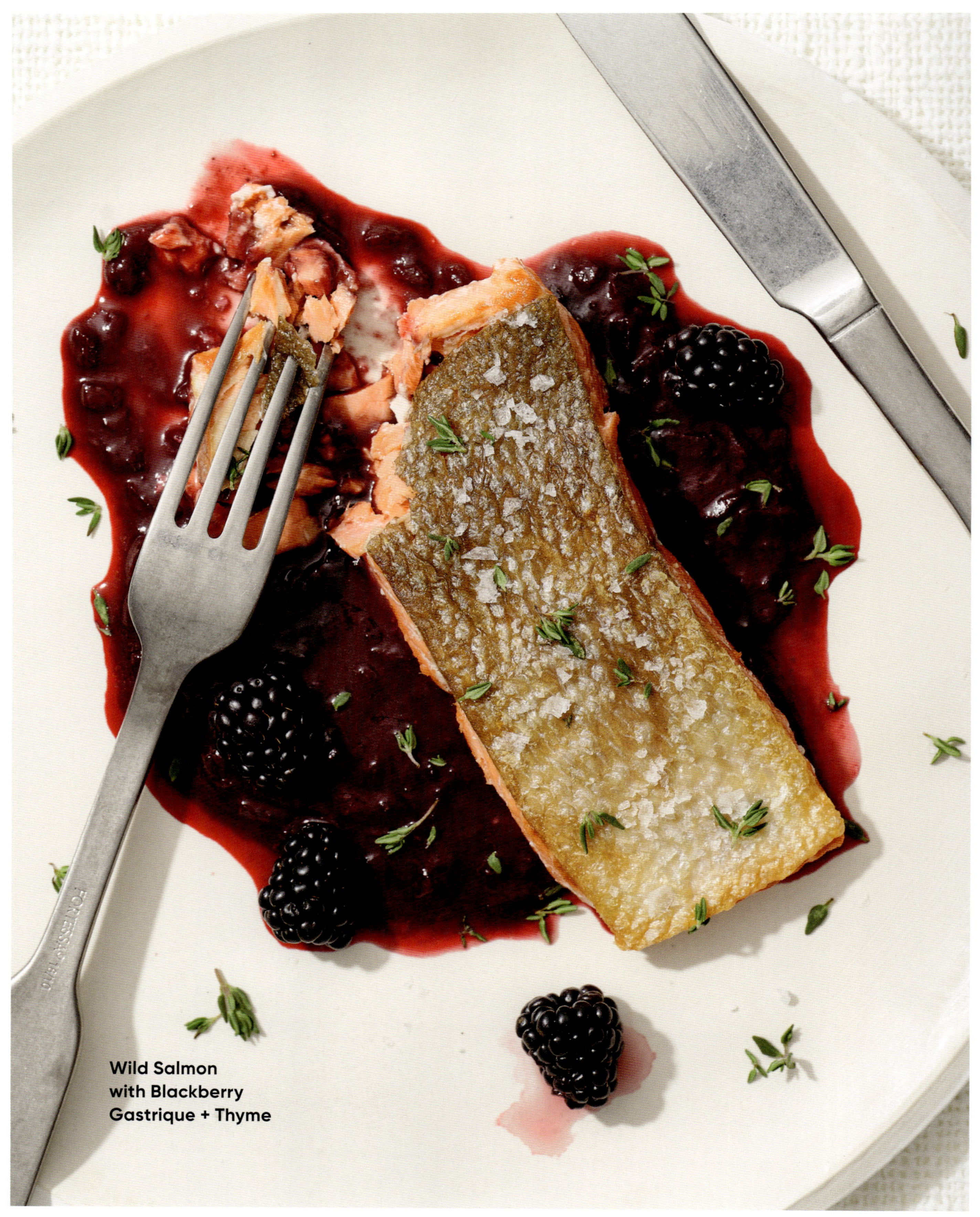

Wild Salmon
with Blackberry
Gastrique + Thyme

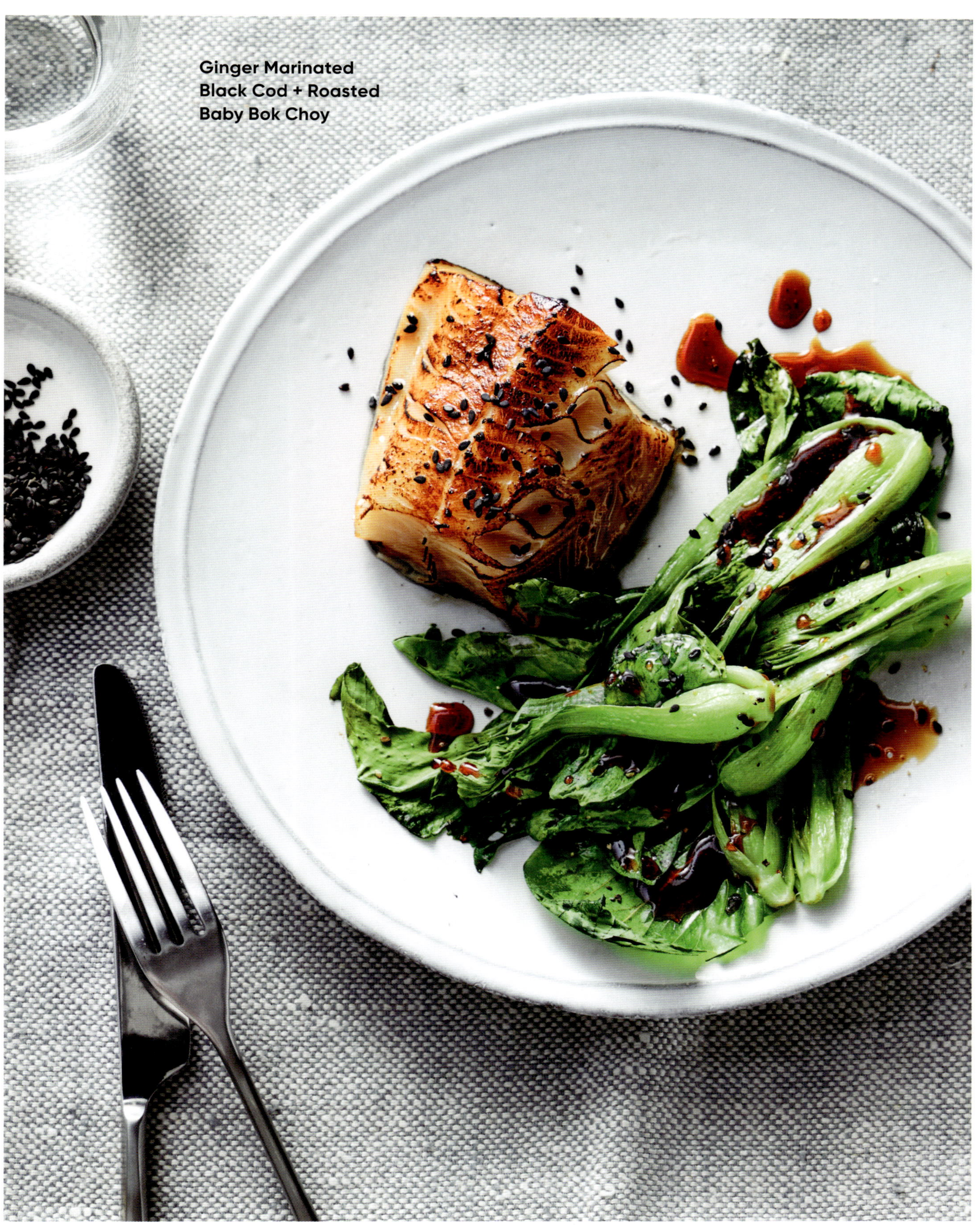
Ginger Marinated Black Cod + Roasted Baby Bok Choy

Black cod has a unique silky texture, a rich, buttery flavor, and the highest content of healthy omega-3 fatty acids of any white fish. Also known as sablefish, it is not actually a member of the cod family. The closest equivalent to black cod would be Chilean sea bass. Plan to marinate the fish for 24 hours in advance.

Ginger Marinated Black Cod + Roasted Baby Bok Choy

SERVES 4

Marinade

1 garlic clove, grated

3 tablespoons freshly squeezed lime juice (see Note)

3 tablespoons honey

2 tablespoons coconut aminos (see Note)

1 tablespoon Red Boat fish sauce

1 teaspoon freshly grated ginger

Black cod

1 (1½-lb/680-g) black cod, cut into 4 fillets

4–8 baby bok choy, depending on the size, halved lengthwise

Extra-virgin olive oil, for brushing

Pink salt, for sprinkling

1 tablespoon black sesame seeds

Marinade Combine all marinade ingredients in a 9 × 13-inch (23 × 33-cm) baking dish, just large enough to accommodate the fish. Whisk the mixture to combine.

Black cod Arrange black cod fillets, flesh-side down, in the marinade. Cover and refrigerate for at least 24 hours.

Remove the marinated black cod from the fridge and place fillets, skin-side down, on a rimmed baking sheet lined with aluminum foil (parchment paper will burn under the broiler). Don't discard the marinade! Allow 30 minutes for the fish to come to room temperature.

Meanwhile, pour the leftover marinade into a small saucepan and simmer over medium heat until syrupy and reduced in volume. Transfer sauce to a small bowl to cool.

Position the top oven rack about 6 inches (15 cm) below the broil element. (In my oven, that's the second notch from the top.) Preheat oven to broil. Broil fish for 6–10 minutes, until it's deeply golden with bits of char around the edges and flakes easily with a fork. Set aside for a few minutes to firm up. Reduce oven temperature to 450°F.

Next, arrange bok choy, cut side up, on a rimmed baking sheet lined with parchment. Using a pastry brush, brush each one with oil, then sprinkle them with salt. Bake on the middle rack for 6–10 minutes, until leaves are crispy and stems are tender.

To serve, plate bok choy alongside a black cod fillet. Drizzle each one with the reduction sauce and sprinkle with black sesame seeds.

NOTES

Sometimes limes can be dry and produce very little juice. I recommend getting 3 limes and using a citrus reamer to extract all the juice.

Look for a brand of coconut aminos that only contains coconut nectar, water, and salt.

This simple pan-seared halibut is adorned with a flavorful golden crust on top and finished with a punchy horseradish-lime aioli. With its mild flavor and firm, meaty texture, Pacific halibut is a guaranteed crowd-pleaser. However, its leanness can make it prone to overcooking. To avoid this, use an instant-read thermometer for perfectly tender, flaky results every time.

Everything Seasoning Encrusted Halibut + Horseradish Aioli

SERVES 4

Aioli

½ cup (117 g) mayonnaise

2 tablespoons prepared horseradish

Zest of ½ lime

1 tablespoon freshly squeezed lime juice

¼ teaspoon pink salt

Halibut

4 (6-oz/170-g) skinless wild-caught halibut fillets

⅓ cup (41 g) everything bagel seasoning (I like Trader Joe's)

Olive oil, for the pan

Chopped chives, for garnish (optional)

Aioli Combine all aioli ingredients in a small bowl. Cover and refrigerate for at least 1 hour so flavors can develop.

Halibut Bring halibut to room temperature by removing it from the fridge and setting aside for 30 minutes. This ensures even doneness.

Assembly Preheat oven to 450°F. Position a rack in the center.

Pat dry halibut. Pour seasoning onto a plate. Place a fillet on top of the seasoning, pressing down firmly with your hand so the seasoning adheres to the fish. Transfer to a plate, then repeat with the remaining fillets.

Heat a generous splash of oil in a large nonstick, oven-proof skillet over medium-low heat until shimmering hot. Add fillets, seasoned side down, and pan-fry for 2 minutes, untouched, until each one forms a golden crust. Be sure to set a timer so the seasoning doesn't burn.

Using tongs, pick fillets up by the sides and flip them. Slide skillet into the oven and roast fillets for 5–7 minutes, until an instant-read thermometer inserted into the thickest part of the fish registers 130°F. Transfer fillets to a plate. Be careful with the hot handle of the skillet!

Garnish with chopped chives, if desired, and serve with aioli.

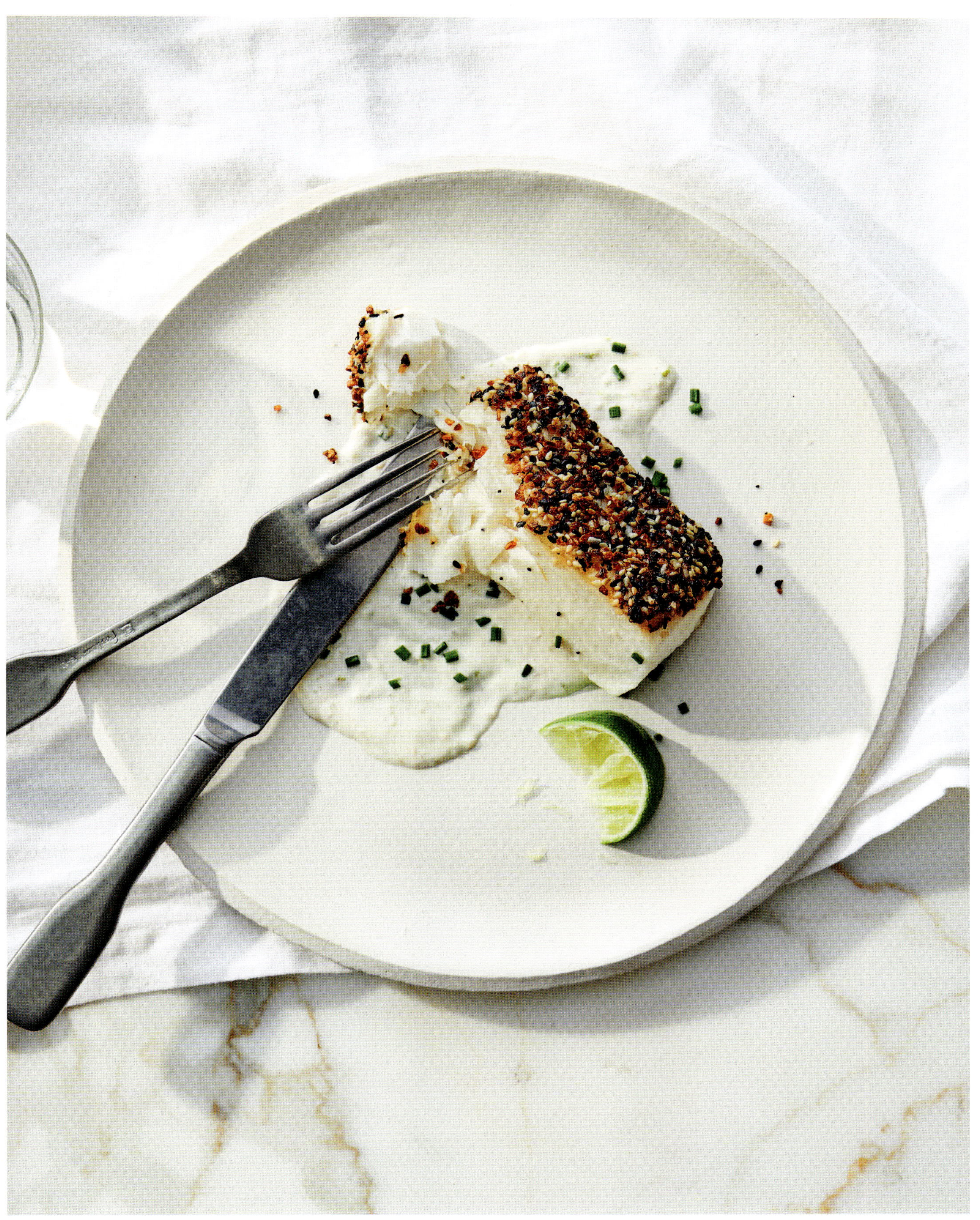

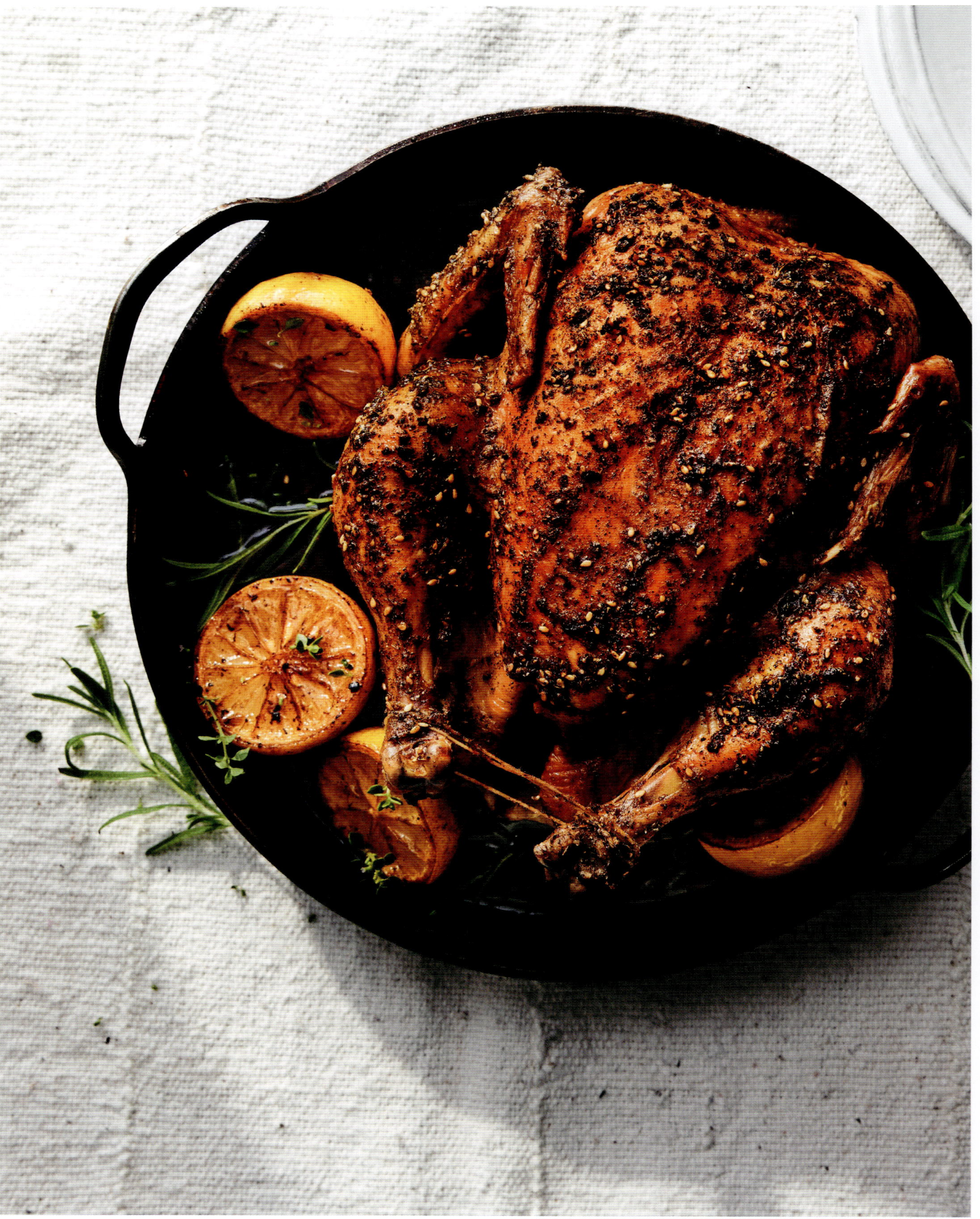

Everyone should master the art of roasting a chicken! There's just something about a whole roasted chicken and the way it perfumes our home with the scent of nostalgia. Not to mention the comfort and nourishment it provides.

A perfectly roasted chicken isn't just delicious—it's versatile, practical, and reminds us of simpler times and simpler pleasures. Whether you serve it in all its golden, crispy-skinned glory, carve it up on a platter, or shred it to stretch across several meals, having a strategy that fits your needs is a game changer. Here, I'm sharing my go-to method, a utilitarian approach that makes life both easier and tastier.

Roast Chicken: A Utilitarian Approach

SERVES 4–6

1 (4–5-lb/1.8–2.3-kg) whole chicken (never frozen), giblets removed

Pink salt and freshly cracked black pepper, to taste

Variation

1 (4–5-lb/1.8–2.3-kg) whole chicken (never frozen), giblets removed

2 tablespoons za'atar

2 tablespoons extra-virgin olive oil

2 teaspoons pink salt

Preheat oven to 375°F. Position a rack in the center.

Rinse chicken inside and out, then pat dry. Using kitchen shears, trim off any extra fat around the cavity opening.

Place chicken in a 9 × 13-inch (23 × 33-cm) Pyrex-style baking dish. Sprinkle with salt and pepper. I don't bother with tying the legs together (known as trussing) because an untrussed chicken cooks faster.

Roast for 55–60 minutes, until an instant-read thermometer inserted into the thickest part of the chicken registers 155°F–160°F. Allow it to rest for 20 minutes (carryover cooking will bring the temperature up to 165°F). Transfer to a cutting board or platter, then slice.

Variation: Za'atar Roast Chicken Za'atar is a savory Middle Eastern spice blend traditionally made with hyssop, an herb believed to have numerous health benefits. I don't care for versions where thyme or oregano are used as substitutes for hyssop. I recommend The Spice Way's traditional Lebanese za'atar with hyssop, which can be found online. For another delicious way to enjoy za'atar, check out the Little Gem Salad with Grapes recipe (page 85).

Place whole chicken on a wire baking rack, set over a rimmed baking sheet so the air can circulate. Combine za'atar, oil, and salt and mix well. Rub the mixture over the chicken, working it into all the cracks and crevices. Follow the roasting instructions for roast chicken.

During the warmer months when our grills are out in full force, we can't get enough of this simple flank steak that relies on coconut aminos as a stand-in for soy sauce. I give it a twenty-four-hour flavor bath and then it's onto a scorching hot grill for a quick sear. Flank steak is a particularly lean and flavorful cut of beef and readily available at any grocer. Make this your new summer staple!

SERVES 4

Grilled Flank Steak

- 3 garlic cloves, grated
- 1 tablespoon balsamic vinegar
- 1 tablespoon pure maple syrup
- ¼ cup (75 g) coconut aminos (see Note)
- 1 (1½-lb/680-g) flank steak
- Maldon flake salt and freshly cracked black pepper, to taste

Combine garlic, vinegar, maple syrup, and coconut aminos in a large zip-top bag. Add steak and swoosh it around until it's entirely coated. Press the air out of the bag, seal it shut, and place it on a plate to catch any drips. Refrigerate for at least 24 hours, turning midway to ensure the other side gets its share of the marinade.

To cook, take the steak out of the fridge 30 minutes in advance so it can come to room temperature. Preheat an outdoor grill over high heat. (Alternatively, use a grill pan over medium-high heat.)

Add the steak to the hot grill and grill for 4–6 minutes per side, until an instant-read thermometer inserted into the center of the meat reaches 135°F–140°F. (Flank steak tends to get chewier the longer it's cooked, so grilling to medium-rare is ideal.) Let it rest for 5–10 minutes so the juices can redistribute.

To serve, slice steak against the grain. This is critical to keeping a cut like flank nice and tender. Sprinkle it liberally with salt and pepper.

NOTE

Look for a brand of coconut aminos that only contains coconut nectar, water, and salt.

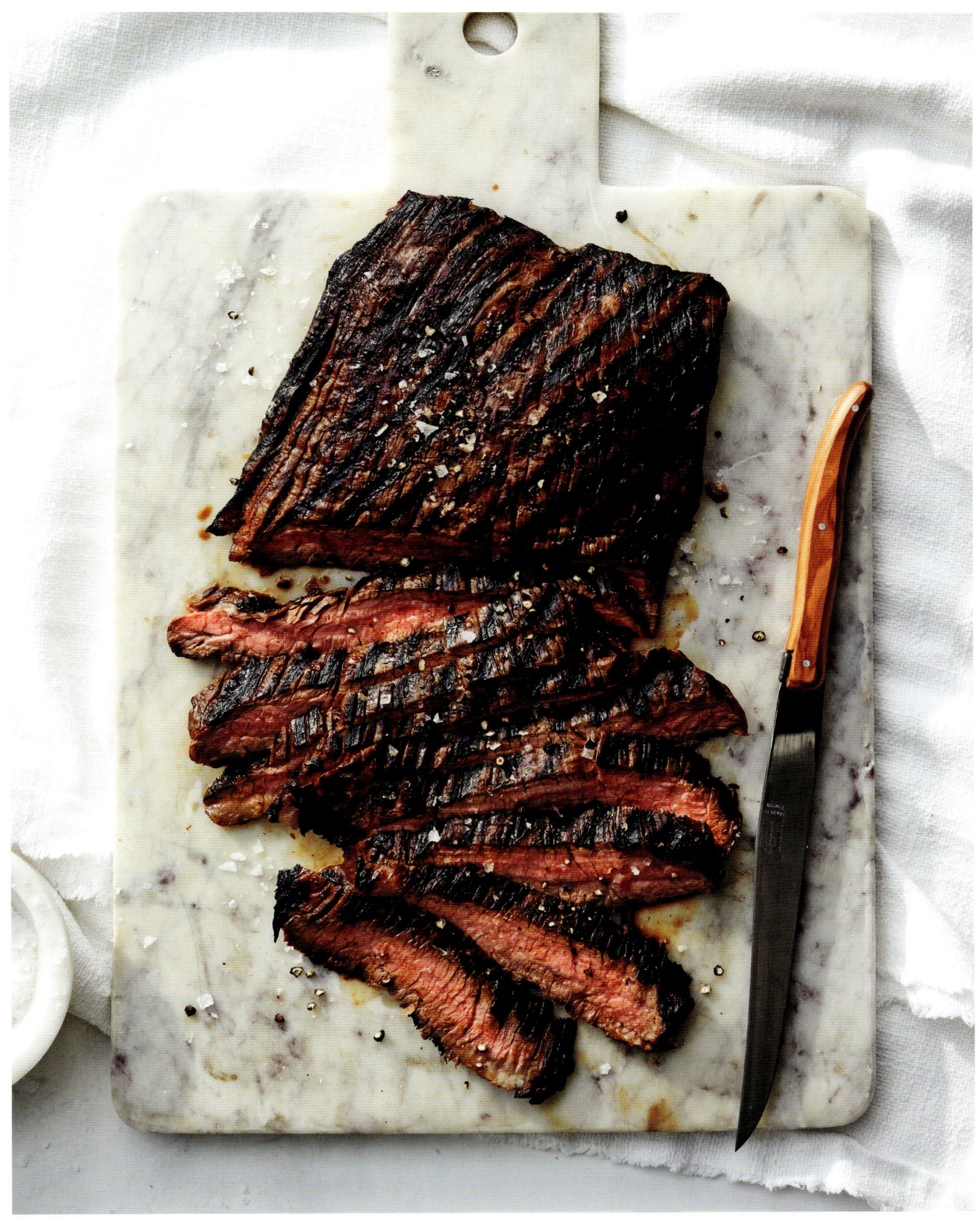

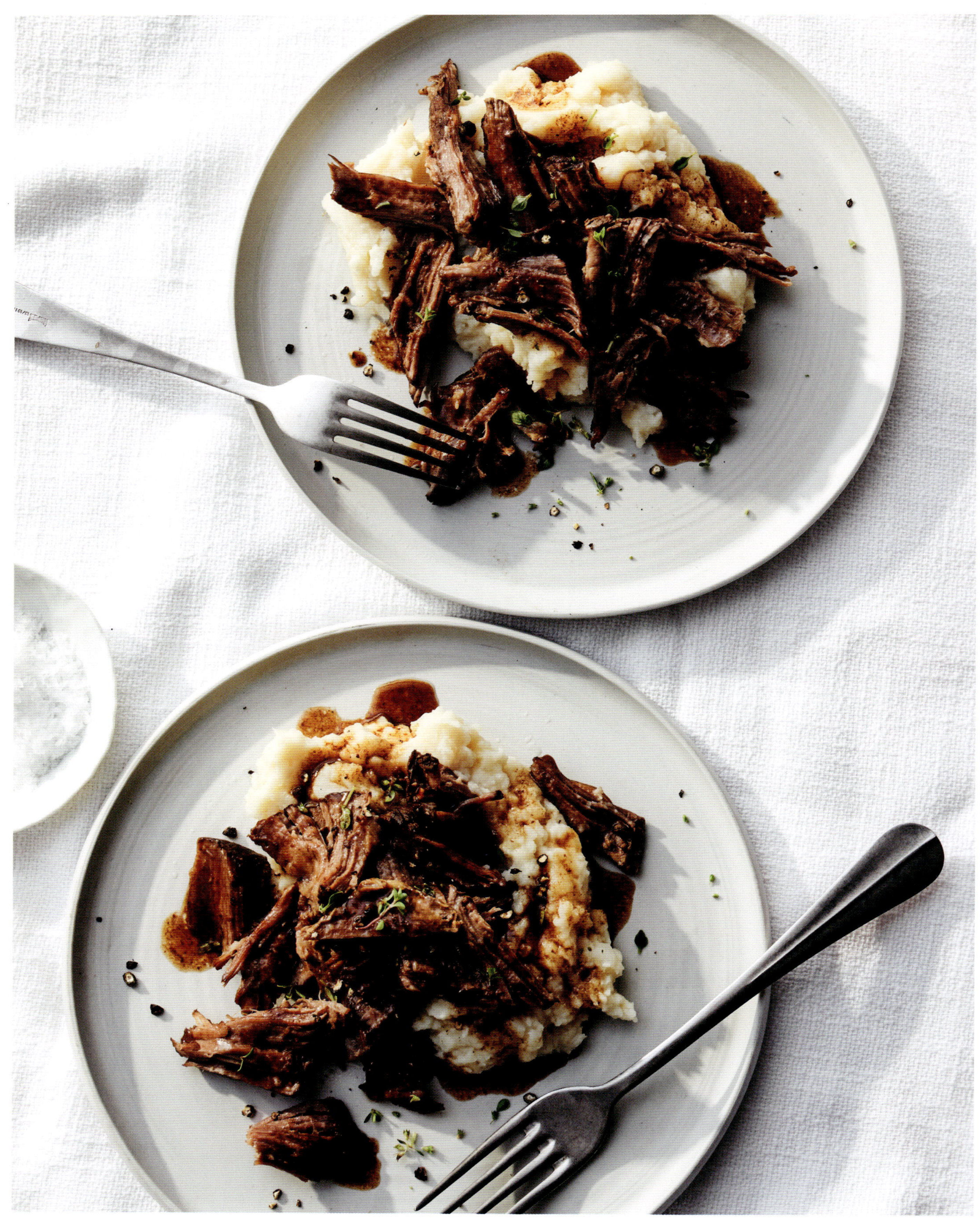

This hearty beef dish, paired with your favorite vegetable mash, is as simple as it is comforting. It fills your home with the warm, inviting aroma of French onion soup and provides essential nutrients that can be lacking if red meat isn't part of your regular rotation. Low-effort yet high-volume, it's a meal you can enjoy for several days in a row or freeze for a quick, satisfying dinner down the line.

SERVES 10

Savory French Onion Beef

- ½ red onion, thinly sliced on a mandoline (see Note)
- 1 yellow onion, thinly sliced on a mandoline (see Note)
- 10 garlic cloves, minced
- 1 tablespoon pink salt
- 1 tablespoon apple cider vinegar
- 4 lbs (1.8 kg) boneless beef chuck roast, twine removed
- Chopped chives, for garnish (optional)
- Maldon flake salt, for sprinkling
- Vegetable mash of choice, to serve

Combine all ingredients, except chives and flake salt, in a slow cooker in the order listed, with the chuck roast sitting on top. Cover, set it to high, and cook for 3 hours.

Use a pair of tongs to flip over the roast, then cook for another 3 hours.

Using 2 forks, break roast into smaller chunks so it will cook evenly and absorb all the other flavors. Cook for another 2 hours.

Pick out any undesirable tendons or fat and discard. Using 2 forks, shred beef so it combines with the juices.

Serve beef over the vegetable mash of your choice. Garnish with chives and sprinkle with flake salt, if desired.

NOTES

The ingredients fit perfectly into a 3.5-quart slow cooker.

It's important to slice the onions paper-thin so they eventually disappear into the beef.

This recipe delivers the comforting, homey vibe of classic meatloaf, but with a twist: It's made with bison! Leaner and higher in protein than beef, bison makes for a wholesome and delicious alternative. For the best results, prepare the meatloaf a few hours ahead of time to let the flavors meld beautifully. Don't skip the extra step of straining the pan juices through a fine-mesh sieve—it's packed with flavor and absolutely worth it.

SERVES 6

Bison Meatloaf + Jus

- Extra-virgin olive oil, for the pan
- 2 small–medium carrots, grated
- 1 yellow onion, finely chopped
- 5 garlic cloves, finely chopped
- 1 large egg
- ⅓ cup (10 g) finely chopped flat-leaf parsley
- 2 tablespoons Dijon mustard
- 1 tablespoon Red Boat fish sauce
- 2 teaspoons pink salt
- 2½ lbs (1.14 kg) ground bison (see Note)

Heat a splash of oil in a large skillet over medium-low heat. Add carrots, onion, and garlic and sauté for 15 minutes, until softened but not browned. Remove from the heat and let the mixture cool to room temperature.

In a large mixing bowl, combine the cooled vegetable mixture, egg, parsley, Dijon mustard, fish sauce, and salt, and mix to combine. Add bison and gently fold it into the mixture until well combined. Be careful not to overwork it.

Transfer the mixture to a 9 × 13-inch (23 × 33-cm) Pyrex-style baking dish and use your hands to form it into a loaf. Cover and refrigerate until ready to bake.

Preheat oven to 375°F.

Bake the meatloaf for 60–65 minutes, until an instant-read thermometer inserted into the center reaches 160°F. Transfer the meatloaf to a platter. Pour pan juices through a fine-mesh sieve into a small bowl. Let the meatloaf rest for 15 minutes, then slice. Spoon jus over each slice of meatloaf.

NOTE

I find 2½-lb (1.14-kg) packs of bison at Costco.

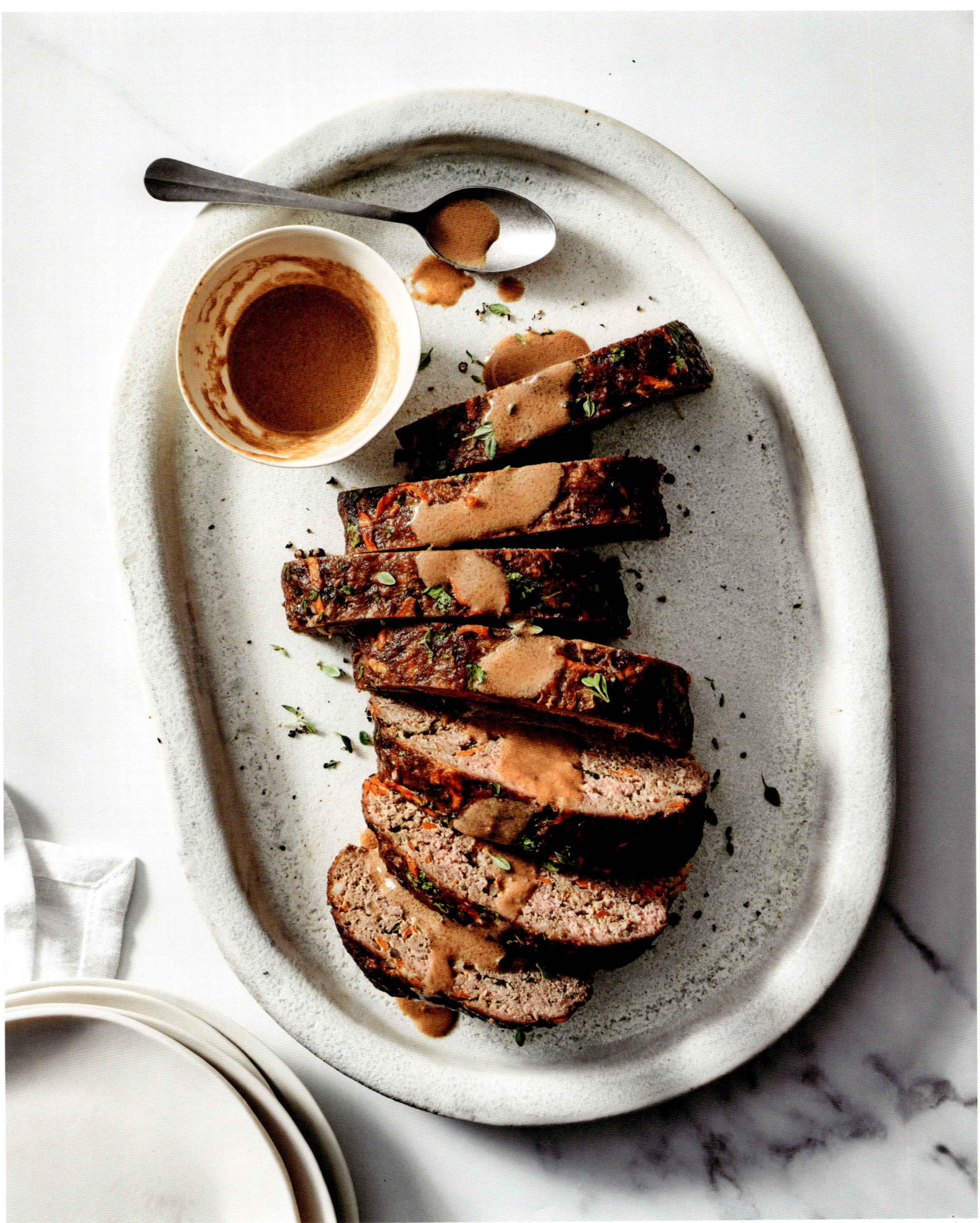

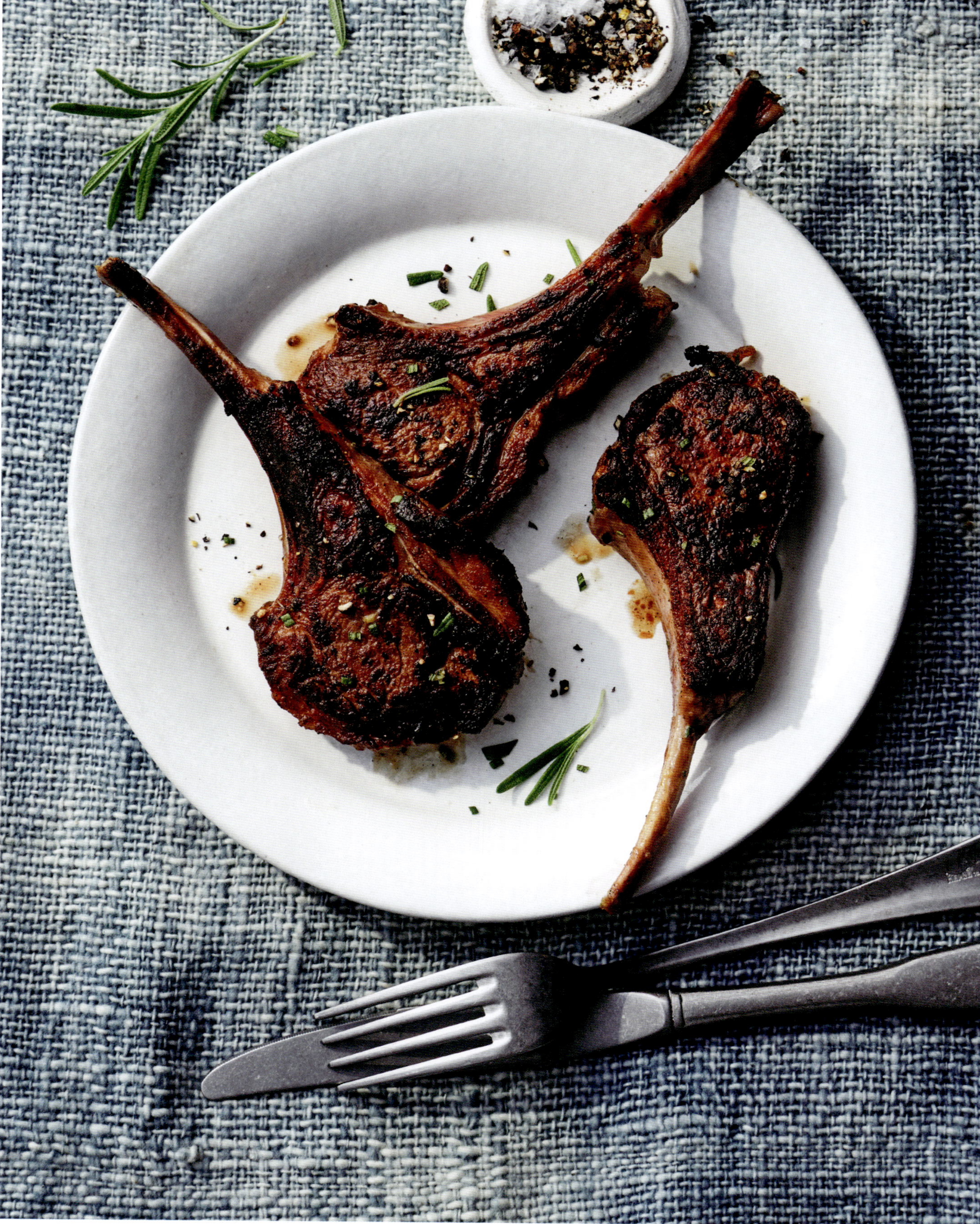

These succulent lamb lollipops are simply individual chops cut from a rack of lamb. You can either cut them yourself by slicing between each rib or ask your butcher to do it. For a slightly more elegant look, they can be frenched, which means the meat and fat along the bone have been cut away, leaving just the medallion of meat at one end.

Pan-Seared Lamb Lollipops with Rosemary, Maple + Dijon

SERVES 2

- 1 rack of lamb, cut into 8 chops
- 2 garlic cloves, grated
- 1 tablespoon finely chopped rosemary
- 3 tablespoons pure maple syrup
- 2 tablespoons Dijon mustard
- Extra-virgin olive oil, for the pan
- Pink salt, to taste

Plan to marinate the chops 24 hours in advance.

In a large zip-top bag, combine garlic, rosemary, maple syrup, and Dijon mustard. Add lamb chops and work mixture until everything is combined and chops are coated. Press the air out of the bag, seal it shut, and refrigerate for 24 hours.

To cook, take the lamb chops out of the fridge 30 minutes in advance so they can come to room temperature. Transfer them to a paper towel–lined plate to soak up any excess marinade. Pat them mostly dry so the sugars in the maple syrup don't scorch.

Heat a splash of oil in a skillet over medium-high heat. Sprinkle the chops generously with salt and sear them on each side until they're deep golden brown and the internal temperature reaches 135°F on an instant-read thermometer. Serve immediately.

NOTE

Use a skillet rather than a grill pan because the ridges prevent the chops from making full contact with the surface of the pan.

This fresh and flavorful leaf-wrapped burger is topped with creamy avocado and a drizzle of bright lemony aioli. I've also been known to turn it into a salad by chopping the lettuce and crumbling the burgers. Making the aioli and the lamb mixture a few hours in advance gives the flavors time to develop.

Lettuce Wrapped Lamb Burgers + Lemon Aioli

SERVES 4

Aioli

½ cup (117 g) mayonnaise

Zest of 1 lemon

1 tablespoon freshly squeezed lemon juice

2 garlic cloves, grated

⅛ teaspoon pink salt

Burgers

2 garlic cloves, minced

¼ cup (35 g) finely chopped red onion

¼ cup (7 g) finely chopped parsley

2 tablespoons finely chopped mint

1 tablespoon extra-virgin olive oil

¾ teaspoon pink salt

½ teaspoon ground cinnamon

¼ teaspoon freshly cracked black pepper

⅛ teaspoon ground cumin

1 lb (454 g) ground lamb

For serving

Red or green leaf lettuce

Avocado slices

Thinly sliced English cucumber

Thinly shaved red onion

Aioli Combine all aioli ingredients in a small bowl and refrigerate until ready to use.

Burgers Mix all burger ingredients, except lamb, together in a medium bowl. Add the lamb, folding gently into the herb mixture until well combined. Avoid overworking the meat. Refrigerate until ready to use.

Form the lamb mixture into 4 patties.

Heat a splash of olive oil in a nonstick skillet over medium heat. Add the patties and cook on each side for 4–5 minutes, until the internal temperature reaches 160°F on an instant-read thermometer inserted into the center.

Assembly Wrap each burger in a large lettuce leaf and drizzle with aioli. Top with avocado slices, cucumber, and red onion.

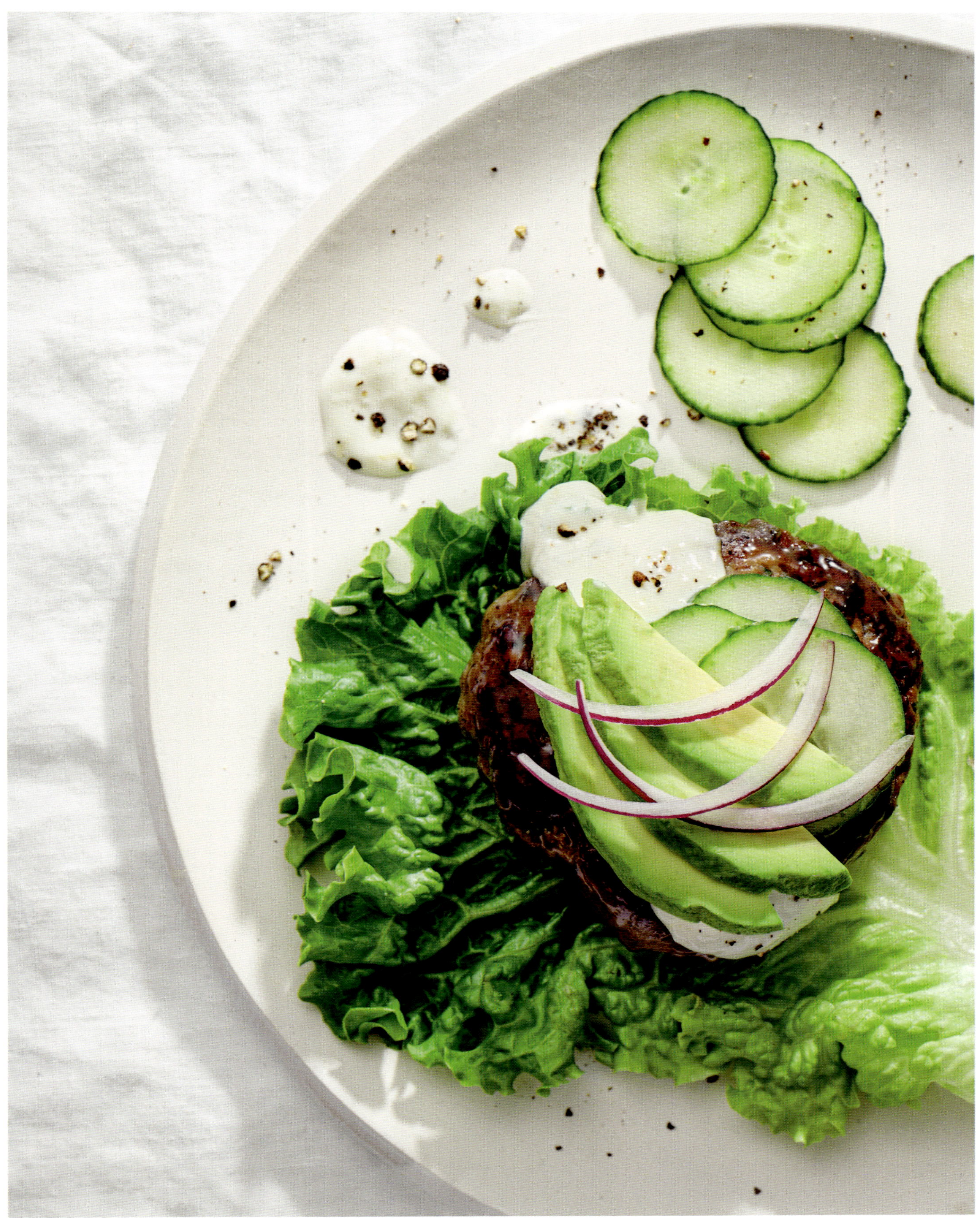

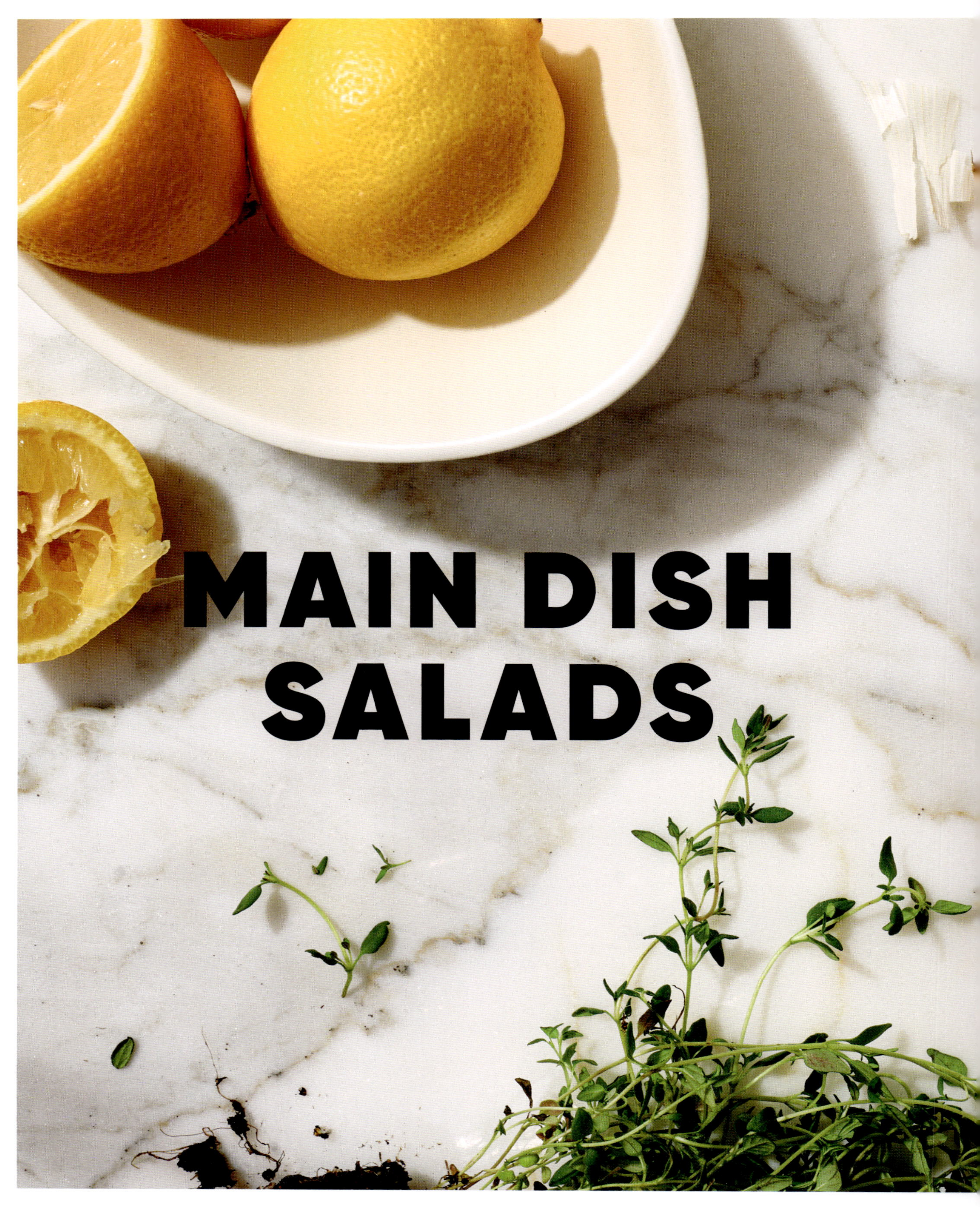

MAIN DISH SALADS

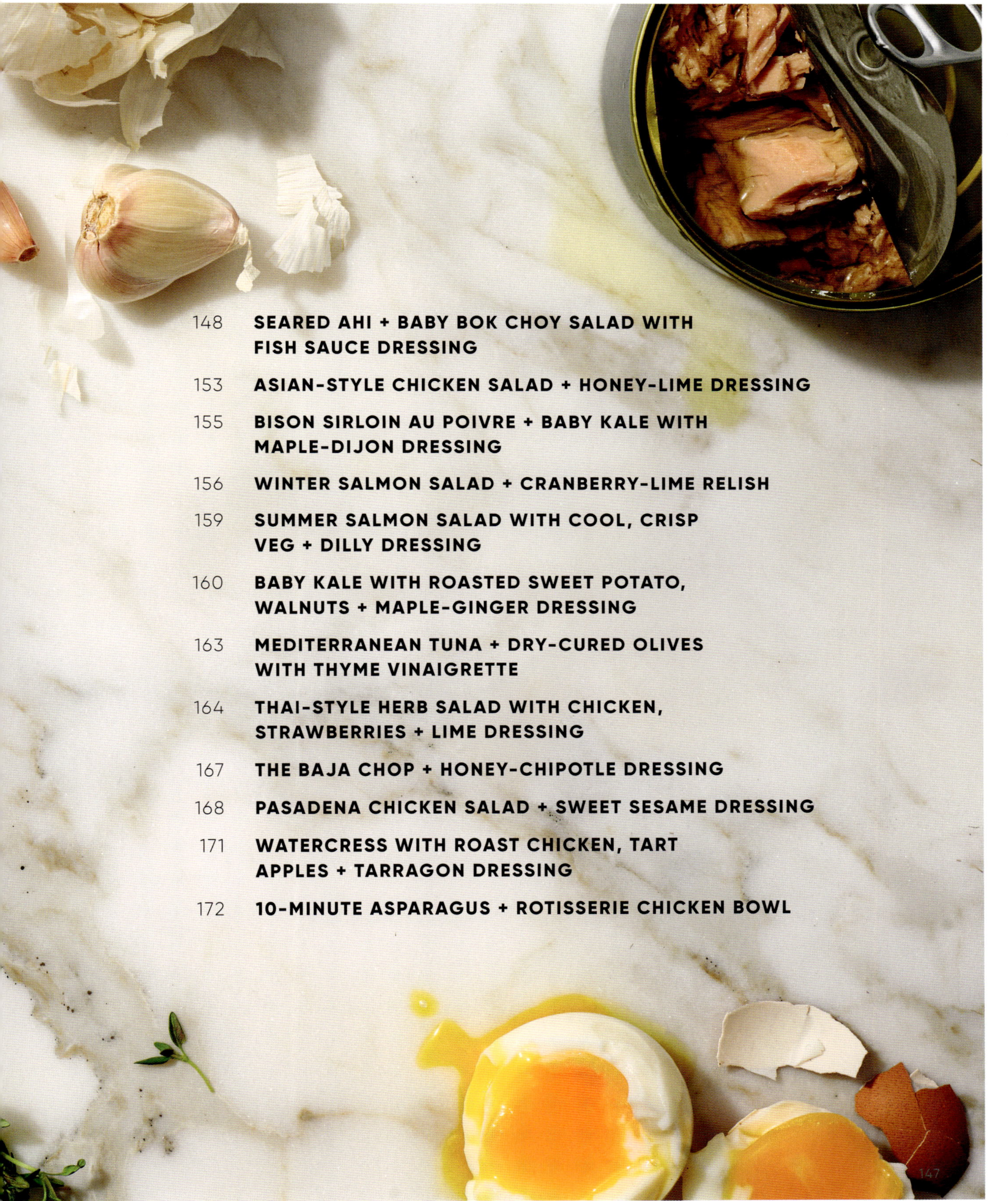

148 SEARED AHI + BABY BOK CHOY SALAD WITH FISH SAUCE DRESSING

153 ASIAN-STYLE CHICKEN SALAD + HONEY-LIME DRESSING

155 BISON SIRLOIN AU POIVRE + BABY KALE WITH MAPLE-DIJON DRESSING

156 WINTER SALMON SALAD + CRANBERRY-LIME RELISH

159 SUMMER SALMON SALAD WITH COOL, CRISP VEG + DILLY DRESSING

160 BABY KALE WITH ROASTED SWEET POTATO, WALNUTS + MAPLE-GINGER DRESSING

163 MEDITERRANEAN TUNA + DRY-CURED OLIVES WITH THYME VINAIGRETTE

164 THAI-STYLE HERB SALAD WITH CHICKEN, STRAWBERRIES + LIME DRESSING

167 THE BAJA CHOP + HONEY-CHIPOTLE DRESSING

168 PASADENA CHICKEN SALAD + SWEET SESAME DRESSING

171 WATERCRESS WITH ROAST CHICKEN, TART APPLES + TARRAGON DRESSING

172 10-MINUTE ASPARAGUS + ROTISSERIE CHICKEN BOWL

I was on the hunt for an alternative to salad greens and turned to the adorable and vibrant yet sorely underrated crucifer: baby bok choy. Regular bok choy can be on the bitter side, but baby bok choy, even when raw, is so tender and sweet. And it deserves its reputation as a nutritional powerhouse because it's loaded with vitamins A, C, and K, and it's an excellent source of minerals. However, like leeks, bok choy often traps dirt and grit between its layers, so a thorough rinse is a must.

Seared Ahi + Baby Bok Choy Salad with Fish Sauce Dressing

SERVES 4

Dressing

- 1 garlic clove, grated
- ¼ cup (80 g) pure maple syrup
- ¼ cup (50 g) extra-virgin olive oil
- 3 tablespoons unseasoned rice vinegar
- 2 tablespoons Red Boat fish sauce
- 1 tablespoon toasted sesame oil
- ⅛ teaspoon red pepper flakes (optional; see Note)

Salad

- 4–6 baby bok choy, depending on the size

Ahi

- 4 (6-oz/170-g) ahi tuna steaks
- Extra-virgin olive oil, for brushing
- Pink salt, for sprinkling

Dressing Make the dressing a few hours (up to a day) in advance so the flavors can meld. Whisk all dressing ingredients in a small bowl together until combined and emulsified. Refrigerate until ready to use.

Salad Clean baby bok choy by submerging it in water and swishing it around a bit to loosen any dirt or grit trapped between its layers. If you have a salad spinner, use it to wash and spin bok choy dry. Slice bok choy thinly crosswise, then slice all the dark green leaves into thin ribbons. Transfer it to a large serving bowl. Add the dressing just before serving, as the bok choy will wilt slightly and drop some liquid.

Ahi Remove the ahi steaks from the fridge 30 minutes in advance to come to room temperature.

Pat them dry with a paper towel, coat in oil, and sprinkle liberally with salt. Heat a skillet on medium-high until *very* hot. Add steaks and sear for 1 minute, undisturbed. Flip them over, then cook for another 1 minute, until cooked to rare.

Toppings

4 scallions, white and green parts, thinly sliced

2/3 cup (87 g) toasted slivered almonds

1 heaping tablespoon black sesame seeds

Assembly Add scallions and toasted almonds to the bowl of bok choy. Dress the salad with a very generous amount of vinaigrette and toss until everything is well coated. Divide the salad among 4 plates and top each one with a sliced ahi steak. Sprinkle each one with black sesame seeds and serve immediately.

Variation: Shredded Chicken This salad is as fantastic with shredded chicken breast as it is with ahi, if that's your preference. Simply replace the tuna with 1 lb (454 g) cooked, shredded chicken breast and add it to the salad with the scallions and toasted almonds.

NOTE

If you're avoiding nightshades, omit the red pepper flakes.

Baby bok choy is a charming and verdant, yet often overlooked, crucifer. A true nutritional powerhouse, it is tender and subtly sweet, even in its raw form.

Seared Ahi + Baby Bok Choy Salad with Fish Sauce Dressing

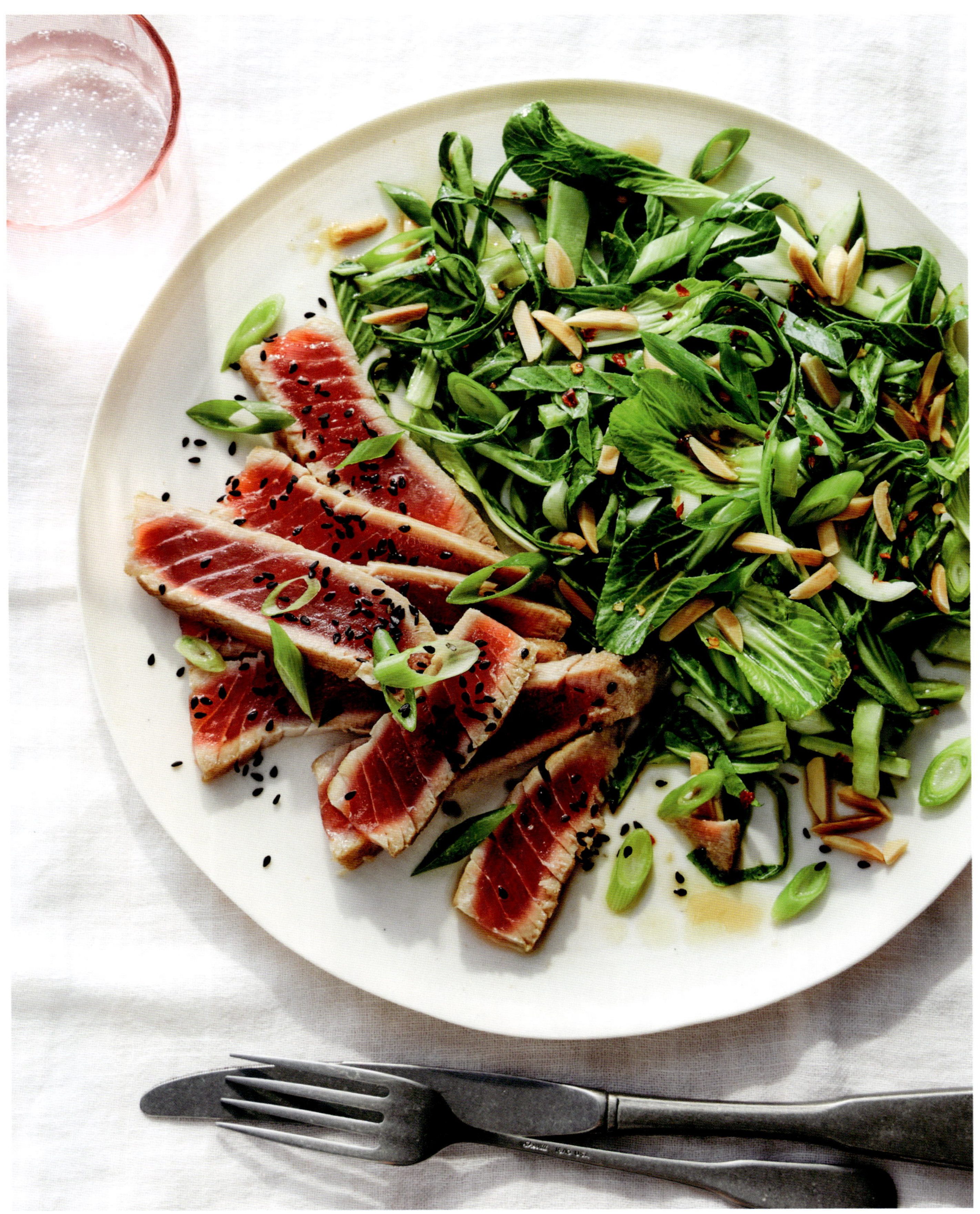

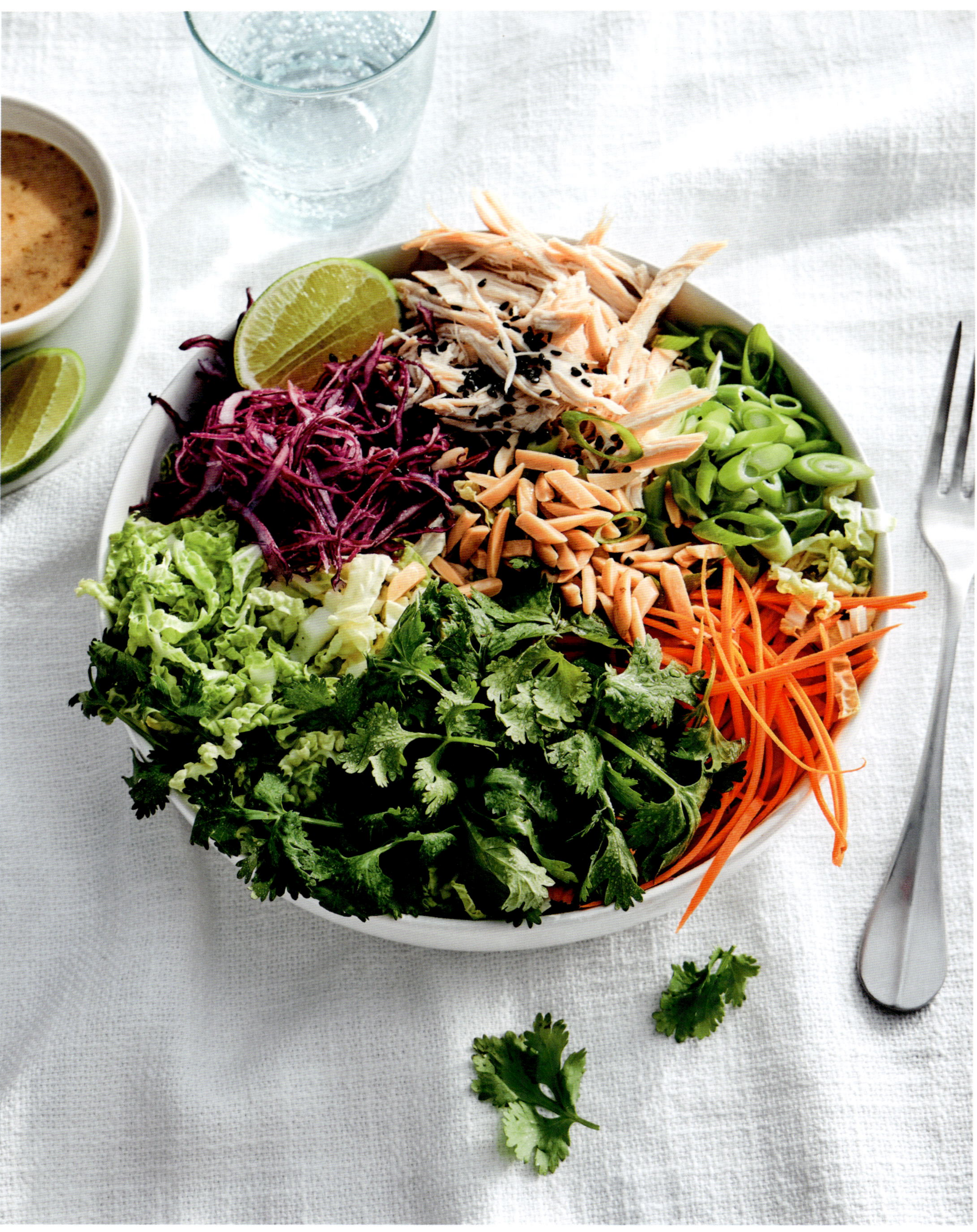

This crisp and refreshing medley of vegetables features cool, crunchy Napa cabbage, which is considered a superfood! Napa cabbage contains higher levels of vitamins A and B3, iron, and copper than regular cabbage. The sweet citrus dressing pulls it all together and can be made a day in advance.

Asian-Style Chicken Salad + Honey-Lime Dressing

SERVES 4

Dressing

2 garlic cloves

⅓ cup (67 g) extra-virgin olive oil

1 tablespoon toasted sesame oil

3 tablespoons honey

Zest of 1 lime

2 tablespoons freshly squeezed lime juice (see Note)

1 tablespoon unseasoned rice vinegar

1 tablespoon coconut aminos (see Note)

1 teaspoon pink salt

Salad

½ Napa cabbage

1 large carrot, cut into matchsticks (see Note)

1 cup (15 g) roughly chopped cilantro leaves with tender stems

½ cup (66 g) toasted slivered almonds

1 lb (454 g) cooked chicken breast, shredded

4 scallions, green and white parts, sliced diagonally

1 cup (60 g) finely shredded red cabbage (optional)

Black sesame seeds, for sprinkling

Maldon flake salt, for sprinkling

Dressing Add garlic to the bowl of a mini food processor and pulse to mince. Add the remaining dressing ingredients and process until combined and creamy. Transfer to a small bowl and refrigerate until ready to use.

Salad Cut cabbage in half lengthwise, then thinly slice into ribbons. Reserve the other half for another use. Combine salad ingredients in a large mixing bowl and toss to combine. Pour the dressing over the salad and toss until thoroughly coated.

Divide among 4 plates or shallow bowls and sprinkle with black sesame seeds and flake salt.

NOTES

I usually have an extra lime on hand in case one of them is dry.

Look for a brand of coconut aminos that contains only coconut nectar, water, and salt.

Rather than hand-cutting the carrot into matchsticks, make quick work of the process by using an OXO Good Grips julienne peeler, available online.

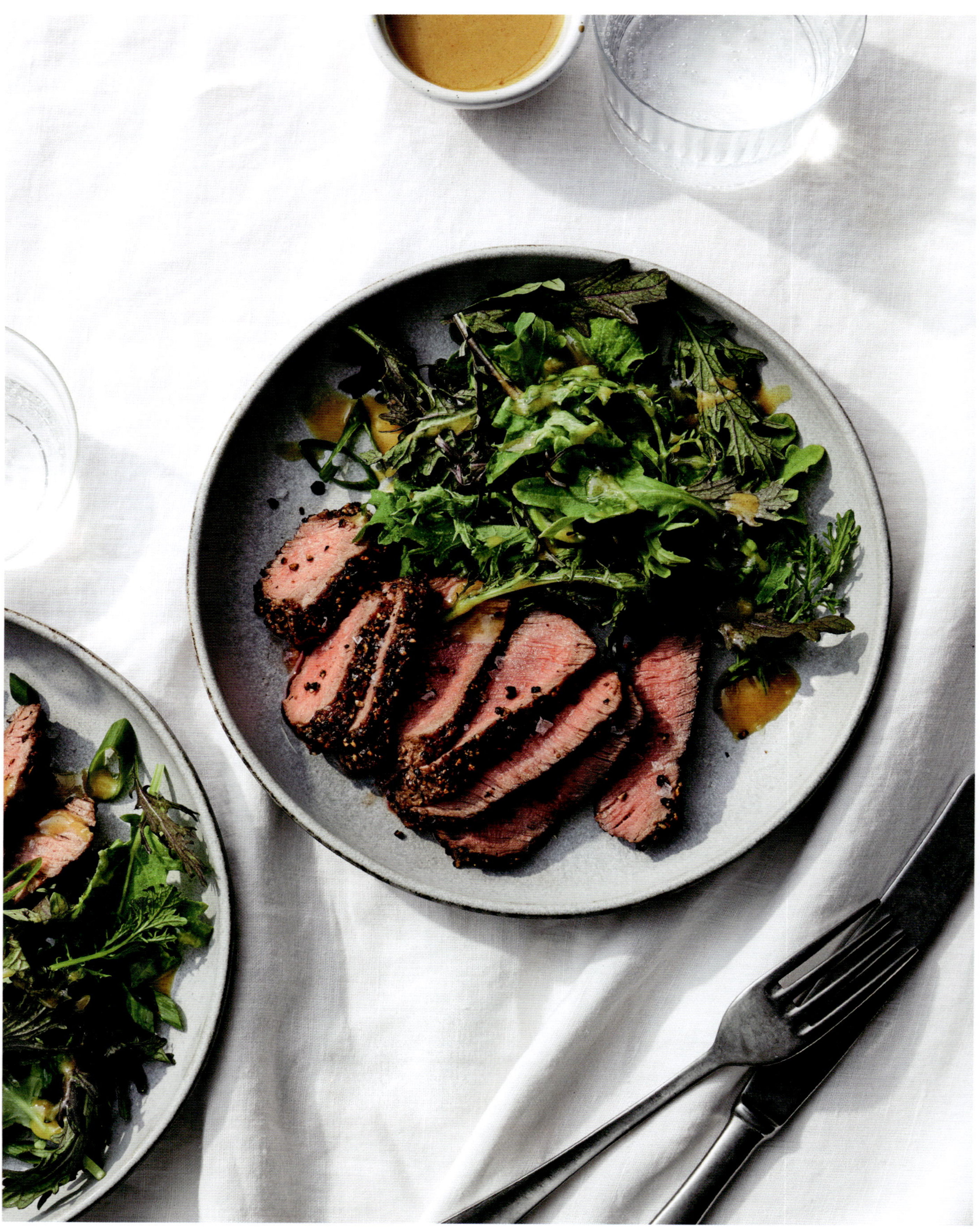

The fastest, easiest weeknight (or weekend!) dinner you'll want in regular rotation. Bison contains more protein than beef and is high in vitamin B12, iron, selenium, and zinc. Mixing the dressing a few hours in advance gives the flavors a chance to mingle. My favorite bison sirloin steaks are from Great Range Premium Bison, available at Whole Foods. We also enjoy the Bison Sirloin au Poivre without the accompanying salad and instead pair it with either the Summer Kale + Strawberry Salad (page 74) or the Garlic Mashed Cauliflower (page 112).

Bison Sirloin au Poivre + Baby Kale with Maple-Dijon Dressing

SERVES 2

Dressing

1 small garlic clove, grated

¼ cup (50 g) extra-virgin olive oil

1 tablespoon pure maple syrup

1 tablespoon Dijon mustard

⅛ teaspoon truffle salt or pink salt (see Note)

Bison

2 (6-oz/170-g) bison sirloin steaks

1 tablespoon Maldon flake salt

2 tablespoons freshly cracked, coarsely ground black pepper

Extra-virgin olive oil, for the pan

Salad

1 (5-oz/142-g) bag baby kale or arugula

2 scallions, green parts only, sliced diagonally

NOTE

My favorite truffle salt is Casina Rossa Truffle & Salt.

Dressing Whisk all dressing ingredients together in a small bowl. Refrigerate until ready to use.

Bison Remove the steaks from the fridge 30 minutes in advance so they can come to room temperature.

Preheat oven to 400°F.

Pat the steaks dry with paper towels. Dial your pepper mill to the coarsest setting before measuring the pepper. (Alternatively, whole peppercorns can be smashed with the bottom of a heavy pan.) Combine salt and pepper on a plate. Set steaks on top of the mixture, pressing firmly so seasonings will adhere. Only coat one side.

Heat a generous splash of oil in a nonstick, ovenproof skillet over medium-high heat until it's shimmery hot. Add steaks, peppercorn side down, and sear for 2 minutes. Using tongs, carefully flip the steaks, trying not to break the peppercorn crust, and sear for another 2 minutes. Slide the skillet into the oven and roast for 4 minutes, or until an instant-read thermometer inserted into the center of the meat reaches 145°F. Be careful of the hot handle on the skillet! Transfer the steaks to a cutting board and allow them to rest for 5 minutes.

Salad Toss kale in enough dressing to coat it, then divide it between 2 plates. Top each salad with scallions. Slice each bison steak crosswise against the grain, then arrange them over the plated greens.

Wild salmon season is just May through September, but I want to reap its nutritional benefits year-round. To brighten up frozen wild salmon during the winter months—when frozen sockeye is most widely available—I turn to a bold, flavorful relish. Sockeye has a more assertive flavor than other varieties, but this relish stands up to it perfectly and is packed with antioxidants! Make the relish at least a few hours in advance—you'll notice that time really softens the bite of the red onion.

Winter Salmon Salad + Cranberry-Lime Relish

SERVES 4

Relish

1 (12-oz/340-g) package fresh cranberries

½ small red onion, roughly chopped

½ teaspoon lime zest

1 tablespoon freshly squeezed lime juice

½ cup (157 g) pure maple syrup

¼ teaspoon pink salt

3 grinds of freshly cracked black pepper

Salmon

4 (6-oz/170-g) wild-caught salmon fillets

Pink salt, for sprinkling

Salad

1 (5-oz/142-g) bag mixed baby greens

1 tablespoon extra-virgin olive oil

Maldon flake salt, for finishing

Relish Rinse cranberries, discarding any that are rotten or squishy. Pat them dry with a paper towel so they don't make the relish too juicy. Combine all relish ingredients in a food processor and pulse until the cranberries are finely chopped. Transfer to a small bowl and refrigerate until ready to use.

Salmon Bring salmon to room temperature by removing it from the fridge 30 minutes in advance—this ensures even doneness.

Pat the fillets dry and sprinkle generously with pink salt. Arrange skin-side down in a cool, dry (no oil) nonstick skillet—you may need to do this in batches. Cook undisturbed on medium heat for 8–10 minutes, until the skin is golden and crispy. Briefly press down with a spatula to ensure the fillet is making full contact with the pan. Flip them over and cook for 1–2 minutes, until an instant-read thermometer inserted in the center registers 125°F–130°F.

Salad In a large bowl, gently toss salad greens with a sprinkle of flake salt and oil to lightly coat. Divide greens among 4 plates and top each one with a salmon fillet. Add a couple spoonfuls of cranberry lime relish. Sprinkle with flake salt and serve.

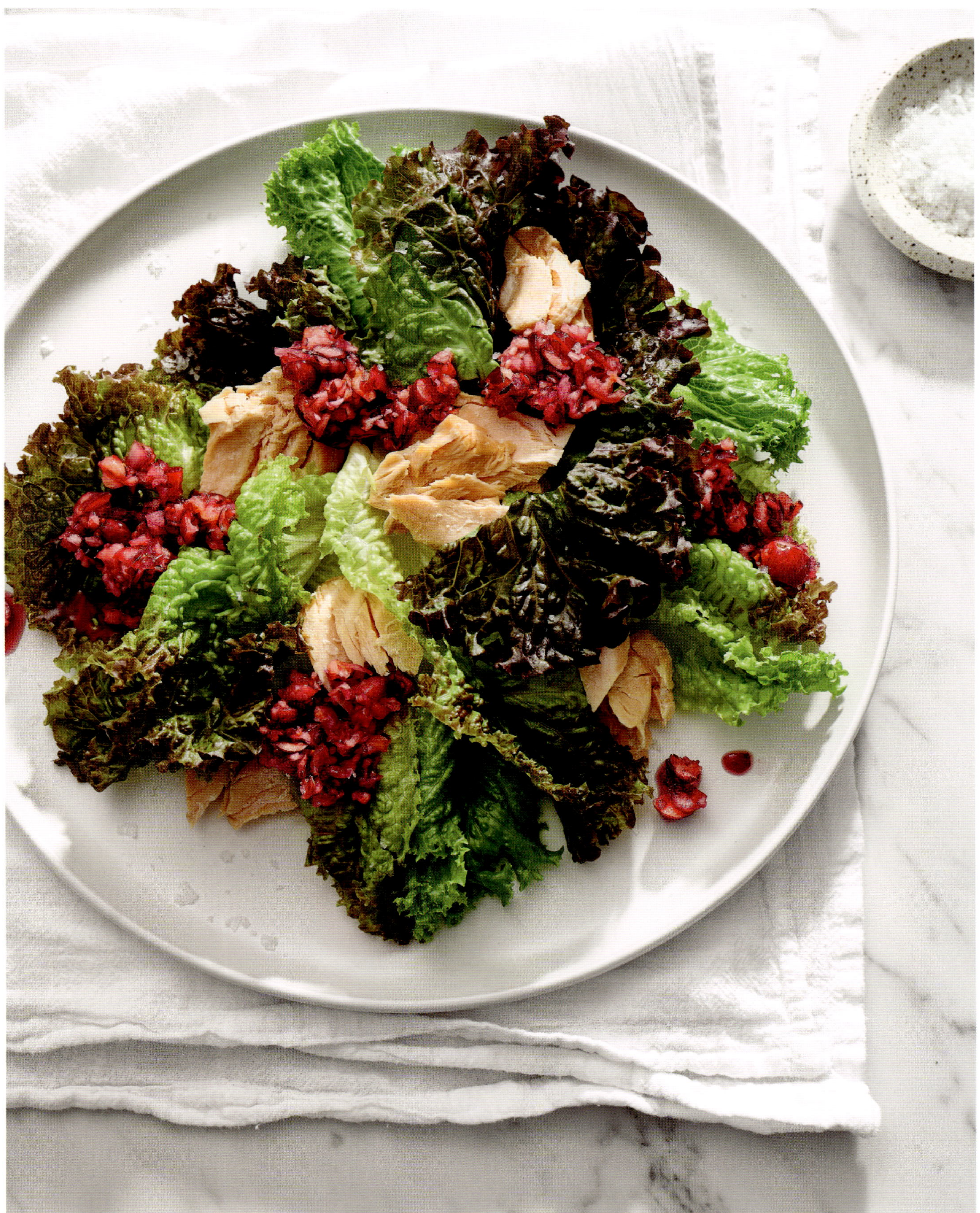

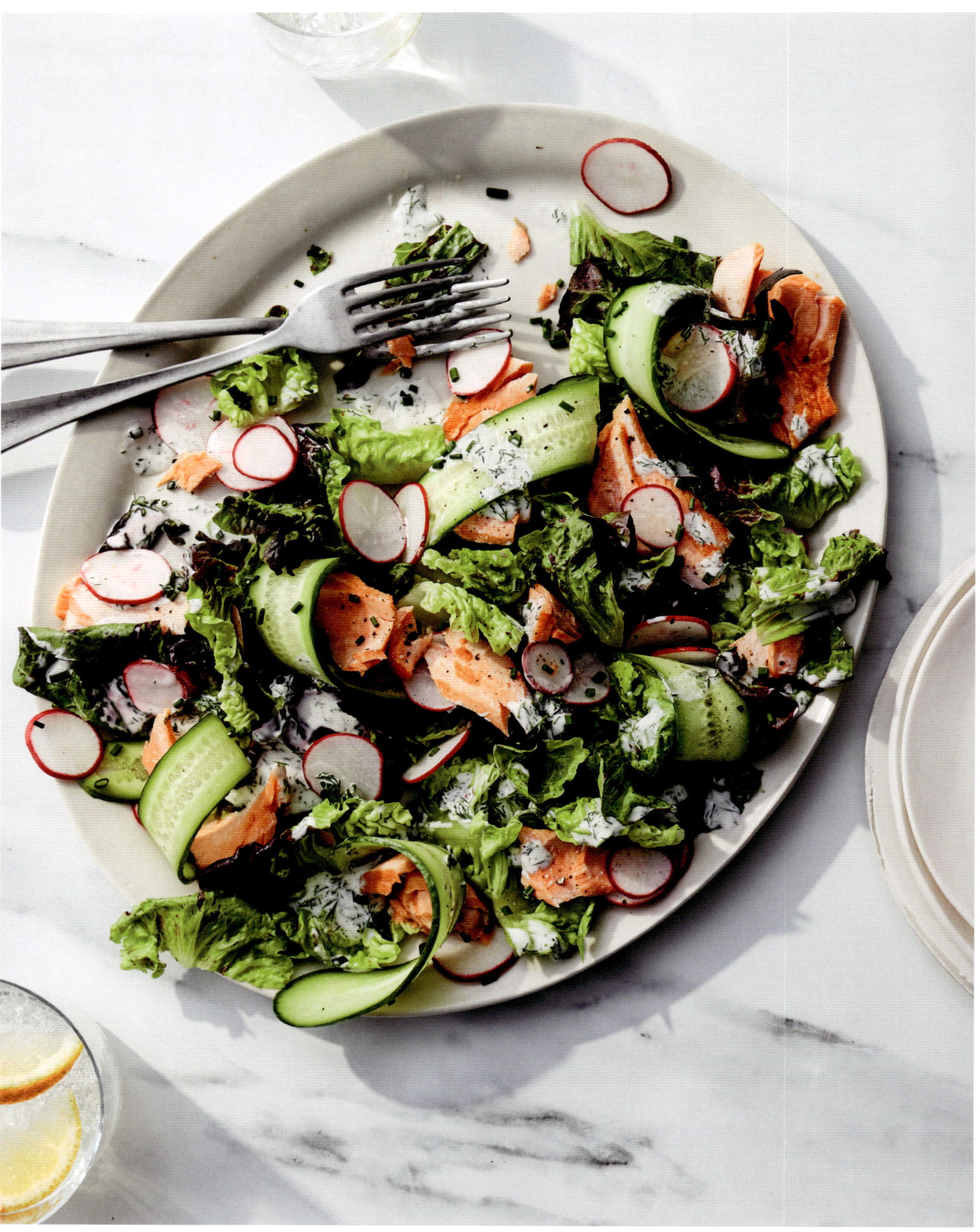

Paired with crisp greens, cool cucumbers, and peppery radishes—this simple, healthful salad can be enjoyed all summer! It's all about a succulent fillet of salmon and this dilly dressing, so always keep a jar in the fridge. Assemble your salad with whatever mild summer greens you spot at the market or your favorite farm stand. Summer fare is all about simplicity and peak ripeness. When it comes to keeping your fresh salmon fillet as silky and unctuous as possible, simply *do not overcook*.

SERVES 4

Summer Salmon Salad with Cool, Crisp Veg + Dilly Dressing

Dressing

1 cup (235 g) mayonnaise

⅓ cup (8 g) lightly packed finely chopped dill fronds

1 tablespoon freshly squeezed lemon juice

1 garlic clove, grated

½ teaspoon pink salt

Salmon

4 (6-oz/170-g) fresh, wild-caught salmon fillets

Extra-virgin olive oil

Pink salt, for sprinkling

Salad

Mild greens of choice, such as spring mix or Little Gem lettuce

¼ English cucumber, thinly sliced on a mandoline

4 radishes, thinly sliced on a mandoline

Handful of chopped chives

Dressing Mix all dressing ingredients in a small bowl and refrigerate until ready to use. Making it a couple hours in advance gives the flavors a chance to develop. It will keep in the fridge for up to a week.

Salmon Bring the salmon to room temperature by removing it from the fridge 30 minutes in advance—this ensures even doneness.

Preheat outdoor grill over medium-high heat.

Pat dry each fillet, coat each one with oil, and generously sprinkle with salt. Grill salmon, skin-side down, until golden, crisp, and nearly cooked through. Flip over and grill for another 1–2 minutes, until an instant-read thermometer inserted in the thickest part of the fillet registers 125°F–130°F. (Alternatively, arrange fillets skin-side down in a cool, dry [no oil] nonstick skillet—you may need to do this in batches. Cook undisturbed on medium heat for 8–10 minutes, until the skin is golden and crispy. Briefly press down with a spatula to ensure the fillet is making full contact with the pan. Flip them over and cook for 1–2 minutes.)

Salad Layer the salad ingredients on 4 individual plates or a large platter, beginning with the greens. Add cucumber, radishes, and chunks of salmon, and then sprinkle with chives. Drizzle the dressing generously and serve immediately.

This enticing contrast of flavors and textures has that hearty, seasonal vibe we seek as summer fades into autumn. It's got a ginger punch and is chock full of roasted veg and toasty walnuts. I love the simplicity of baby kale—no stripping woody stalks or massaging fibrous leaves as is the case with adult varieties. If you store your ginger in the freezer, you'll always have some at the ready, and it will grate up nice and fluffy instead of the fibers gumming up your Microplane.

Baby Kale with Roasted Sweet Potato, Walnuts + Maple-Ginger Dressing

SERVES 4

Dressing

- 1 large garlic clove, grated
- 2 teaspoons freshly grated ginger
- ¼ cup (50 g) extra-virgin olive oil
- ¼ cup (60 g) unseasoned rice vinegar
- ¼ cup (80 g) pure maple syrup
- ¼ teaspoon pink salt
- 4 grinds of freshly cracked black pepper

Salad

- 2 orange-fleshed sweet potatoes, cut into ½-inch (12-mm) cubes
- ½ small red onion, thinly sliced into half moons
- Extra-virgin olive oil, for drizzling
- Pink salt, for sprinkling
- 1 (5-oz/142-g) bag baby kale or arugula
- ¾ cup (80 g) toasted walnuts, roughly chopped
- 1 lb (454 g) cooked chicken breast, shredded
- Maldon flake salt, for sprinkling

Dressing Whisk all dressing ingredients together in a small bowl until combined and refrigerate until ready to use. Making the dressing a few hours in advance allows the flavors to develop.

Salad Preheat oven to 400°F. Line a rimmed baking sheet with parchment paper.

Place sweet potatoes and onions on the prepared baking sheet. Drizzle them with oil, sprinkle with pink salt, and toss with your hands until everything is well coated. Spread them out evenly.

Roast on the center rack for 20 minutes. Stir, then roast for another 5–15 minutes, until vegetables are tender with a bit of color.

Combine all salad ingredients in a large bowl. Drizzle with a generous amount of dressing and toss until well coated. Divide among 4 plates, sprinkle with flake salt, and enjoy.

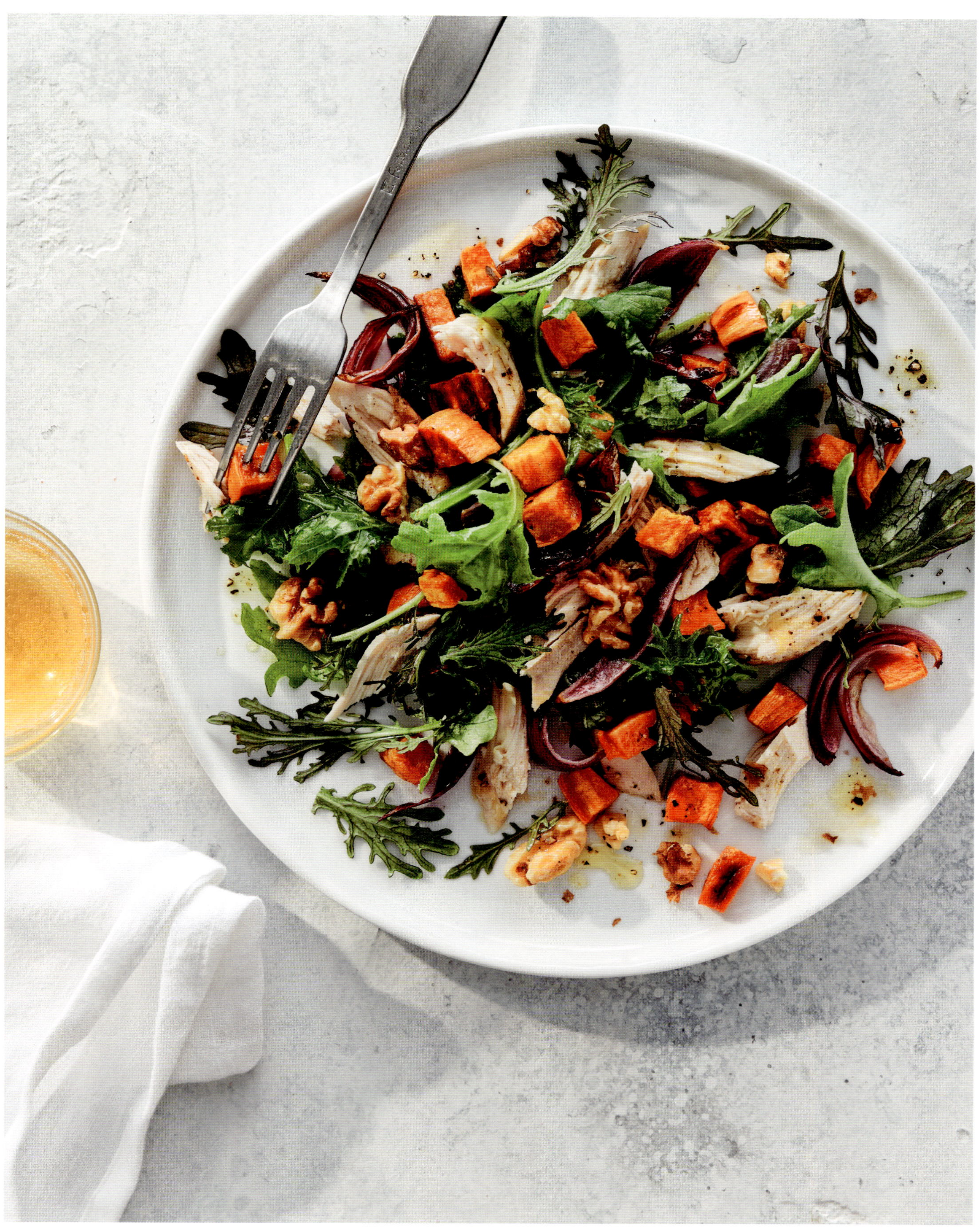

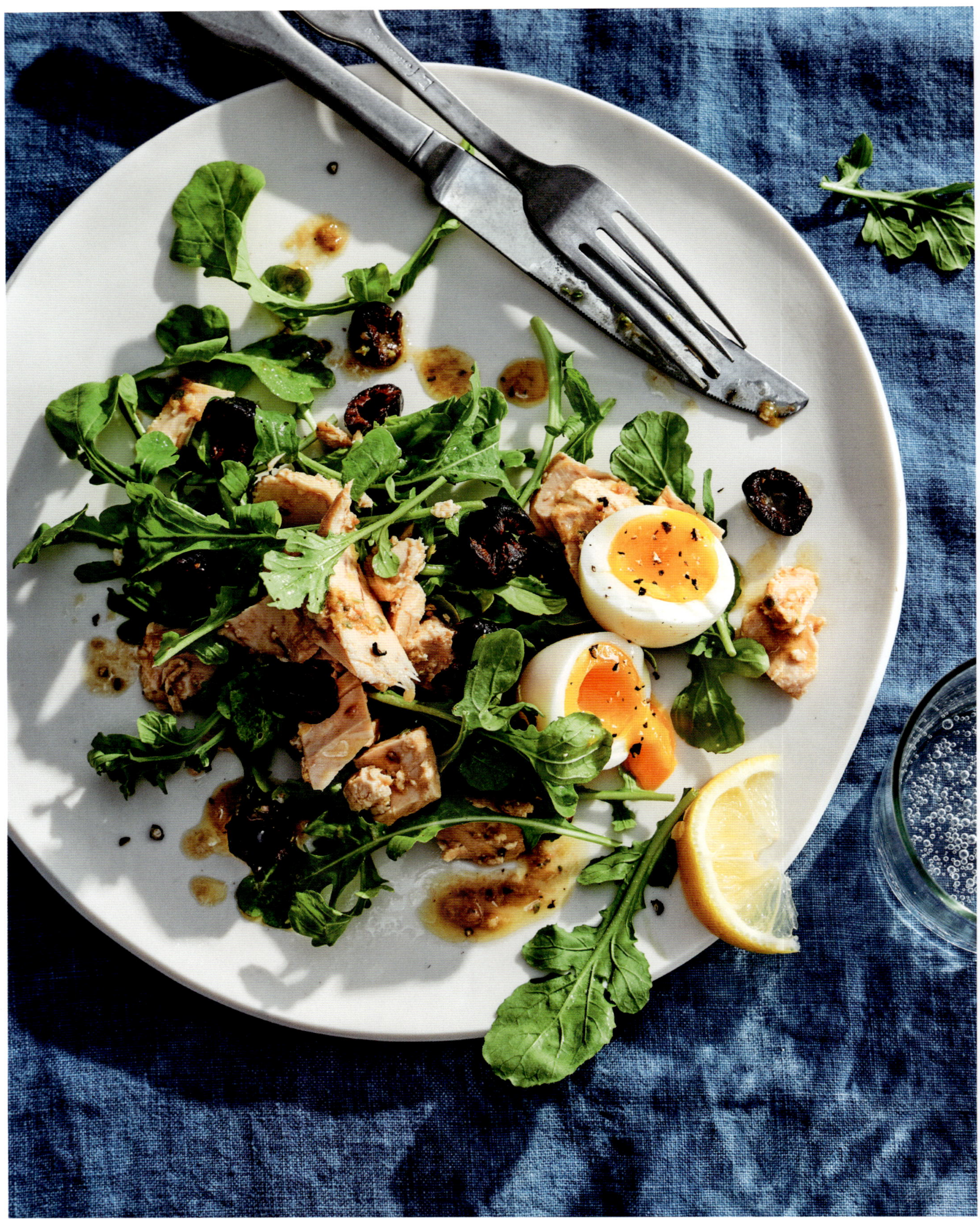

This hearty salad is super savory and satisfying, relying on just a handful of pantry items and fresh arugula. Peppery greens paired with tuna and jammy eggs come together with the Mediterranean flavors of the vinaigrette to make a spectacular lunch for friends. The dry-cured olives, also known as oil-cured, dial up the flavor, so I don't recommend subbing those out for another type.

Mediterranean Tuna + Dry-Cured Olives with Thyme Vinaigrette

SERVES 4

- 2 garlic cloves
- 4 oil-packed anchovy fillets
- Zest of 1 lemon
- 2 tablespoons freshly squeezed lemon juice
- ⅓ cup (67 g) extra-virgin olive oil, plus extra for drizzling
- 2 tablespoons vinagre de Jerez sherry vinegar
- 2 teaspoons thyme leaves
- ¼ teaspoon pink salt
- 2 (5-oz/142-g) cans wild albacore tuna (see Note)
- 4 large eggs
- 1 (5-oz/142-g) bag arugula
- ½ cup (87 g) dry-cured black olives, pitted and torn in half
- Maldon flake salt, for finishing

In the bowl of a mini food processor, pulse garlic until minced. Add anchovies, lemon zest, and juice and pulse a couple times, until anchovies have broken down. Add oil, vinegar, thyme, and pink salt and pulse until well combined.

Transfer the mixture to a medium-sized bowl, then add tuna and its liquid. Using a fork, break the tuna into chunks and toss to coat. Cover and refrigerate for at least a few hours, or overnight.

To make jammy soft-boiled eggs, bring a small saucepan of water to a boil. Gently lower eggs into the water and set the timer for 8 minutes. When time is up, quickly drain off the hot water and rinse twice in cold water, then add cold water and ice to the saucepan. Set aside for 5 minutes until the eggs are cool. Refrigerate the eggs until ready to use.

To serve, divide the arugula among 4 plates. Top each one with the tuna mixture and olives. Peel eggs, then cut them in half. Add them to each plate and sprinkle each salad with flake salt. Drizzle lightly with olive oil, then serve.

NOTE

I use Wild Planet tuna for this salad because it's packed in its own juice, without added water or oil.

This boldly herbaceous salad begs to be kept a bit wild and unfussy, as summer things should be! Tangles of cilantro stems nest among the basil and mint leaves, ripe juicy strawberries mingle with toasty flaked coconut, and it's all brought together with a sweet and savory citrus dressing. This is an adaptation of a *Sunset* magazine recipe.

Thai-Style Herb Salad with Chicken, Strawberries + Lime Dressing

SERVES 4

Dressing

1 teaspoon lime zest

⅓ cup (80 g) freshly squeezed lime juice

1 tablespoon Red Boat fish sauce

2 tablespoons extra-virgin olive oil

3 tablespoons honey

½ teaspoon pink salt

Salad

1 cup (40 g) unsweetened coconut flakes

1 lb (454 g) cooked chicken breast, shredded

2 cups (30 g) lightly packed cilantro sprigs (see Note)

2 cups (30 g) lightly packed basil leaves (see Note)

2 cups (16 g) lightly packed mint leaves (see Note)

1 lb (454 g) strawberries, hulled and quartered

Maldon flake salt, for finishing

Dressing Make the dressing a few hours in advance so the flavors can develop. Whisk all dressing ingredients together in a small bowl. Refrigerate until ready to use.

Salad Preheat oven to 350°F.

Toast coconut for 4–5 minutes, until lightly golden around the edges. Keep an eye on it because it can go from golden to dark very quickly.

Combine all salad ingredients in a large bowl. Drizzle with the dressing, then toss gently to thoroughly coat. Divide among 4 plates, sprinkle with flake salt, and serve.

NOTE

For accuracy, when measuring by weight, weigh out the herbs before you wash them.

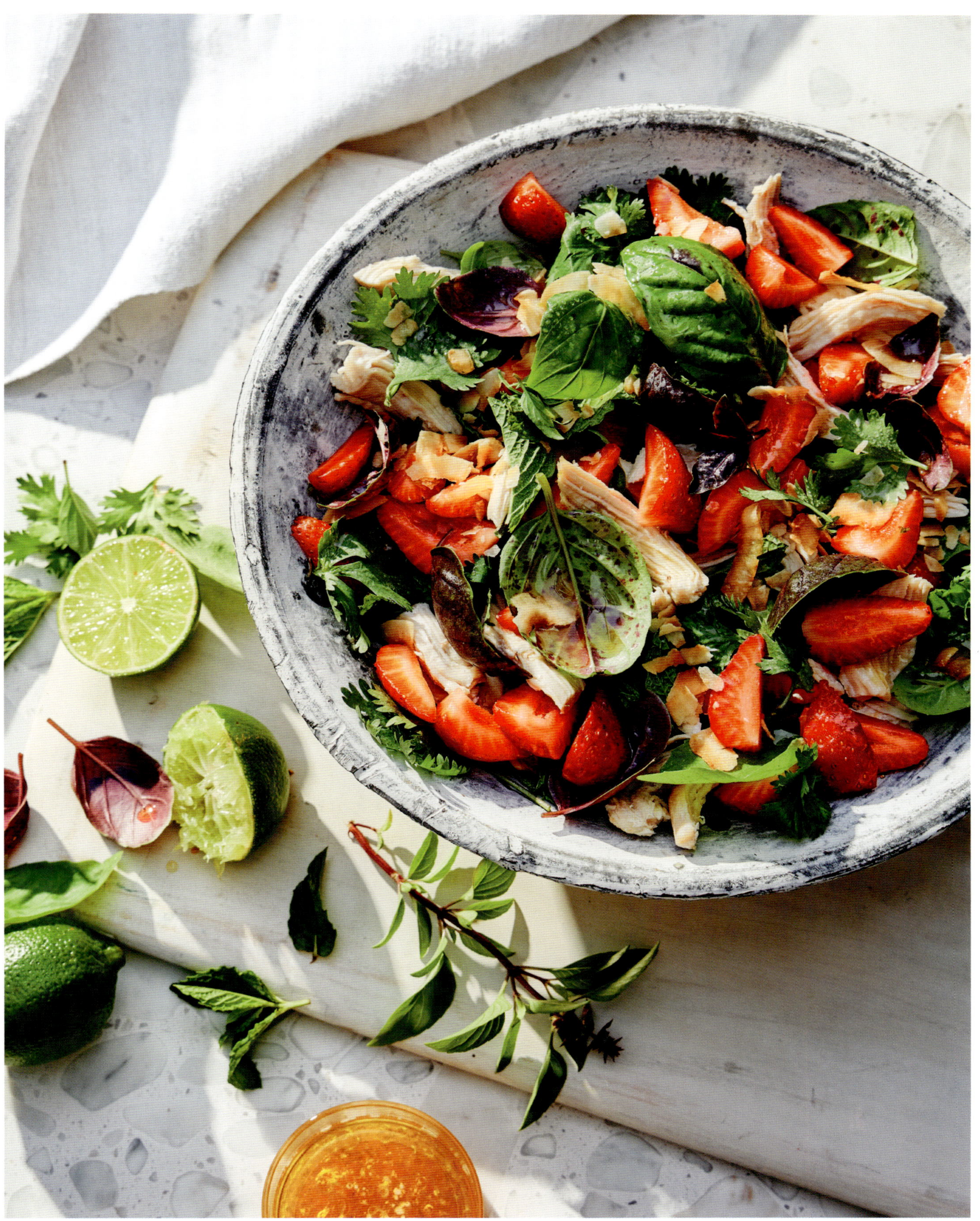

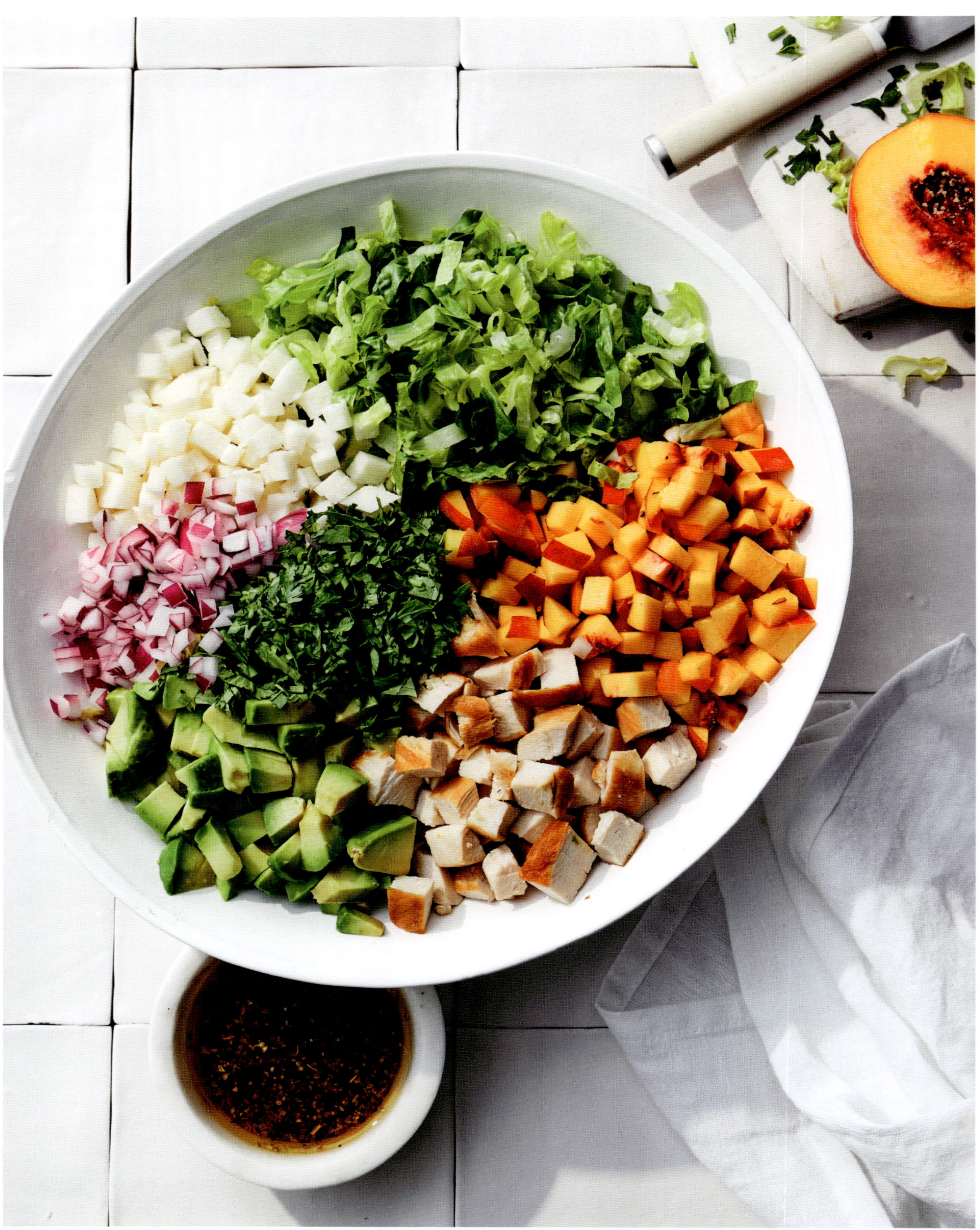

This salad was built from the jicama up. I wanted to work more of it into my diet because jicama, which is native to Mexico, is high in a prebiotic fiber called inulin that makes it good for digestion and has unique properties that can be good for glucose management. I love a chopped salad because you get all the flavors and textures in each bite! Jicama skin is toxic, so be sure to cut it all away.

The Baja Chop + Honey-Chipotle Dressing

SERVES 4

Dressing

1 garlic clove, grated

1/4 cup (50 g) extra-virgin olive oil

1/4 cup (85 g) honey

1/4 cup (55 g) apple cider vinegar

1/4 teaspoon chipotle powder (optional; see Note)

1/4 teaspoon dried oregano

1/8 teaspoon ground cumin

1 teaspoon pink salt

3 grinds of freshly cracked black pepper

Salad

1 lb (454 g) cooked chicken breast, diced

1–2 romaine hearts, depending on size, finely chopped

1 ripe avocado, diced

1/2 cup (70 g) finely diced red onion

1 cup (20 g) chopped cilantro leaves with tender stems

1 cup (150 g) finely diced jicama

1 peach, nectarine, or mango (whichever is in season), diced

Dressing Make the dressing a few hours in advance so the flavors can develop.

Whisk all dressing ingredients together in a small bowl and refrigerate until ready to use.

Salad Combine all salad ingredients in a large bowl and toss to combine. Add the dressing and toss until everything is well coated. Serve immediately.

NOTE

If you are avoiding nightshades, omit the chipotle powder.

Inspired by the popular Pasadena salad at Trader Joe's, my cleaned-up version is a staple worthy of your regular rotation. It's sweet and crunchy, and the scallions give it a subtle bite. Let rotisserie chicken do the heavy lifting, making this your go-to assembly-only salad for effortless weeknight meals.

Pasadena Chicken Salad + Sweet Sesame Dressing

SERVES 4

Dressing

¼ cup (60 g) unseasoned rice vinegar

2 tablespoons toasted sesame oil

2 tablespoons honey

2 tablespoons pure maple syrup

1 tablespoon freshly squeezed lemon juice

1 garlic clove, grated

½ teaspoon pink salt

½ teaspoon freshly cracked black pepper

Salad

1–2 romaine hearts, depending on size, thinly sliced

1 lb (454 g) cooked chicken breast, shredded

4 scallions, green and white parts, thinly sliced

⅔ cup (87 g) toasted slivered almonds

2 tablespoons black sesame seeds (divided)

1 ripe avocado, sliced (optional)

Dressing Whisk all dressing ingredients together in a small bowl. Refrigerate until ready to use. Making it a few hours in advance gives the flavors time to develop.

Salad In a large bowl, combine romaine, chicken, scallions, almonds, and 1 tablespoon of the black sesame seeds and toss to mix. Add the dressing and toss again until well coated.

Sprinkle with remaining tablespoon of sesame seeds and top with sliced avocado, if desired. Serve immediately.

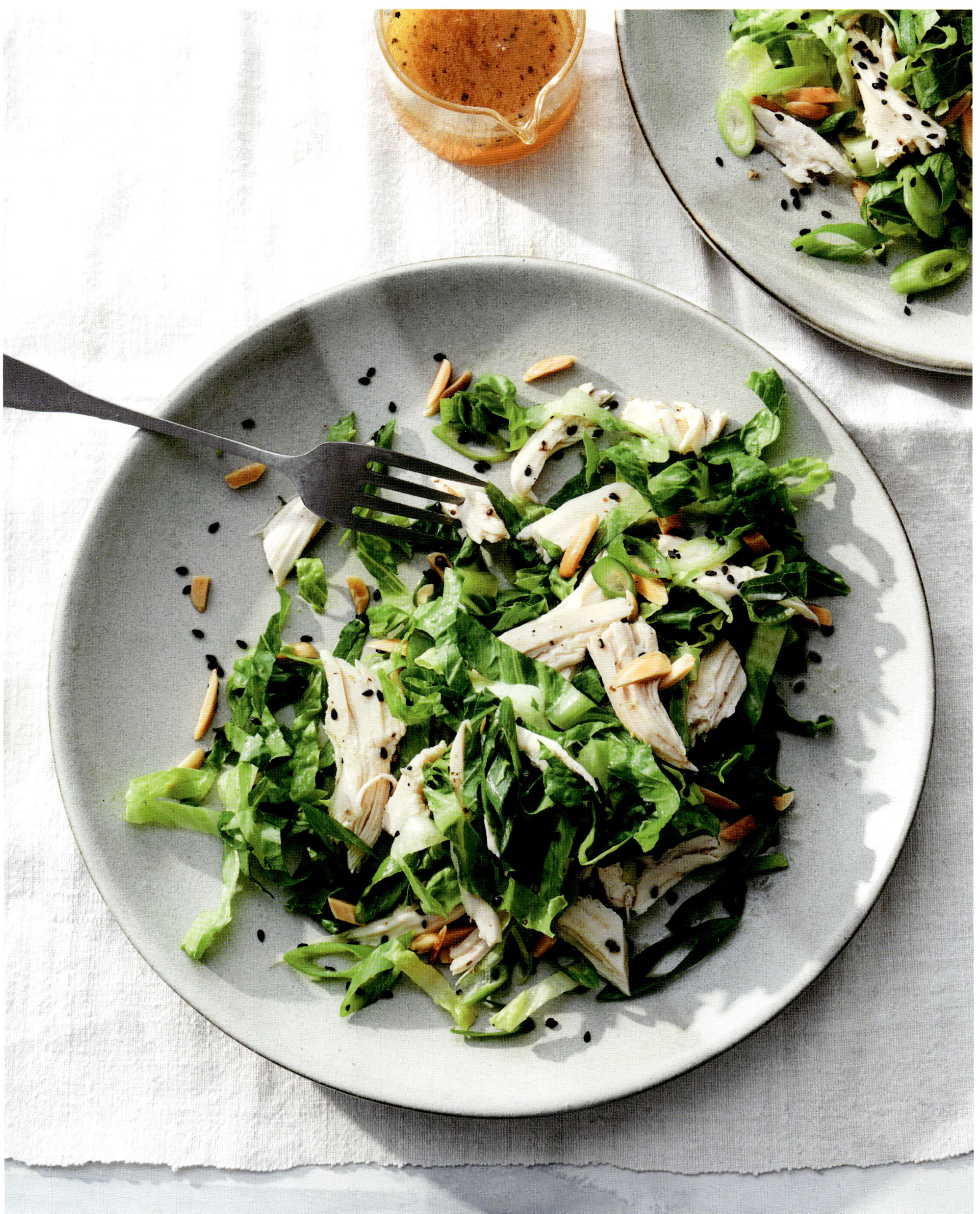

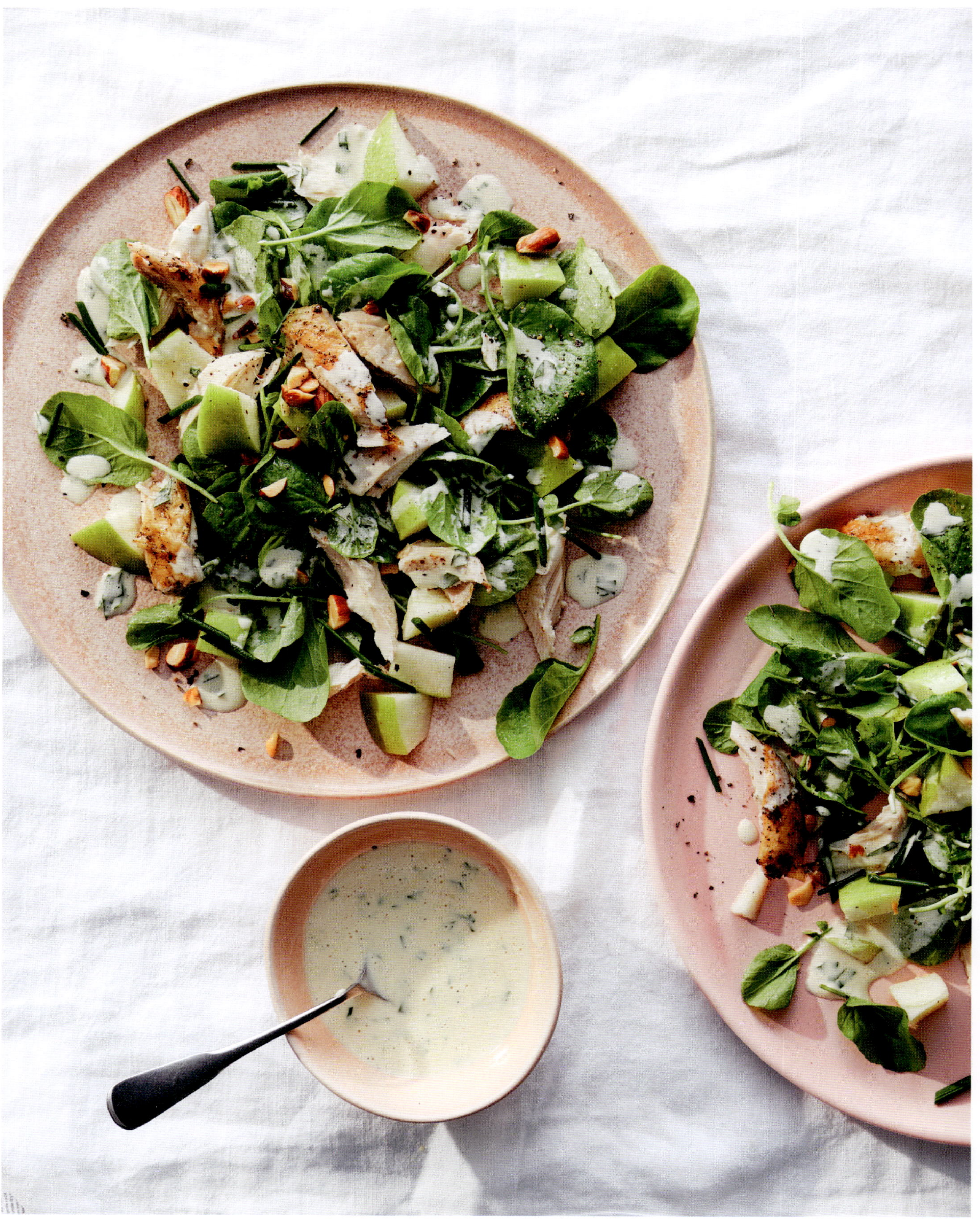

Watercress is considered the most nutrient-dense vegetable you can eat! It has a punchy flavor—the more mature a bunch of watercress, the more intense the flavor is likely to be. I go for a younger, milder, tenderer variety such as upland cress or hydro-cress, which is usually sold with the root ball still attached. Bagged baby watercress is available too.

Watercress with Roast Chicken, Tart Apples + Tarragon Dressing

SERVES 4

Dressing

- 2/3 cup (156 g) mayonnaise
- 1 tablespoon chopped tarragon
- 2 tablespoons Champagne vinegar
- 2 tablespoons Dijon mustard
- 1 tablespoon honey
- 1 large garlic clove, grated
- 1/4 teaspoon pink salt
- 1/2 teaspoon freshly cracked black pepper

Salad

- 4 servings of watercress, baby watercress, or upland cress
- 1 lb (454 g) cooked chicken breast, shredded
- 1/4 cup (10 g) chopped chives or thinly sliced scallions
- 1 Granny Smith apple, cored and chopped
- 1/3 cup (40 g) unsalted, dry-roasted almonds, roughly chopped
- Maldon flake salt, for sprinkling
- Freshly cracked black pepper, for sprinkling

Dressing Whisk all dressing ingredients together in a small bowl. Refrigerate until ready to use. Make a few hours or up to a day ahead, so the flavors can develop.

Salad Combine all salad ingredients, except flake salt and black pepper, in a large bowl. Dress it generously and toss to coat. Divide salad among 4 plates, then sprinkle with the salt and pepper.

This oh-so-lemony chicken and asparagus bowl comes together in minutes. It's quick, easy, and on heavy rotation at home—it meets my nightly nutritional goals of 4 ounces (114 g) of lean protein and lots of veg. Bonus: Shallots, packed with quercetin and richer in essential nutrients than onions, add a flavorful boost. I usually make two extra bowls to refrigerate and enjoy chilled the next day.

10-Minute Asparagus + Rotisserie Chicken Bowl

SERVES 2

- Zest and juice of 1 large, juicy lemon
- 1 small shallot, finely chopped
- Bunch of asparagus, trimmed
- ½ teaspoon pink salt
- 2 tablespoons mayonnaise
- 8 oz (227 g) rotisserie chicken breast, shredded
- Maldon flake salt, to taste

Divide lemon zest and juice (use a citrus reamer to get it all!) between 2 dinner bowls. To each bowl, add shallots and mix. Allow shallots to sit in the freshly squeezed lemon juice while prepping the other ingredients so it can soften their bite.

Position an oven rack 6 inches (15 cm) from the broil element. (In my oven that's the second notch from the top.) Preheat oven to broil. Line a baking sheet with parchment paper.

Arrange asparagus (dry) on a parchment paper–lined baking sheet in a single layer. Broil for 3–5 minutes, until tender and slightly charred.

Meanwhile, divide pink salt and mayonnaise between the bowls. Stir to combine. Chop the asparagus spears into fours. Add chicken and asparagus to bowls and mix well (the asparagus is not kept separate as pictured). Season to taste with flake salt if desired—I like lots! Serve either warm or chilled.

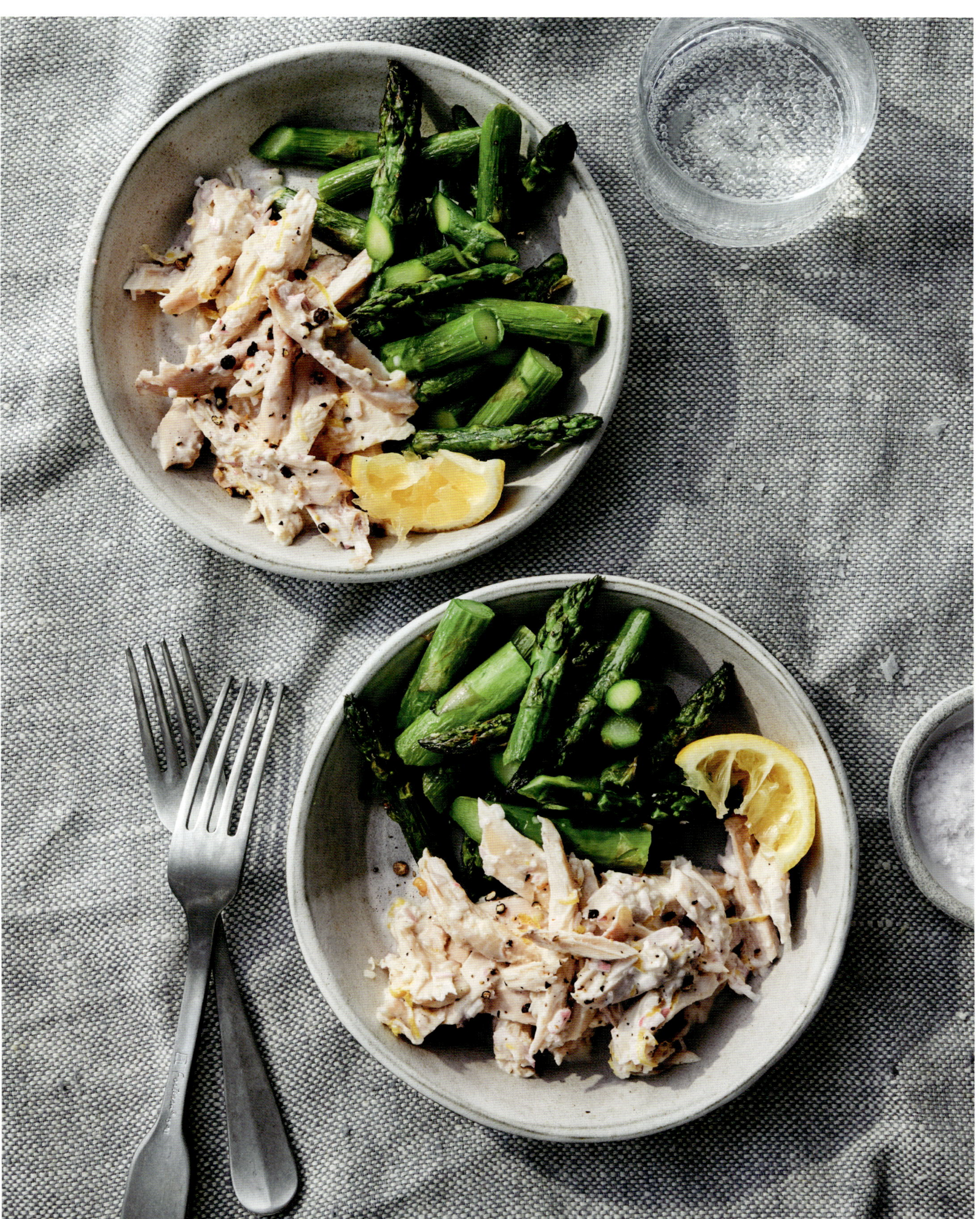

SWEETS

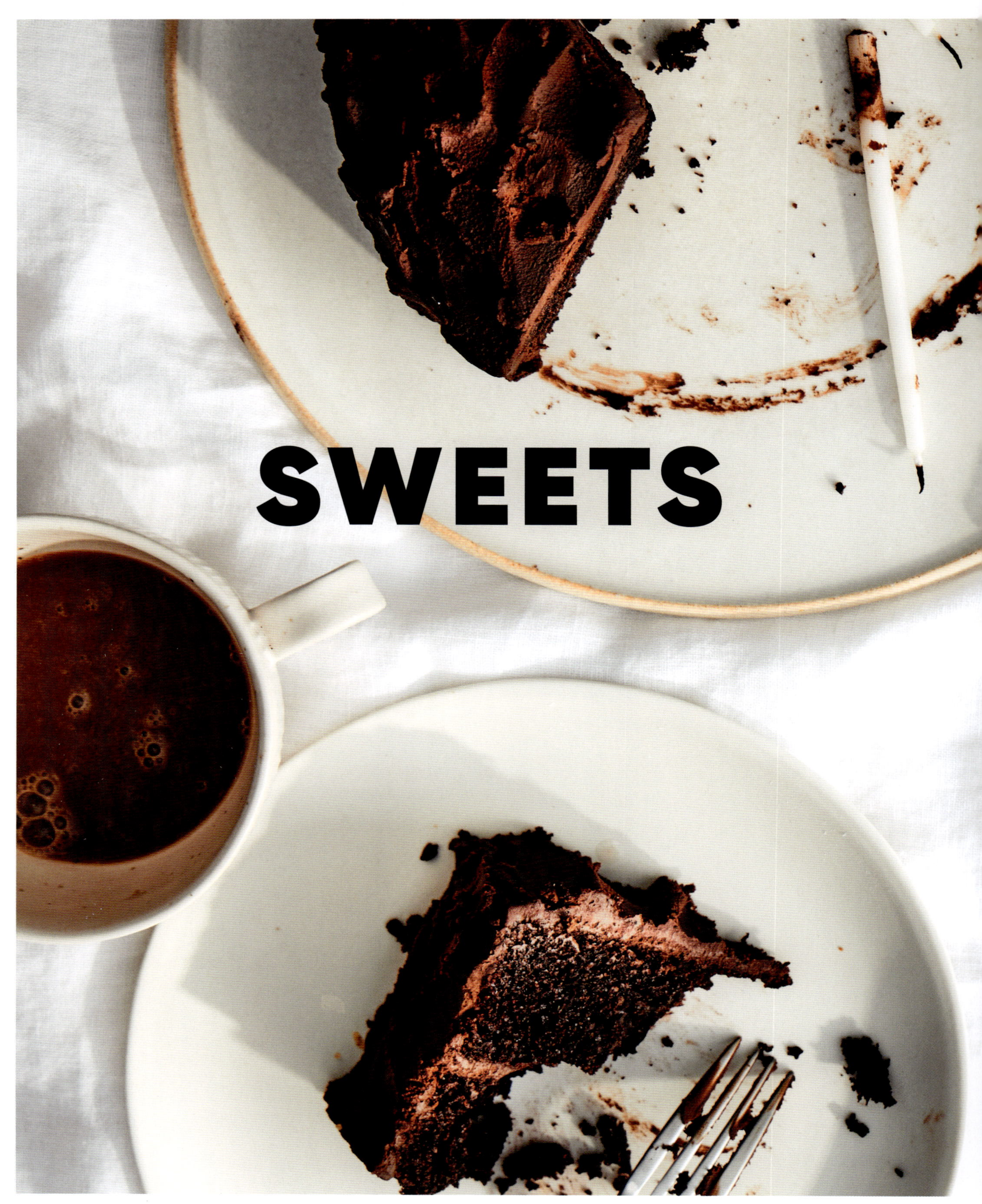

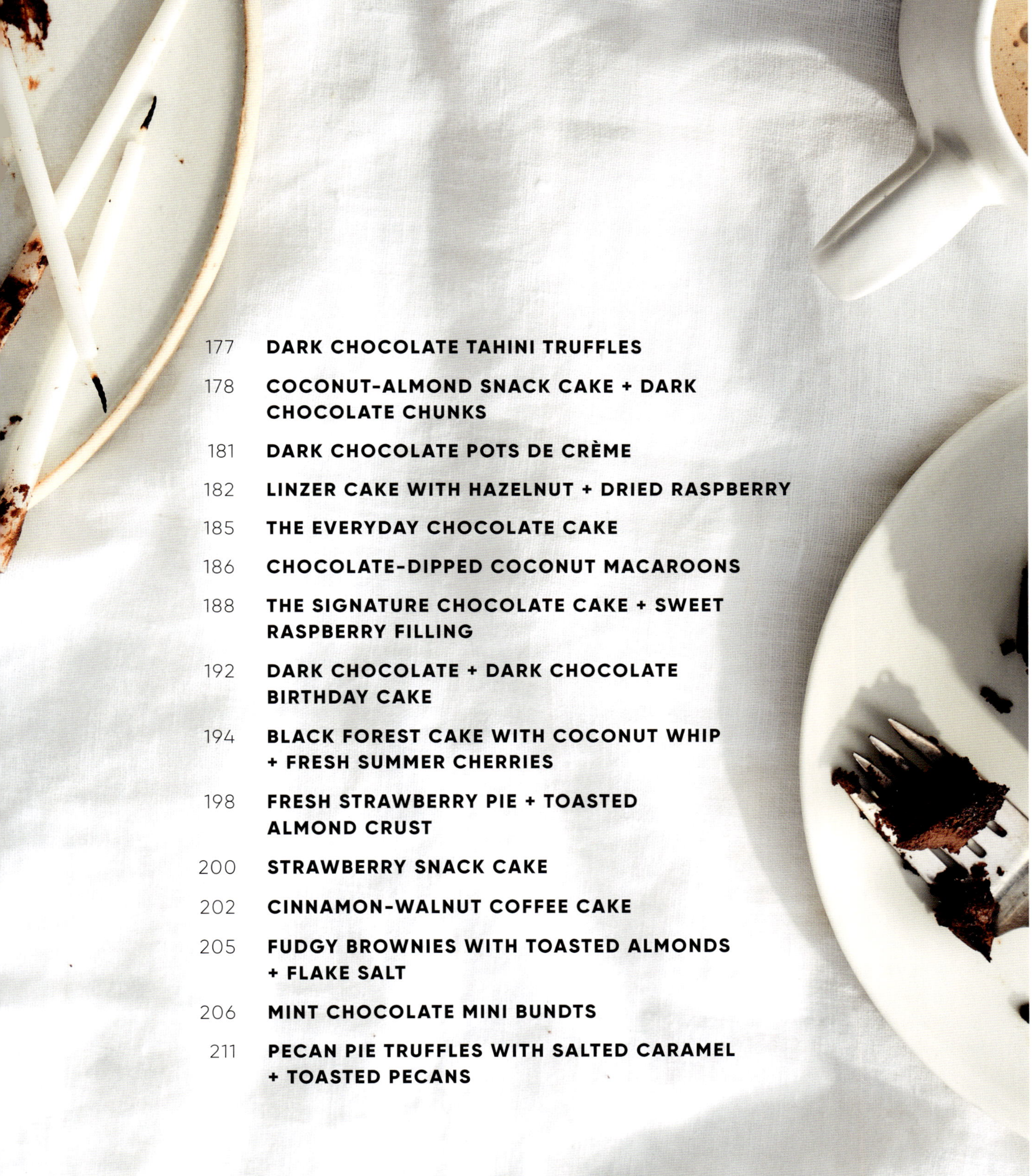

177 DARK CHOCOLATE TAHINI TRUFFLES

178 COCONUT-ALMOND SNACK CAKE + DARK CHOCOLATE CHUNKS

181 DARK CHOCOLATE POTS DE CRÈME

182 LINZER CAKE WITH HAZELNUT + DRIED RASPBERRY

185 THE EVERYDAY CHOCOLATE CAKE

186 CHOCOLATE-DIPPED COCONUT MACAROONS

188 THE SIGNATURE CHOCOLATE CAKE + SWEET RASPBERRY FILLING

192 DARK CHOCOLATE + DARK CHOCOLATE BIRTHDAY CAKE

194 BLACK FOREST CAKE WITH COCONUT WHIP + FRESH SUMMER CHERRIES

198 FRESH STRAWBERRY PIE + TOASTED ALMOND CRUST

200 STRAWBERRY SNACK CAKE

202 CINNAMON-WALNUT COFFEE CAKE

205 FUDGY BROWNIES WITH TOASTED ALMONDS + FLAKE SALT

206 MINT CHOCOLATE MINI BUNDTS

211 PECAN PIE TRUFFLES WITH SALTED CARAMEL + TOASTED PECANS

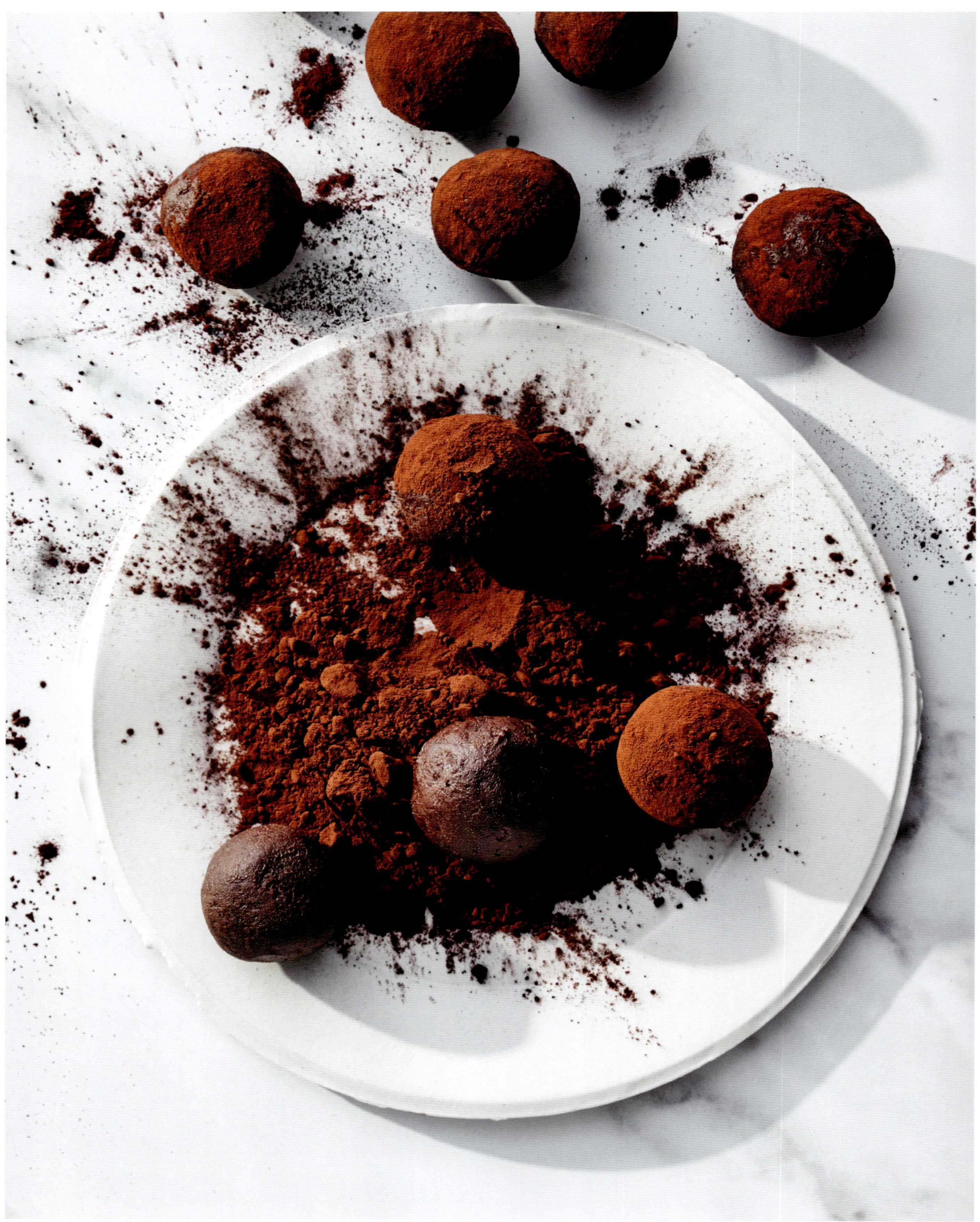

These simple but rich and voluptuous truffles elevate any occasion, and the everyday. Pile them high on a dessert table or share them as gifts. I like their toothy texture cold—straight from the fridge!

Dark Chocolate Tahini Truffles

MAKES 24 TRUFFLES

- 6 oz (170 g) 100% unsweetened chocolate, chopped (see Note)
- 3 tablespoons virgin coconut oil
- ¾ teaspoon pink salt
- 1 cup (240 g) well-stirred tahini (see Note)
- ⅔ cup (210 g) pure maple syrup
- 2 tablespoons Valrhona cocoa powder (divided; see Note)

Bring a small saucepan filled with an inch of water to a gentle simmer. Combine chocolate, coconut oil, and salt in a medium heatproof bowl, then set it over the saucepan. Whisk periodically until the chocolate has melted—don't let any water come in contact with the chocolate or it will seize.

Move the bowl to a work surface lined with a kitchen towel. Whisk in the tahini, maple syrup, and 1 tablespoon of cocoa powder until well incorporated. Cover and refrigerate mixture for at least 4 hours or overnight, until firm enough to scoop.

Line a small rimmed baking sheet with parchment paper. Use a medium (size 40) cookie scoop to portion mixture, and roll into balls. Place the balls on the prepared baking sheet and refrigerate, uncovered, for 1 hour, until very firm. Transfer the chilled balls to an airtight container. Add 1 tablespoon of cocoa powder to the container, close it, and give it a quick shake to coat all the truffles at once. Store in the fridge—they will hold up beautifully for weeks.

NOTES

Guittard 100% cacao unsweetened baking bars come in a 6-oz (170-g) box and work perfectly in this recipe.

For the best flavor, look for a tahini that's made with toasted sesame seeds rather than raw seeds.

Valrhona cocoa is my cocoa powder of choice for its rich flavor and deep, velvety hue.

Marzipan lovers, this one's for you! Nutrient-dense almond flour contains more protein than other gluten-free flours. It's also denser and therefore less forgiving, so I don't recommend any substitutions. Please see my notes on measuring and sourcing almond flour (pages 18 and 25) to ensure it turns out perfectly! This cake will hold in the fridge for up to a week—simply reheat each slice for 15 seconds in the microwave to return it to fresh-baked status.

Coconut-Almond Snack Cake + Dark Chocolate Chunks

SERVES 8

- 2½ cups (260 g) super-fine blanched almond flour
- ¾ cup (75 g) finely shredded unsweetened coconut
- 1 teaspoon baking powder
- ½ teaspoon baking soda
- ¾ teaspoon pink salt
- 4 large eggs, room temperature (see Note)
- 2 tablespoons melted coconut oil, plus extra for greasing
- ⅔ cup (210 g) pure maple syrup
- 1½ teaspoons almond extract
- 5 oz (142 g) coarsely chopped dark chocolate (see Note)
- ½ cup (62 g) sliced almonds, for the topping

Preheat oven to 350°F. Grease a 9-inch (23-cm) nonstick springform pan and line the bottom with a parchment paper round.

In a medium mixing bowl, whisk together almond flour, coconut, baking powder, baking soda, and salt, breaking up any lumps. Add the eggs, coconut oil, maple syrup, and almond extract and whisk until the ingredients are well combined and the batter is smooth.

When you get to the chocolate, swap your whisk for a rubber spatula and fold the chocolate into the batter until it's evenly distributed. Pour the batter into the springform pan and spread it toward the edges. Tap the pan on the counter to level the batter. Sprinkle the sliced almonds evenly over the top, with the goal of covering all the batter.

Bake on the center rack for 30 minutes. Cool before transferring to a serving plate.

Variation: Coconut-Almond Muffins Prepare a muffin tin with 12 paper liners. Make the batter as directed. Use a spoon to divide the batter among the 12 muffin cups. (Cups will be full because almond flour doesn't rise as much as all-purpose flour.) Sprinkle the tops with the sliced almonds, covering as much of the batter as possible. Bake on the center rack for 23 minutes.

NOTES

Use room temperature eggs, as cold eggs may cause the coconut oil to solidify.

You may be tempted to use chocolate chips instead of chopped dark chocolate, but they won't produce the same luxurious puddles of melted chocolate.

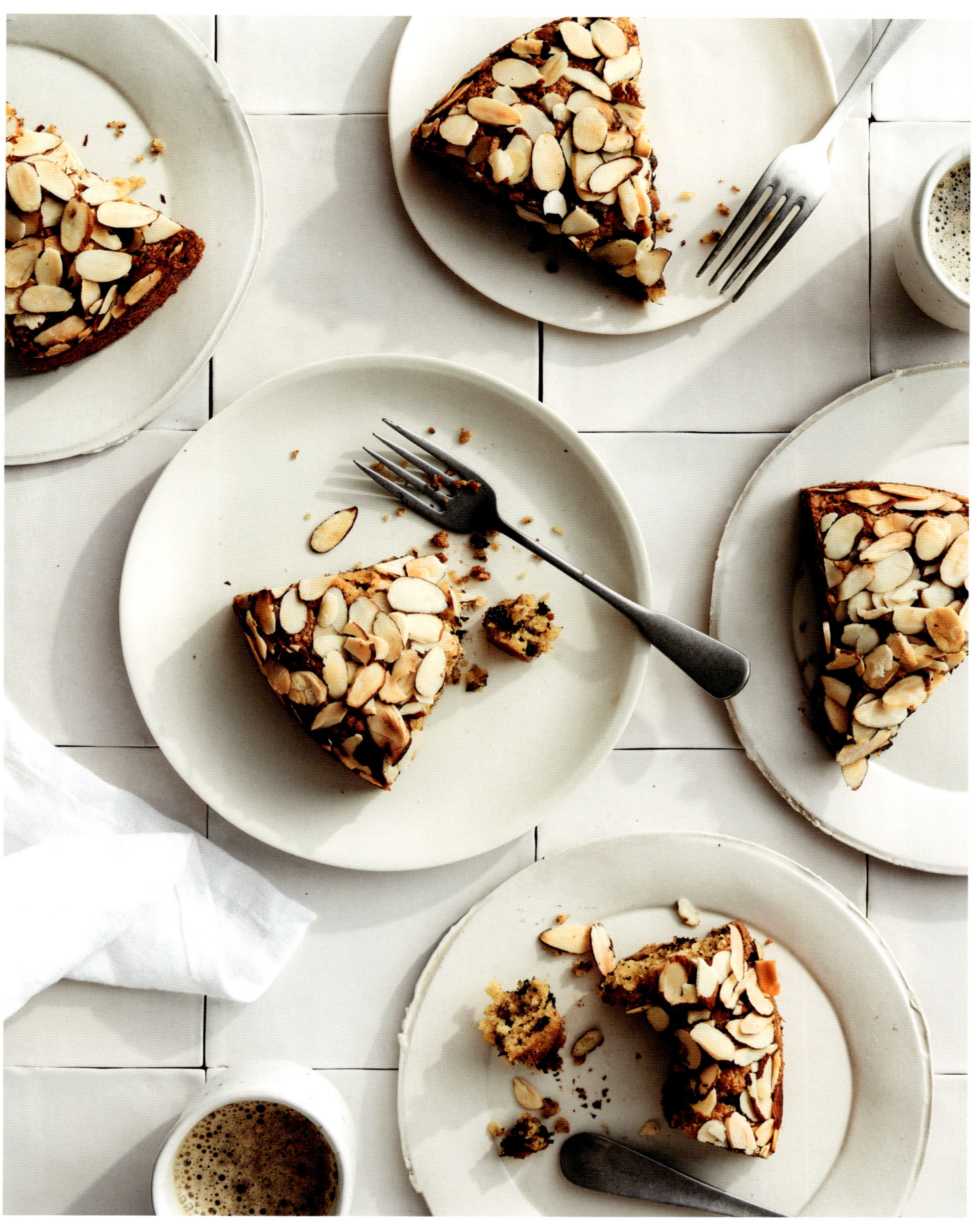

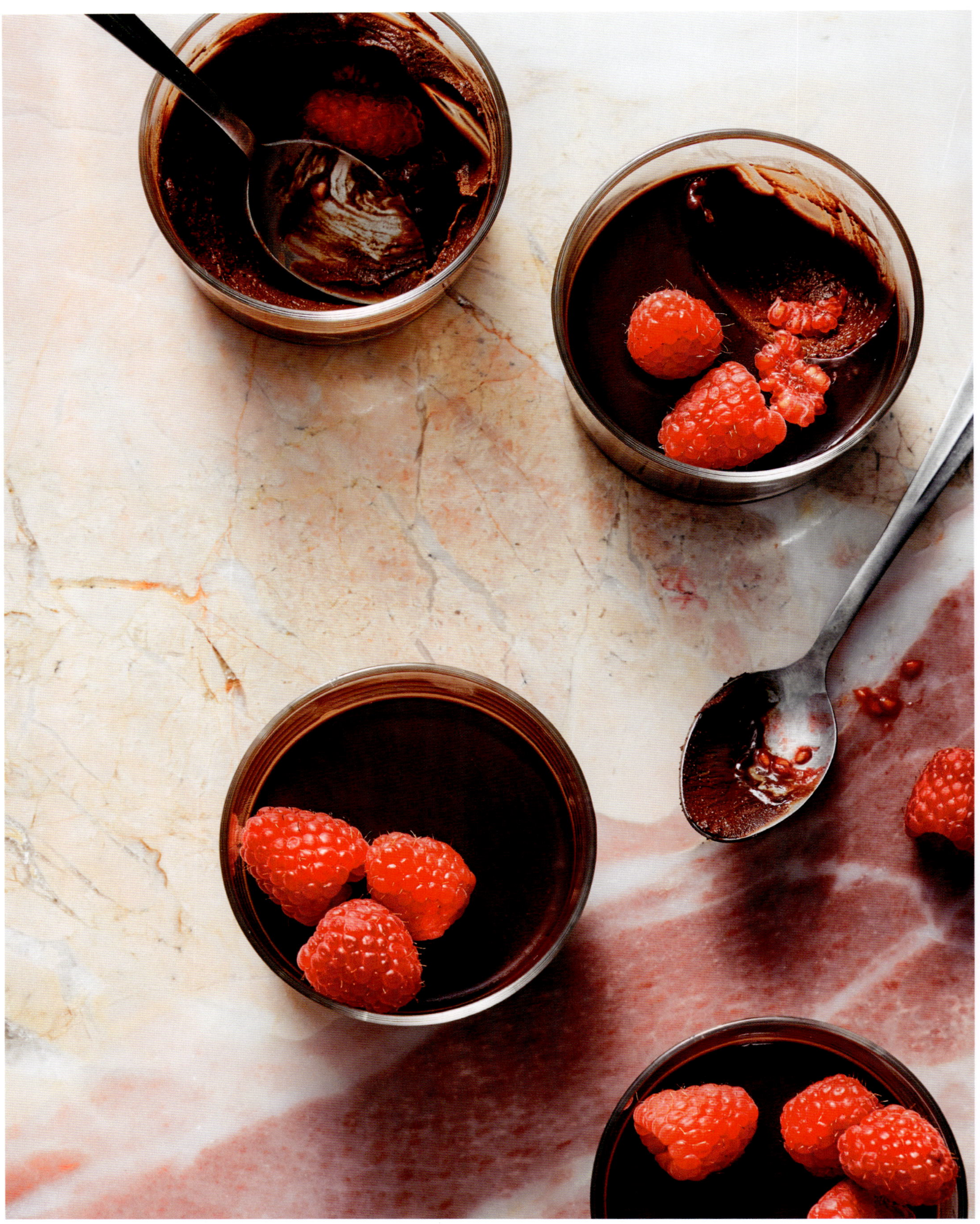

Chocolate and raspberry are a classic coupling! These irresistible pots of creamy dark chocolate are ridiculously easy to make and the perfect way to punctuate a meal. I go off script a bit here by using regular sugar-sweetened chocolate—but I wanted to include it because it was the very first recipe I developed after changing my diet.

Dark Chocolate Pots de Crème

SERVES 6

- 1 (13.5-oz/400-ml) can full-fat, additive-free coconut milk
- 2 tablespoons pure maple syrup
- 1 teaspoon pure vanilla extract
- ¼ teaspoon pink salt
- 10 oz (284 g) dark chocolate, chopped (see Note)
- 6 oz (170 g) raspberries

Place 6 small ramekins or vessels of your choice on a small rimmed baking sheet for easy transfer to the fridge.

In a small saucepan, combine coconut milk, maple syrup, vanilla, and salt. Bring just to a simmer over medium-low heat. Do not allow it to boil. Remove from the heat, add the chocolate, and set it aside for 3 minutes. Whisk gently for about 3 minutes, until chocolate is melted, smooth, glossy, and slightly thickened. Using a rubber spatula, incorporate any chocolate from the bottom of the pan.

For ease of pouring, transfer the mixture to a glass measuring cup with a pour spout. Pour it into the ramekins, leaving enough space at the top for raspberries.

Set aside at room temperature, uncovered, for 1 hour.

Cover with plastic wrap and refrigerate for 3 hours, until fully set.

To serve, top each one with raspberries.

NOTE

I use either Guittard 74% organic bittersweet chocolate baking wafers or, for a more economical option, Trader Joe's Pound Plus dark chocolate bar, which is made by Callebaut. If you're using the Pound Plus bar and don't have a kitchen scale, you'll need 23 squares.

You'll love the sweet-tart quality of the dried raspberries and the subtle complexity the hazelnut flour brings to the mix. This fuss-free cake comes together quickly and holds up for a week in the fridge!

Linzer Cake with Hazelnut + Dried Raspberry

SERVES 6–8

- Virgin coconut oil, for greasing
- 2¼ cups (240 g) super-fine blanched almond flour
- ½ cup (45 g) finely ground hazelnut flour (see Note)
- 2 teaspoons baking powder (see Note)
- ¾ teaspoon pink salt
- ¾ cup (235 g) pure maple syrup
- 3 large eggs, room temperature
- 1 teaspoon vanilla extract
- ½ teaspoon almond extract
- 1 (1.2-oz/34-g) bag freeze-dried raspberries (see Note)

Preheat oven to 350°F. Thoroughly grease a 9-inch (23-cm) nonstick springform pan with coconut oil and line the bottom with parchment paper.

In a medium mixing bowl, whisk the almond flour, hazelnut flour, baking powder, and salt, breaking up any lumps. Add the remaining ingredients, except dried raspberries, and whisk until smooth and well combined. Using a rubber spatula, gently fold in dried raspberries until evenly distributed.

Pour into the prepared springform pan and use the spatula to smooth the top. Bake for 25 minutes on the center rack. Allow it to cool for 20 minutes before transferring to a serving plate.

NOTES

Hazelnut flour has a short shelf life; storing it in the fridge will help extend its freshness.

Be sure to use baking powder (not baking soda) for this recipe, as baking soda seems to react poorly with the dried raspberries.

Inexplicably, Natierra brand raspberries don't work in this cake—this was confirmed by my recipe testers. Trader Joe's freeze-dried raspberries are inexpensive and my favorite—several other brands can be found online.

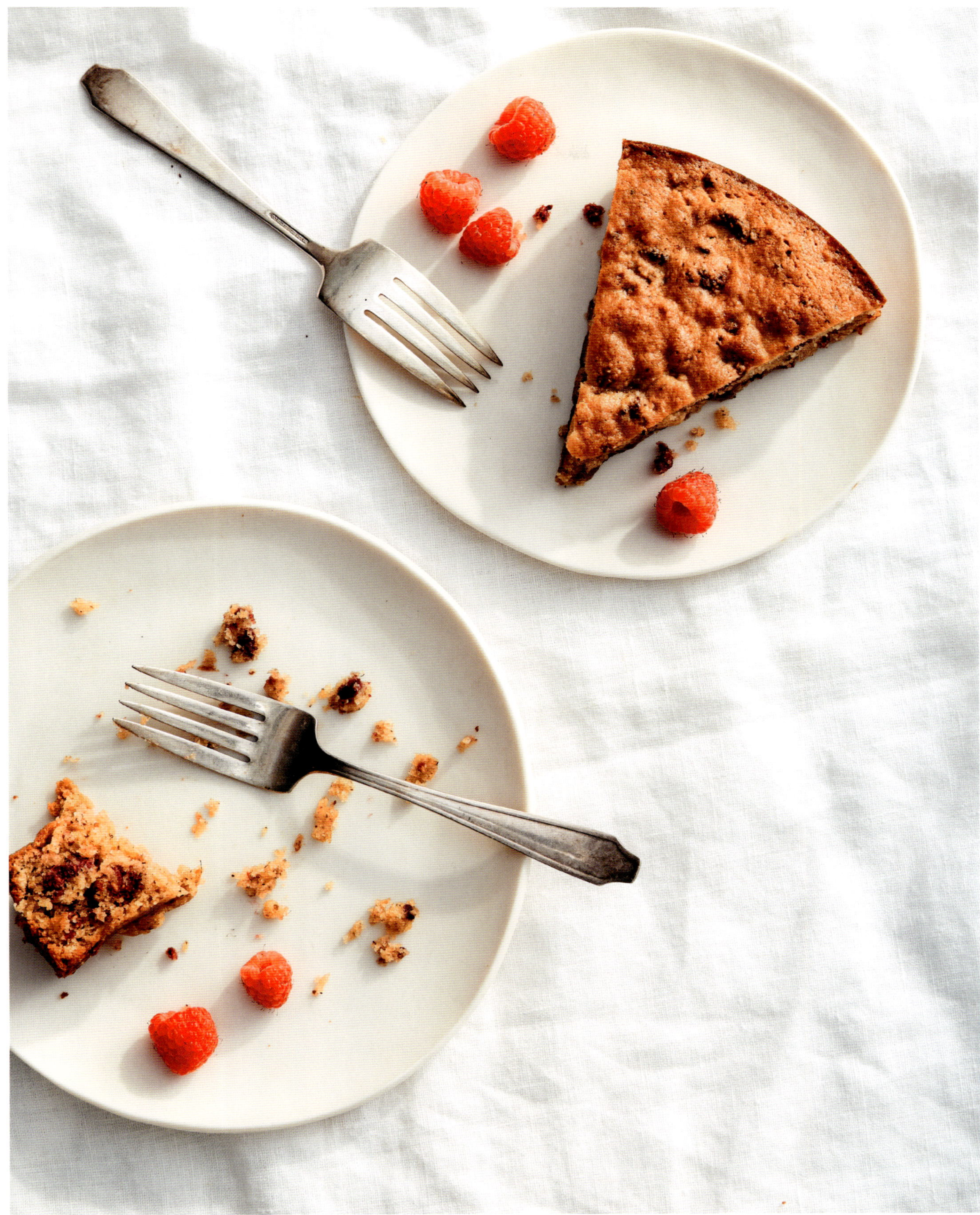

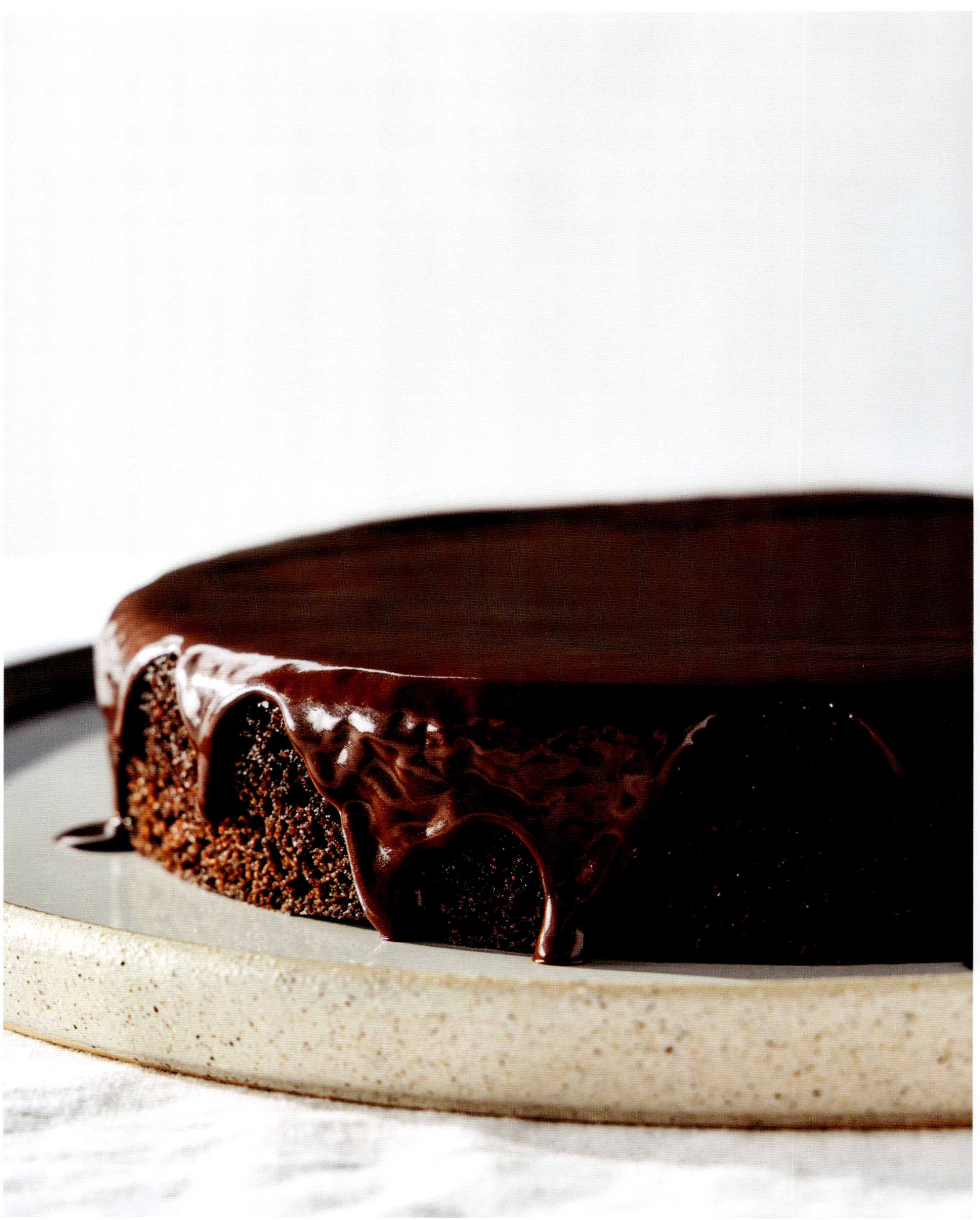

Sweet satisfaction on the daily! This fuss-free cake contains 15 grams of protein per serving, takes a mere ten minutes to get into the oven, and holds up beautifully in the fridge for a whole week. Have a slice for lunch—who's to stop you?

The Everyday Chocolate Cake

SERVES 6

Cake

Virgin coconut oil, for greasing

2½ cups (260 g) super-fine blanched almond flour

¼ cup (30 g) Valrhona cocoa powder

1 teaspoon baking soda

¾ teaspoon pink salt

¾ cup (235 g) pure maple syrup

3 large eggs, room temperature

Ganache

¼ cup (60 g) canned full-fat, additive-free coconut milk (see Note)

2 oz (57 g) 100% unsweetened chocolate (see Note)

2 tablespoons pure maple syrup

⅛ teaspoon pink salt

NOTE

This recipe was developed using Guittard's 100% cacao baking bars and Trader Joe's canned full-fat, additive-free coconut milk. Using coconut milk that contains additives or thickening agents is not advised. Look for a baking bar that contains only cacao beans.

Cake Preheat oven to 350°F. Thoroughly grease a 9-inch (23-cm) nonstick springform pan with coconut oil and line the bottom with parchment paper.

In a medium mixing bowl, whisk together almond flour, cocoa, baking soda, and salt, breaking up any lumps. Add the remaining ingredients and whisk until smooth and well combined. Pour the batter into the springform pan. Using a rubber spatula, spread it toward the edges and tap the pan on the counter to level the batter.

Bake for 25 minutes on the center rack. Cool for 20 minutes, then transfer it onto a serving plate.

Ganache Allow the cake to cool completely before making the ganache.

Combine all ganache ingredients in a small glass or porcelain bowl and microwave for 30 seconds. Using a small whisk, whisk gently for 2–3 minutes, until the chocolate is melted, smooth, glossy, and slightly thickened, but still pourable.

Pour the chocolate ganache onto the top (center) of the cake. Using an offset spatula or the back of a spoon, carefully spread it over the cake, nudging it gently over the edge and allowing it to drip down the sides as much as you like. Tapping the plate on the counter will help the ganache flow down the sides.

Refrigerate, uncovered, for 30 minutes so the ganache can set.

Cover and store at room temperature for up to 3 days, or in the fridge for up to a week.

It's nice to have classics like these macaroons as part of your gluten-, grain-, and dairy-free repertoire. Plus, any excuse to use almond extract! The longer you bake them, the chewier they become, so personal preference comes into play. I like them to be plenty chewy before I give them a dunk in deep, velvety dark chocolate. This was adapted from Laurel and Claire of Sweet Laurel Bakery's macaroon recipe. They have a beautiful grain-free bake shop in Los Angeles!

Chocolate-Dipped Coconut Macaroons

MAKES 24 COOKIES

- 4 large egg whites
- 3⁄4 cup (235 g) pure maple syrup
- 3⁄4 teaspoon pink salt
- 1 teaspoon vanilla extract
- 1 teaspoon pure almond extract
- 1½ cups (165 g) super-fine blanched almond flour
- 3 cups (300 g) finely shredded unsweetened coconut
- 4 oz (114 g) dark chocolate, chopped, for dipping

Preheat oven to 350°F. Line a rimmed baking sheet with parchment paper.

Whisk egg whites in a medium bowl until frothy. Add the remaining ingredients, except chocolate, and mix with a spoon until combined.

Using a medium (size 40) cookie scoop, scoop the dough, scraping it across the lip of the bowl to pack it down. Release each ball onto the prepared baking sheet.

Bake for 16–20 minutes on the center rack, until macaroons reach your desired color and chewiness. Keep a watchful eye, as oven temperatures vary. Cool completely.

Assembly Place chocolate in a small microwave-safe bowl that's slightly larger in diameter than your macaroons. Microwave in 15-second intervals until the chocolate has melted, stirring each time. Be careful not to overheat!

Line the baking sheet with a fresh piece of parchment paper. Dip the macaroons in the melted chocolate. Give each one a little shake before you place it on the baking sheet so the excess chocolate can drip off and you avoid creating a "foot." Cool at room temperature until the chocolate has set.

Macaroons can be covered and stored at room temperature for up to 4 days, but note that the texture is best the day they're baked.

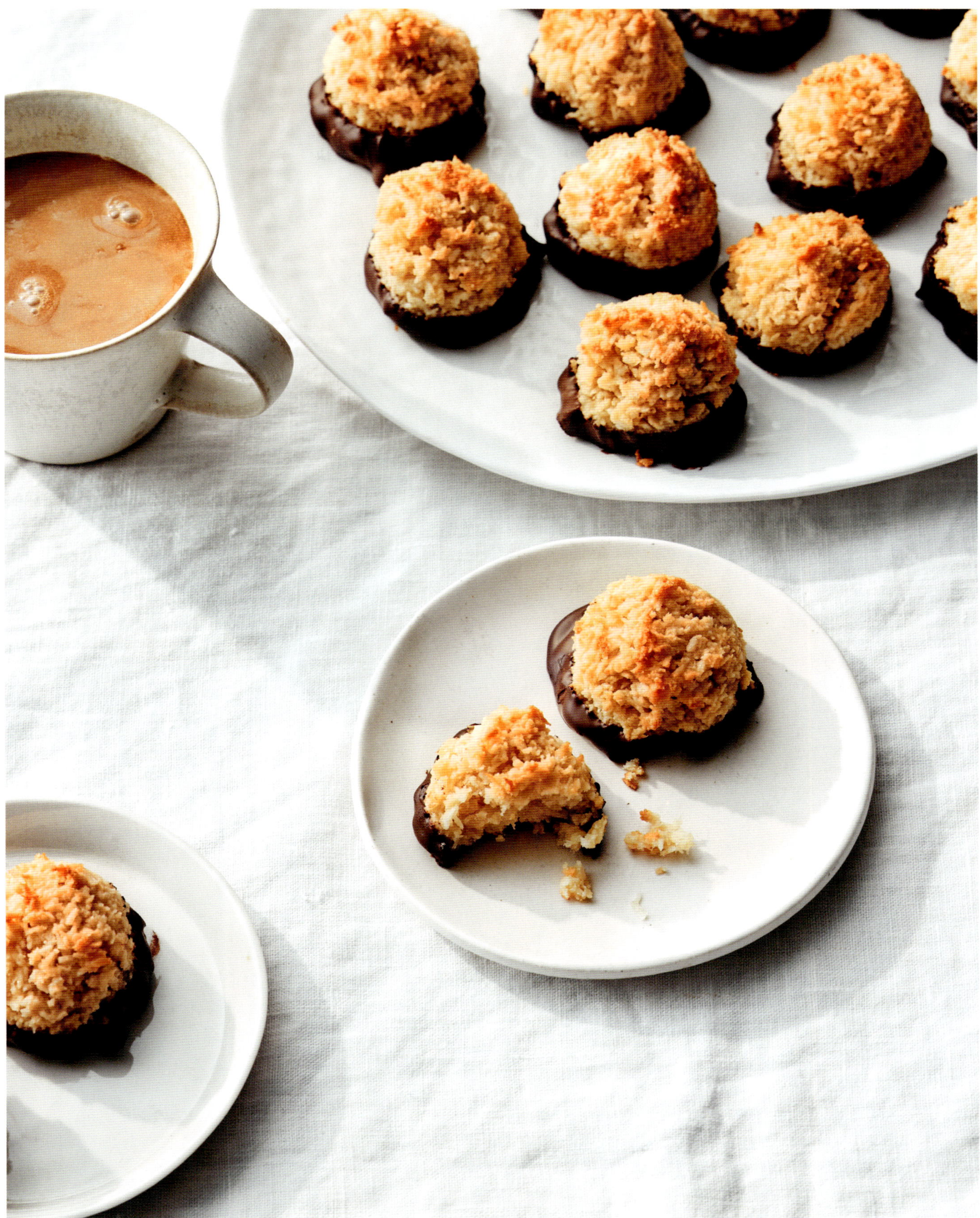

I consider this my signature cake because my friends always ask for it, and it will easily win over any skeptics who don't usually adhere to a gluten-, dairy-, or sugar-free diet. It takes a quick ten minutes to get into the oven, relies on store-bought, fruit-sweetened raspberry jam as the filling, and is finished with a simple dark chocolate ganache that gets drizzled over the top. You will need two 6-inch (15-cm) round cake pans.

The Signature Chocolate Cake + Sweet Raspberry Filling

SERVES 6

Cake

- Virgin coconut oil, for greasing
- 2½ cups (260 g) super-fine blanched almond flour
- ¼ cup (30 g) Valrhona cocoa powder
- 1 teaspoon baking soda
- ¾ teaspoon pink salt
- ¾ cup (235 g) pure maple syrup
- 3 large eggs, room temperature

Cake Preheat oven to 350°F. Thoroughly grease two 6-inch (15-cm) round cake pans with coconut oil and line the bottoms with parchment paper.

In a medium mixing bowl, whisk together almond flour, cocoa, baking soda, and salt until combined, breaking up any lumps. Add the maple syrup and eggs and whisk until smooth and combined.

Divide the batter between the cake pans, using a kitchen scale for accuracy (if you have one). Using a rubber spatula, scrape the batter from the bowl and smooth the top of each cake. Tap each pan on the counter to level the batter. Bake for 25 minutes on the center rack.

Cool cakes in the pans for 20 minutes. Invert the cakes, flat side up, onto a cooling rack and set aside for 1 hour so the excess moisture can evaporate. This ensures the filling will adhere to the cake.

Filling

1/3 cup (100 g) store-bought, fruit-only raspberry jam, such as St. Dalfour Red Raspberry Fruit Spread

Ganache

1/4 cup (60 g) canned full-fat, additive-free coconut milk (see Note)

2 oz (57 g) 100% unsweetened chocolate, chopped (see Note)

2 tablespoons pure maple syrup

1/8 teaspoon pink salt

Filling Arrange a cake layer, flat side up, on a serving plate. Spread raspberry jam over the surface, stopping about ½ inch (12 mm) from the edge of the cake. Top with a second cake layer, domed side up, and press down lightly.

Ganache Combine all ganache ingredients in small glass or porcelain bowl and microwave for 30 seconds. Using a small whisk, whisk gently for 2-3 minutes, until the chocolate is melted, smooth, glossy, and slightly thickened, but still pourable.

Pour the chocolate ganache onto the top (center) of the cake. Using an offset spatula or the back of a spoon, carefully spread it over the cake, nudging it gently over the edge and allowing it to drip down the sides as much as you like. Tapping the plate on the counter will help the ganache flow down the sides.

Refrigerate, uncovered, for 30 minutes so the ganache can set.

Cover and store at room temperature for up to 3 days, or in the fridge for up to a week.

NOTE

This recipe was developed using Guittard's 100% cacao baking bars and Trader Joe's canned full-fat, additive-free coconut milk. Using coconut milk that contains additives or thickening agents is not advised. Look for a baking bar that contains only cacao beans.

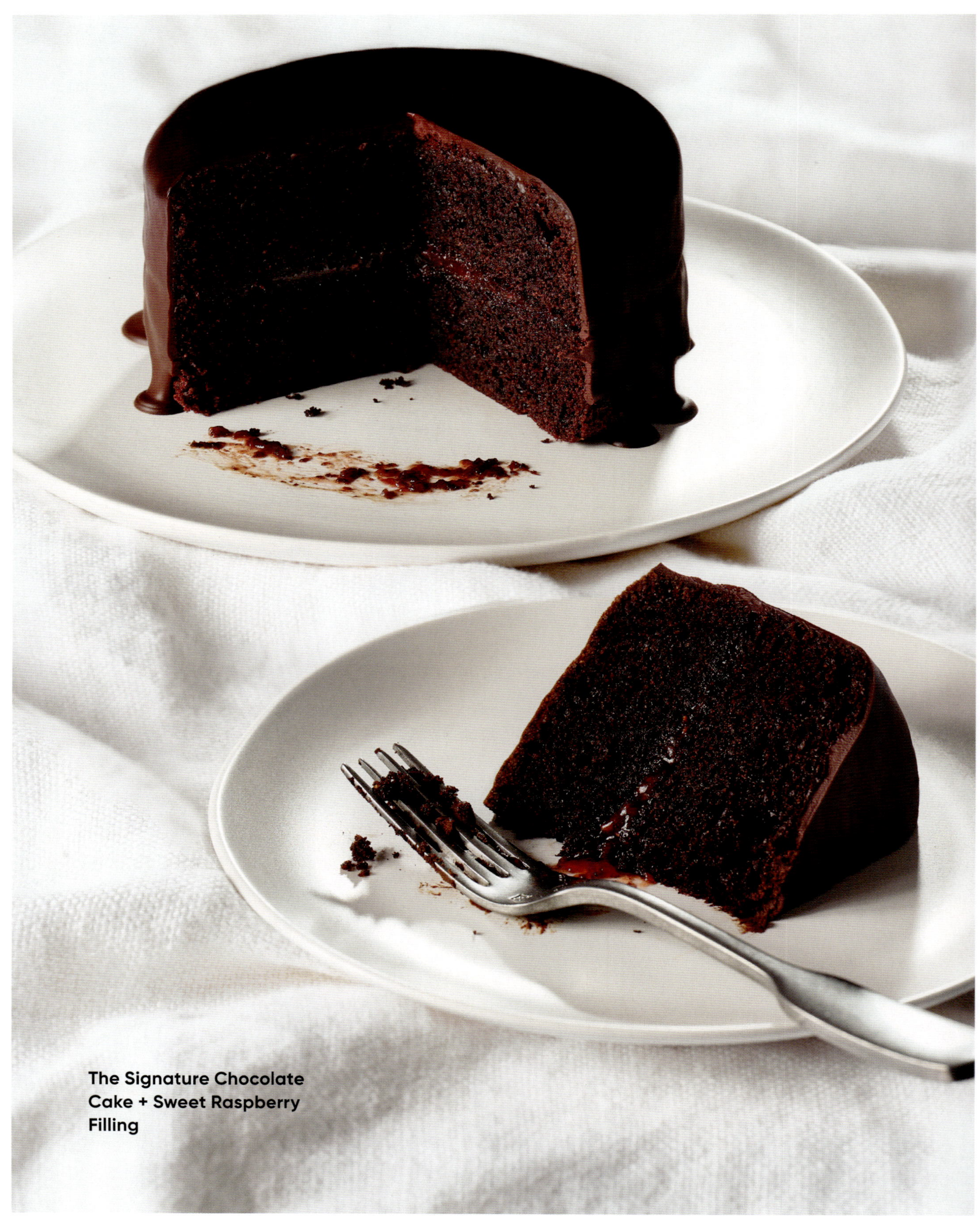

The Signature Chocolate Cake + Sweet Raspberry Filling

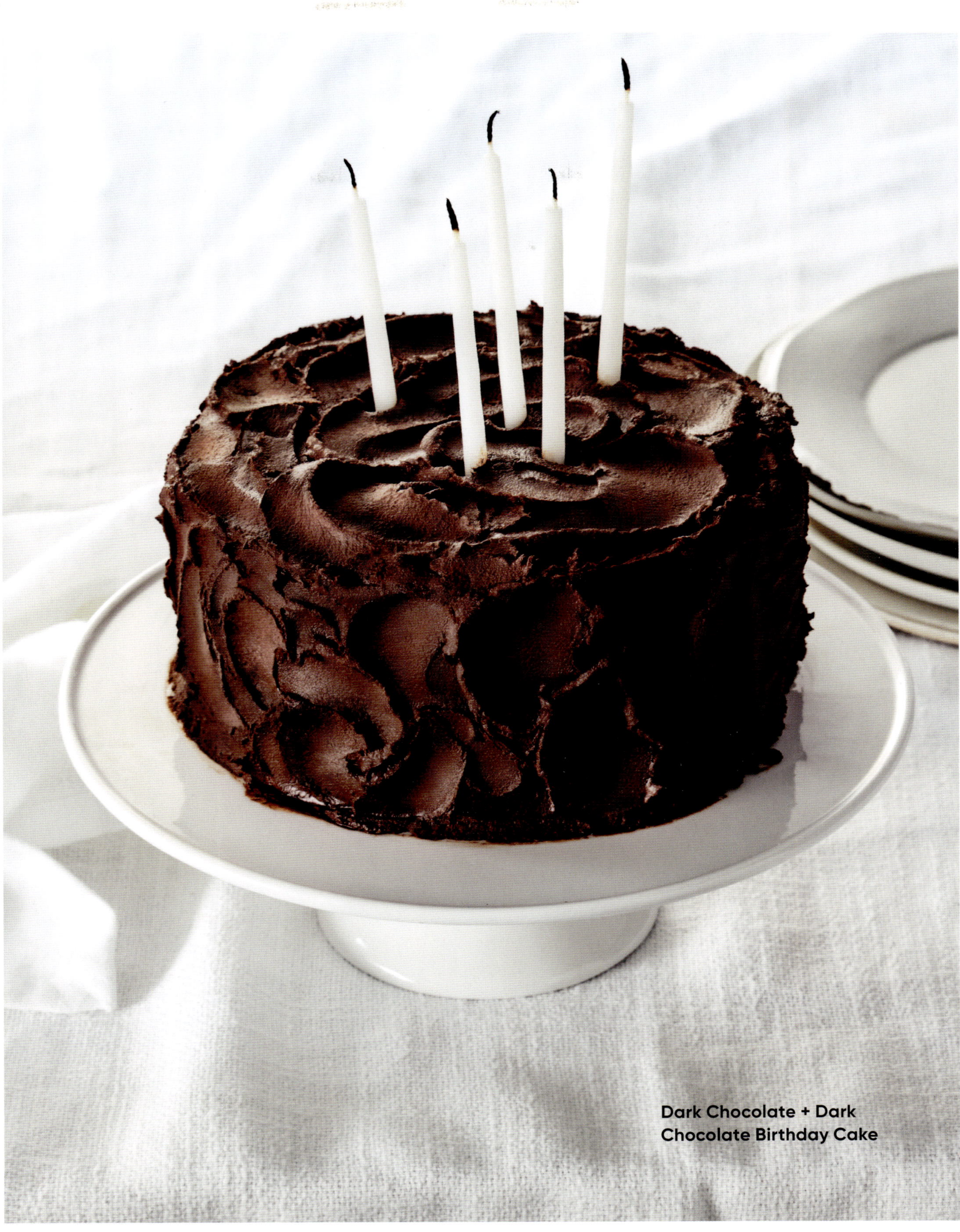

Dark Chocolate + Dark Chocolate Birthday Cake

Yes, you can have your cake and eat it too. I wanted to create a layer cake like the ones I grew up with, so birthdays could be celebrated in a way that felt traditional. Here, The Everyday Chocolate Cake (page 185) is reimagined and made more decadent by making it a layer cake and slathering it in a creamy, thick, and luxurious spreadable ganache. Happy Birthday, or any day that ends in Y! You will need two 6-inch (15-cm) round cake pans for this cake.

Dark Chocolate + Dark Chocolate Birthday Cake

SERVES 8

Cake

- Virgin coconut oil, for greasing
- 2½ cups (260 g) super-fine blanched almond flour
- ¼ cup (30 g) Valrhona cocoa powder
- 1 teaspoon baking soda
- ¾ teaspoon pink salt
- ¾ cup (235 g) pure maple syrup
- 3 large eggs, room temperature

Ganache

- 6 oz (170 g) 100% unsweetened chocolate (see Note)
- ⅓ cup (70 g) virgin coconut oil
- ¼ teaspoon pink salt
- ⅔ cup (160 g) canned full-fat, additive-free coconut milk (see Note)
- ½ cup (157 g) pure maple syrup

Cake Preheat oven to 350°F. Prepare two 6-inch (15-cm) round cake pans by greasing them with coconut oil and lining the bottoms with parchment paper.

In a medium mixing bowl, whisk together almond flour, cocoa, baking soda, and salt until combined, breaking up any lumps. Add the maple syrup and eggs and whisk until smooth and combined.

Divide the batter between the cake pans, using a kitchen scale for accuracy (if you have one). Using a rubber spatula, scrape the batter from the bowl and smooth the top of each cake. Tap each pan on the counter to level the batter. Bake for 25 minutes on the center rack.

Cool cakes in the pans for 20 minutes. Invert the cakes, flat side up, onto a cooling rack and set aside for 1 hour so the excess moisture can evaporate. This ensures the ganache will adhere to the cake.

Ganache Chop the chocolate for easier melting. Bring a small saucepan filled with an inch of water to a gentle simmer. Combine chocolate, coconut oil, and salt in a medium heat-proof bowl, then set it over the saucepan. Whisk periodically until the chocolate has melted—don't let any water come in contact with the chocolate or it will seize.

Move the bowl to a work surface lined with a kitchen towel. Whisk in the coconut milk and maple syrup until smooth, glossy, and slightly thickened—about 2 minutes. Set ganache aside at room temperature for 1½ hours, until set. It will go from the consistency of a pudding to a thick frosting very quickly. Resist the temptation to refrigerate the ganache because it will become stiff and grainy.

Assembly Place the first cake layer on a serving plate, flat side up. Using an offset spatula or tool of choice, spread the first layer with ganache. Top it with the second layer, dome side up, and press down lightly.

Spread the remaining ganache over the top and sides of the cake. Set cake aside to rest at room temperature for 1 hour so the ganache can continue to firm up. Slice, then serve.

Cover leftover cake and store at room temperature for up to 4 days.

NOTE

This recipe was developed using Guittard's 100% cacao baking bars and Trader Joe's organic coconut milk (full fat, not reduced fat). Be sure to use 100% chocolate, which contains only cacao beans and nothing else, and canned coconut milk that is additive-free.

I didn't want this cake to be limited to the seasonality of cherries, so I set out to find a suitable alternative using frozen cherries. I tried roasting them and simmering them into compote, but they just didn't hold a candle to their fresher form. So I suppose, like so many other summer things, the fleeting nature of cherries is part of their charm. Make this cake on repeat when fresh cherries are in season—and be sure to have some coconut cream chilling in the fridge! In a pinch, ready-made coconut whip is available.

Black Forest Cake with Coconut Whip + Fresh Summer Cherries

SERVES 8

Cake

- Virgin coconut oil, for greasing
- 2½ cups (260 g) super-fine blanched almond flour
- ¼ cup (30 g) unsweetened Valrhona cocoa powder
- 1 teaspoon baking soda
- ¾ teaspoon pink salt
- ¾ cup (235 g) pure maple syrup
- 3 large eggs, room temperature

Coconut whip

- 1 (13.5-oz/400-ml) can unsweetened coconut cream, refrigerated overnight (see Note)
- 2 teaspoons pure maple syrup
- 1 teaspoon vanilla extract

Cake Preheat oven to 350°F. Thoroughly grease a 9-inch (23-cm) nonstick springform pan with coconut oil and line the bottom with parchment paper.

In a medium mixing bowl, whisk together almond flour, cocoa, baking soda, and salt, breaking up any lumps. Add the maple syrup and eggs and whisk until smooth and well combined. Using a rubber spatula, pour the batter into the springform pan. Spread it toward the edges and tap the pan on the counter to level the batter. Bake for 25 minutes on the center rack.

Cool for 20 minutes in the pan, then transfer the cake, dome side up, to a serving plate.

Coconut whip Chill a mixing bowl for 10 minutes in the freezer.

Spoon the thickened coconut cream into the chilled bowl, leaving any liquid behind for another use. Using a hand mixer, beat on high for 2 minutes, until soft peaks form. Add the maple syrup and vanilla and whip just long enough to incorporate. Be careful not to overmix—it will not be as light and fluffy as regular dairy whipped cream.

Use immediately or store in the fridge until needed—it does not hold up well at room temperature.

Toppings

Fresh sweet cherries, pitted and sliced in half

Dark chocolate, for shaving

Assembly Plate each slice of cake individually and top each one with a hefty dollop of coconut whip and a handful of sliced cherries. Use a vegetable peeler to shave dark chocolate over the top. Enjoy immediately.

NOTE

I use Savoy coconut cream because it's very thick and additive-free. It can be found in select grocery stores, Asian markets, and online. I also like Let's Do Organic's Organic Heavy Coconut Cream—but it contains more liquid and will only net about half the amount of whipped cream compared to the Savoy, and it has a looser texture once whipped. At this time (vendors may change), I've found Trader Joe's coconut cream to be waxy and grey, which is not suitable for this use.

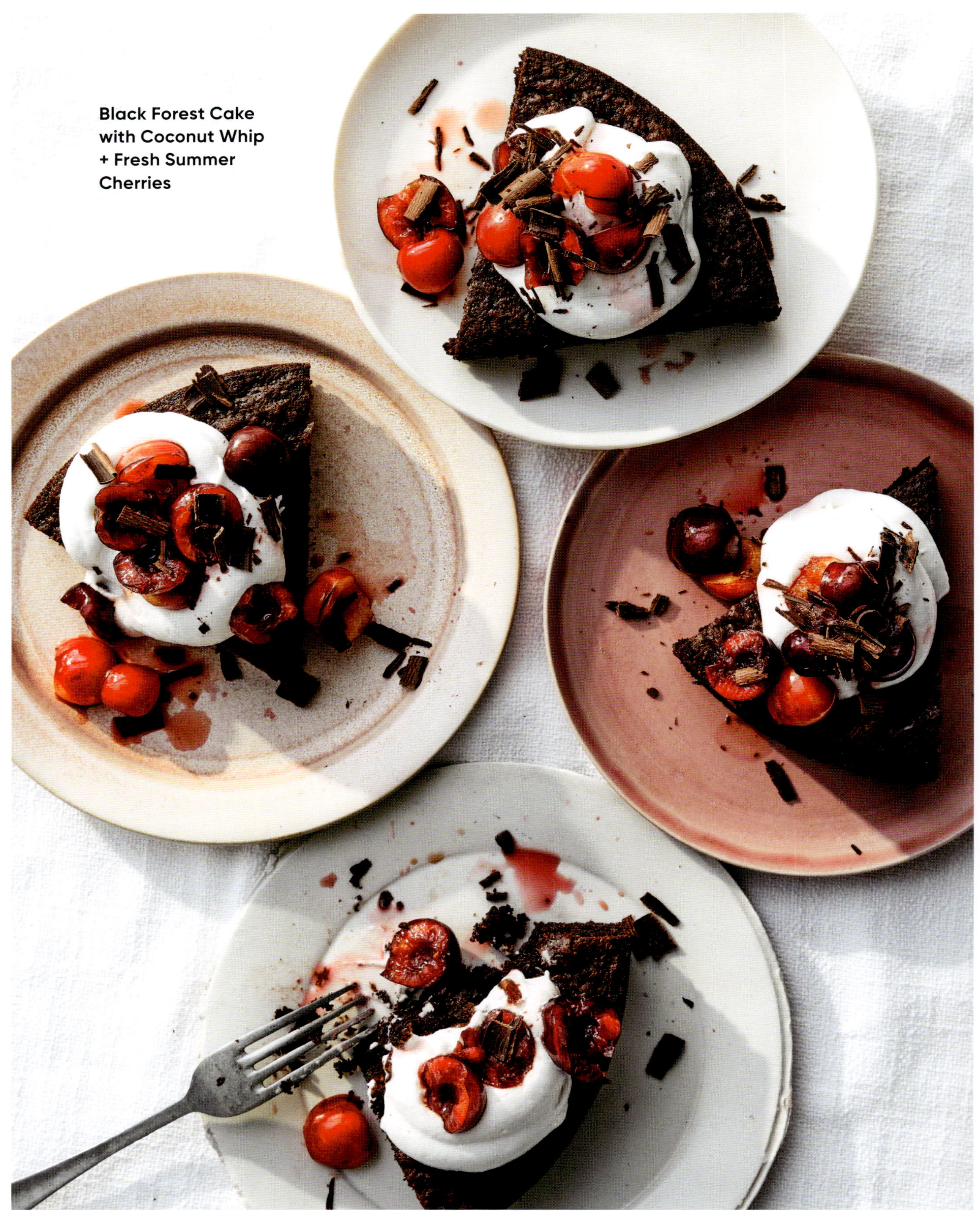

Black Forest Cake with Coconut Whip + Fresh Summer Cherries

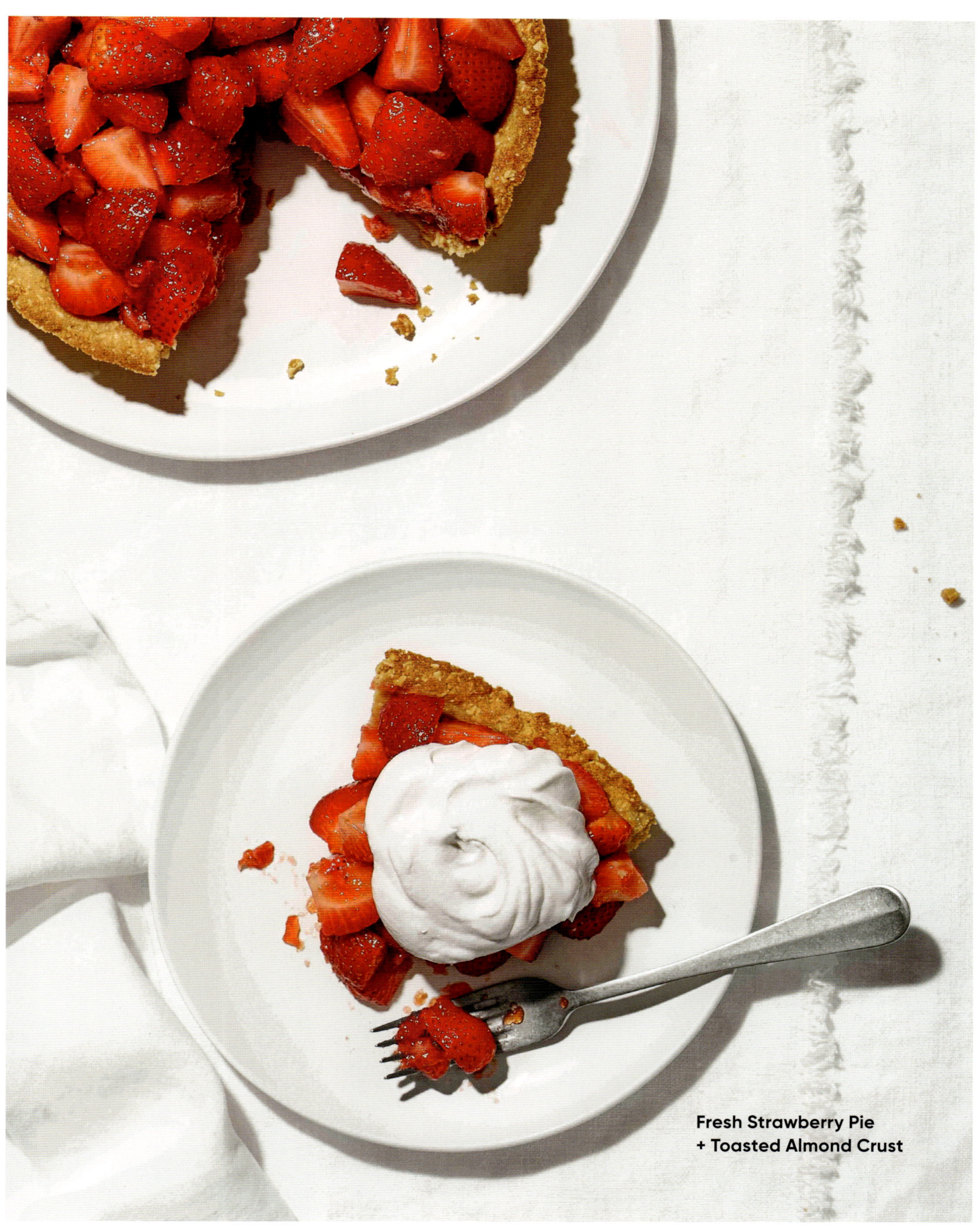

Fresh Strawberry Pie
+ Toasted Almond Crust

Sweet berries juxtaposed with a salty nut crust! I reserve this gorgeous pie for spring and summer when strawberries are at their best: fresh, ripe, and deliciously fragrant. Seasonal ingredients will always have the most flavor and nutrition, so they're worth waiting for. Top it with a pillowy dollop of coconut whipped cream. Ready-made coconut whip is available to use in a pinch.

Fresh Strawberry Pie + Toasted Almond Crust

SERVES 6

Filling

2 lbs (907 g) strawberries, hulled and quartered (divided)

2 tablespoons freshly squeezed lemon juice

¼ cup (80 g) pure maple syrup

2 tablespoons honey

1 (7-g) envelope unflavored gelatin

Zest of 1 orange

Crust

1 cup (130 g) toasted slivered almonds

¾ cup + 1 tablespoon (93 g) super-fine blanched almond flour

3 tablespoons melted unrefined coconut oil, plus extra for greasing

3 tablespoons pure maple syrup

¾ teaspoon pink salt

Filling Add 2 cups (400 g) of the hulled and quartered strawberries to a small saucepan. Using a potato masher, mash them until chunky. Add the lemon juice, maple syrup, and honey, and stir to combine. Sprinkle the gelatin over the top and let it sit for 2 minutes to hydrate. Stir over medium heat until it reaches a gentle simmer—do not boil. Transfer the mixture to a large bowl and allow it to cool. Once cool, stir in the orange zest and remaining hulled and quartered strawberries. Cover and refrigerate for 2–4 hours to set.

Crust Preheat oven to 350°F. Grease a 9-inch (23-cm) nonstick pie pan (this crust will stick to a glass pie pan).

Process the almonds in a mini food processor until well chopped but still slightly chunky. Transfer the chopped nuts to a small bowl, then mix them with the remaining crust ingredients until well combined. Transfer mixture to the prepared pie pan. Press firmly into the bottom and up the sides, keeping the thickness as uniform as possible. Leave the top edge craggy and rustic if you like. Bake on the center rack for 12 minutes, until golden (check on it after 9 minutes and rotate if one side has more color). Set aside to cool.

Coconut whip

1 (13.5-oz/400-ml) can unsweetened coconut cream, refrigerated overnight (see Note)

2 teaspoons maple syrup

1 teaspoon pure vanilla extract

Coconut whip Chill a mixing bowl for 10 minutes in the freezer.

Spoon the thickened coconut cream into the chilled bowl, leaving any liquid behind for another use. Using a hand mixer, beat on high for 2 minutes, until soft peaks form. Add the maple syrup and vanilla and whip just long enough to incorporate. Be careful not to overmix—it will not be as light and fluffy as regular dairy whipped cream.

Use immediately or store in the fridge until needed—it does not hold up well at room temperature.

Assembly Give the strawberry filling a quick stir, then pour it into the prepared pie crust; refrigerate until ready to use. For the crispiest crust, enjoy right away. Serve with coconut whip.

NOTE

I use Savoy coconut cream, which can be found in Asian markets and online, or Let's Do Organic's Organic Heavy Coconut Cream, which is widely available. It contains more liquid and will only net about half the amount of whipped coconut cream compared to the Savoy, and it has a looser texture once whipped. At this time (vendors may change), I have found Trader Joe's coconut cream to be waxy and grey, which is not suitable for this use.

This easy snack cake has a tender crumb and big bursts of strawberry. And you get to choose your own adventure by adding your choice of lime zest, lemon zest, or cardamom to the batter.

SERVES 6

Strawberry Snack Cake

- Virgin coconut oil, for greasing
- 2½ cups (260 g) super-fine blanched almond flour
- Zest of 1 large lime or lemon (see Note) or 1 teaspoon ground cardamom
- 2½ teaspoons baking powder
- ½ teaspoon pink salt
- 3 large eggs, room temperature
- ¾ cup (235 g) pure maple syrup
- 1 teaspoon vanilla extract
- 1 (1.2-oz/34-g) bag freeze-dried strawberries (see Note)

Preheat oven to 350°F. Thoroughly grease a 9-inch (23-cm) nonstick springform pan with coconut oil and line the bottom with parchment paper.

In a medium mixing bowl, whisk together almond flour, zest (or cardamom), baking powder, and salt, breaking up any lumps. Add the remaining ingredients, except freeze-dried strawberries, and whisk until smooth and combined.

Using a rubber spatula, gently fold in strawberries and break up any clumps, until evenly distributed. Pour the batter into the prepared springform pan and use the spatula to spread it toward the edges and smooth the top. Bake for 27 minutes on the center rack.

Cool cake for 20 minutes in the pan, then transfer it to a serving plate.

The cake can be covered and stored at room temperature for up to 3 days.

NOTES

If you're using lemon or lime zest, use a Microplane so it's very finely grated.

Trader Joe's freeze-dried strawberries are the best and most economical option I've found.

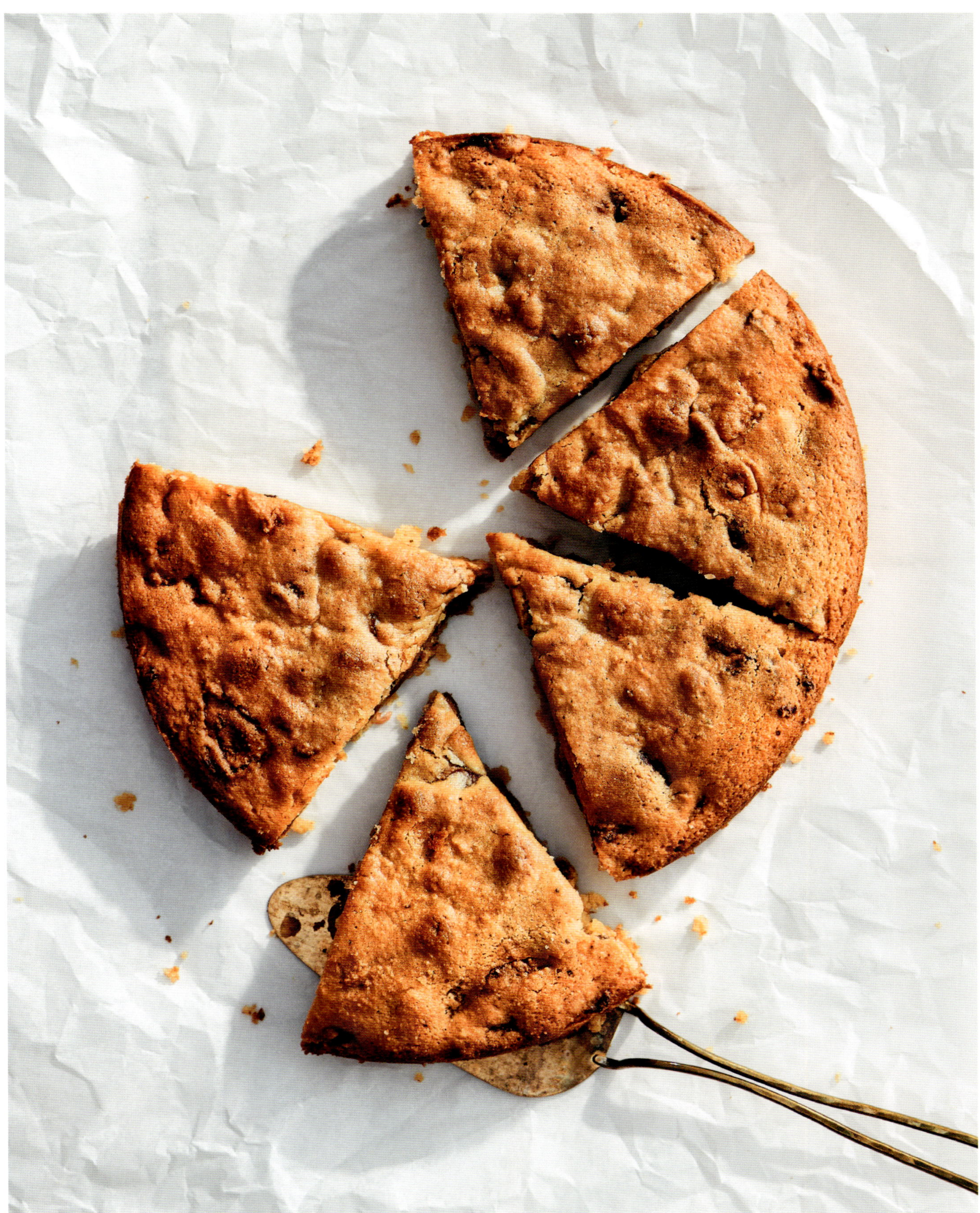

Hearty and satisfying with the warmth of cinnamon and the crunch of toasty walnuts, this classic coffee cake is all cleaned up and should be enjoyed with abandon!

Cinnamon-Walnut Coffee Cake

SERVES 8

Cake

- 2½ cups (260 g) super-fine blanched almond flour
- ¾ cup (75 g) finely shredded unsweetened coconut
- 1 tablespoon ground cinnamon
- 1 teaspoon baking powder
- ¾ teaspoon pink salt
- ½ teaspoon baking soda
- 4 large eggs, room temperature
- ½ cup (157 g) pure maple syrup
- 2 tablespoons melted virgin coconut oil, plus extra for greasing
- 1 tablespoon vanilla extract

Filling

- 2 tablespoons pure maple syrup
- 1 tablespoon ground cinnamon

Topping

- 1 cup (123 g) finely chopped raw walnuts

Cake Preheat oven to 350°F. Thoroughly grease a 9-inch (23-cm) springform pan with coconut oil and line the bottom with a parchment paper round.

In a medium mixing bowl, whisk together almond flour, coconut, cinnamon, baking powder, salt, and baking soda, breaking up any lumps. Add the remaining cake batter ingredients and whisk until smooth and well combined. Pour half of the batter into the prepared springform pan and spread it toward the edges. Tap the pan on the counter to level the batter.

Filling In a small bowl, mix the filling ingredients together to form a thick syrup. Using a spoon, drizzle filling over the first layer of batter. Drop the remaining cake batter in small spoonfuls over the filling, covering as much of the filling as possible. Carefully smooth it out and avoid disturbing the filling as much as possible. Tap the pan on the counter to level the batter.

Topping Sprinkle walnuts over the top, with the goal of covering all the batter. Bake on the center rack for 30 minutes. Cool completely, then transfer cake to a plate. Store at room temperature for up to 4 days.

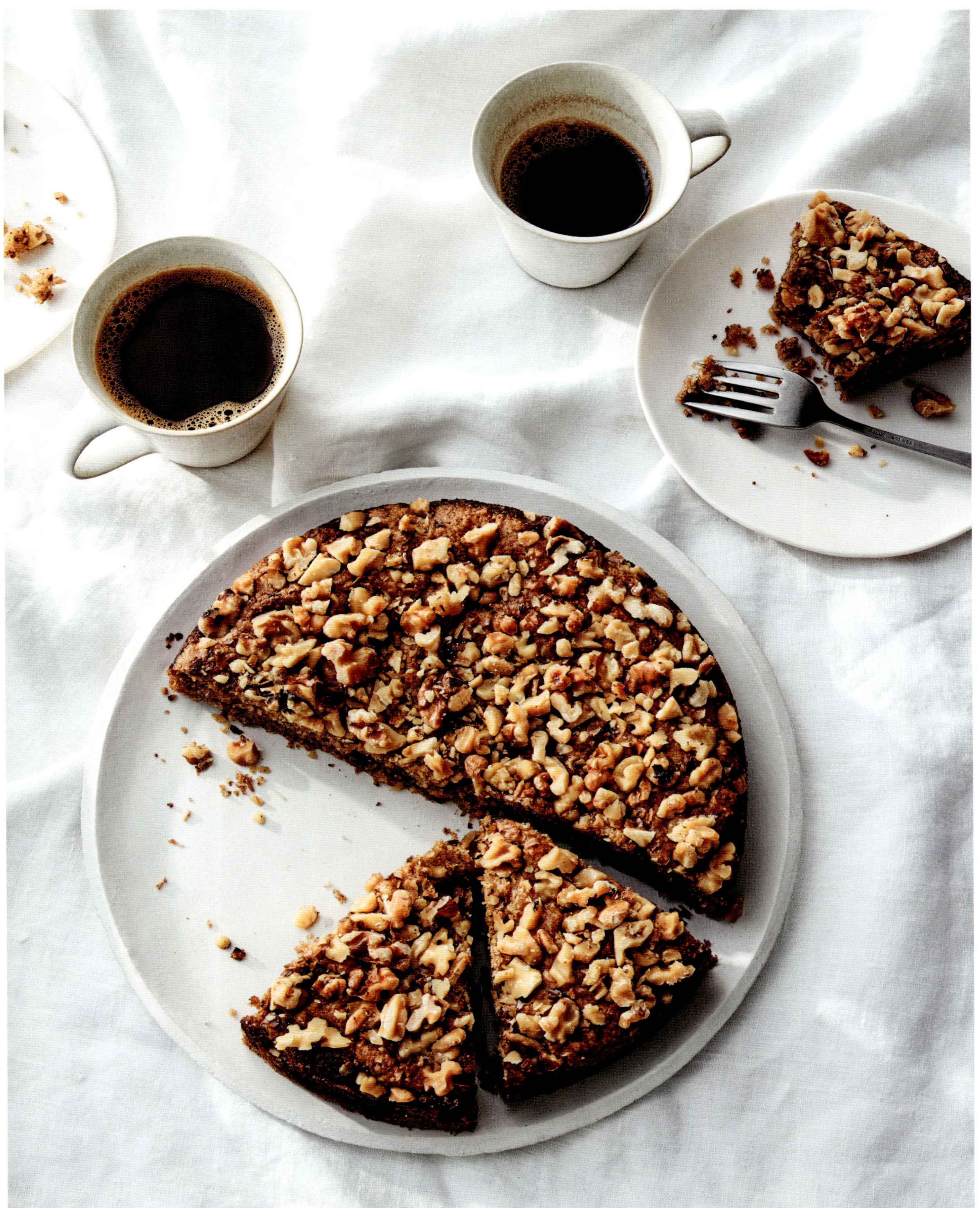

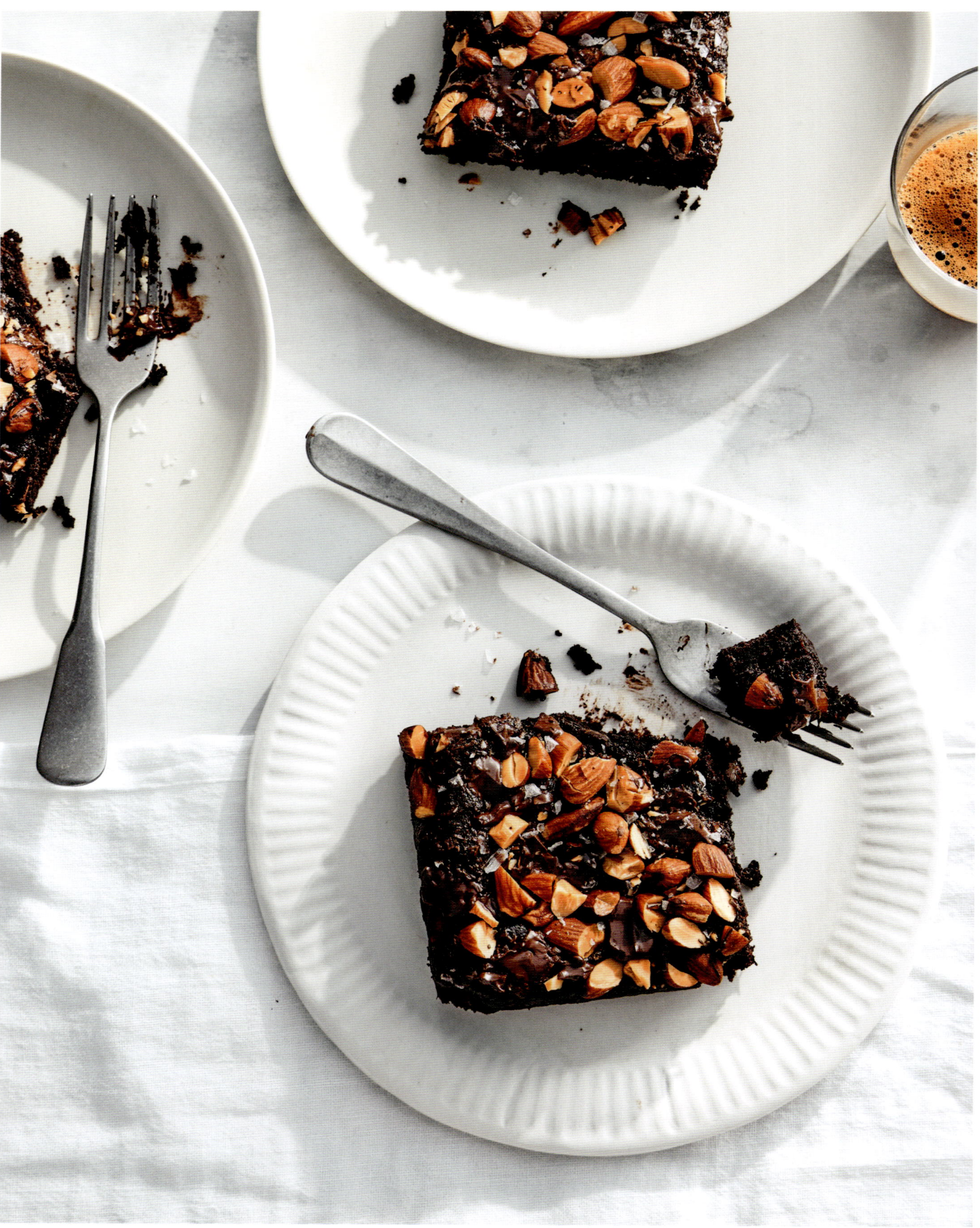

These are the kind of fudge brownies you eat with a fork! They're intensely chocolatey and topped with crunchy almonds and luxurious puddles of molten dark chocolate. These brownies hold up well in the fridge for up to a week, and 20 seconds in the microwave will return your square to its molten glory. If you don't eat eggs, you're in luck: I've included an egg-free variation using flax seeds.

Fudgy Brownies with Toasted Almonds + Flake Salt

SERVES 9

Brownies

3/4 cup (200 g) well-stirred almond butter

1/2 cup (157 g) pure maple syrup

1 large egg, room temperature

3/4 cup (182 g) unsweetened applesauce

1 teaspoon baking soda

3/4 teaspoon pink salt

1/2 cup (60 g) Valrhona cocoa powder (see Note)

3 tablespoons coconut flour (use a knife to level)

Toppings

1/2 cup (3 oz/85 g) coarsely chopped dark chocolate (see Note)

1/2 cup (60 g) unsalted, dry-roasted almonds, coarsely chopped

Maldon flake salt, for sprinkling

Brownies Preheat oven to 350°F. Line an 8-inch (20-cm) square metal baking pan with parchment paper.

In a medium mixing bowl, add each brownie ingredient in the order listed, whisking well after each addition. Pour the batter into the prepared pan. Using a rubber spatula, spread the batter to the edges. Tap the pan on the counter to smooth out the thick batter.

Top with the chopped chocolate and almonds, with the goal of covering all the batter. Add a light sprinkle of flake salt. Bake on the center rack for 30 minutes.

Cool completely in the pan, then transfer to a cutting board and cut into squares.

Variation: Egg-Free Brownies To make these egg-free, you can swap out the egg for ground flax seeds and water. Add 1 tablespoon of ground flax seeds and 3 tablespoons of water to the mixing bowl first. Give it a few minutes to thicken a bit, then proceed with the recipe as written, omitting the egg.

NOTES

Using Valrhona cocoa is critical to the deep chocolatey flavor of this brownie.

You may be tempted to use chocolate chips for the topping but note that they will not produce the same melty puddles as chopped dark chocolate.

If you love a thin mint cookie, this one's for you! These scrumptious little cakes are approved for all audiences and can be dressed according to the occasion. Pictured are both the plain Jane version and the floral version sprinkled with rose petals and cacao nibs.

Make the floral version for a bridal shower or Valentine's Day! I recommend omitting the mint extract when decorating with rose petals, though, because the flavors aren't compatible. Bundt cakes can require bit of negotiation to get them out of the pan, but if you adhere to the directions, you shouldn't have a problem.

Mint Chocolate Mini Bundts

SERVES 6

Cake

- 2½ cups (260 g) super-fine blanched almond flour
- ¼ cup (30 g) Valrhona cocoa powder
- 1 teaspoon baking soda
- ¾ teaspoon pink salt
- 3 large eggs, room temperature
- ¾ cup (235 g) pure maple syrup
- Virgin coconut oil, for greasing

Cake Preheat oven to 350°F.

In a medium mixing bowl, whisk together almond flour, cocoa, baking soda, and salt until combined, breaking up any lumps. Add the eggs and maple syrup and whisk until smooth and well combined.

Grease a nonstick mini bundt (bundtlette) pan by melting a small amount of coconut oil in the microwave and using a silicone pastry brush to reach every crack and crevice. Use a generous amount, and don't forget the center tube.

Using a spoon, carefully divide the batter among the 6 cavities. Tap the pan on the counter to level the batter. Bake for 25 minutes on the center rack.

Set the pan aside for precisely 10 minutes—set a timer! Invert the pan and tap (bang) it against the counter until the cakes release. Let them finish cooling on a cooling rack.

Dark chocolate mint ganache

¼ cup (60 g) canned full-fat, additive-free coconut milk (see Note)

2 oz (57 g) 100% unsweetened chocolate, chopped (see Note)

2 tablespoons pure maple syrup

⅛ teaspoon pink salt

⅛ teaspoon pure peppermint extract, or to taste

Dark chocolate mint ganache Place the mini bundt cakes on a parchment paper–lined baking sheet.

Combine all ganache ingredients in a small glass or porcelain bowl and microwave for 30 seconds. Using a small whisk, whisk gently for 2–3 minutes, until chocolate is melted, glossy, and slightly thickened, but still pourable.

Using a spoon, drizzle the ganache over the bundt cakes, quickly, before it sets up. Tapping the baking sheet on the counter will help the ganache flow down the sides of the cakes.

Allow an hour for the bundts to set. If it's a particularly hot day, you may need to refrigerate them for 15 minutes.

NOTE

This recipe was developed using Guittard's 100% cacao baking bars and Trader Joe's canned full-fat coconut milk. Using coconut milk that contains additives or thickening agents is not advised. Look for a baking bar that contains only cacao beans.

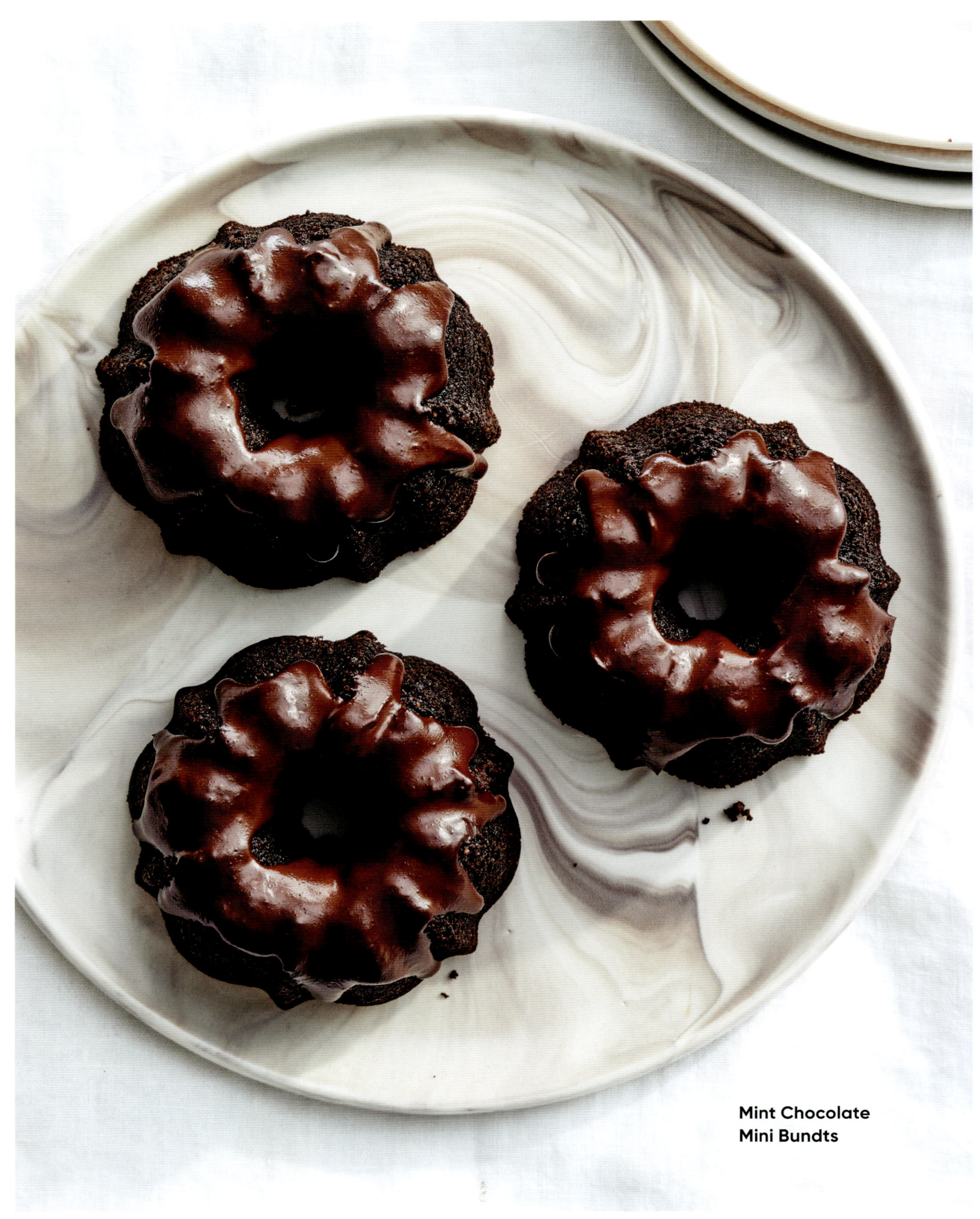

Mint Chocolate
Mini Bundts

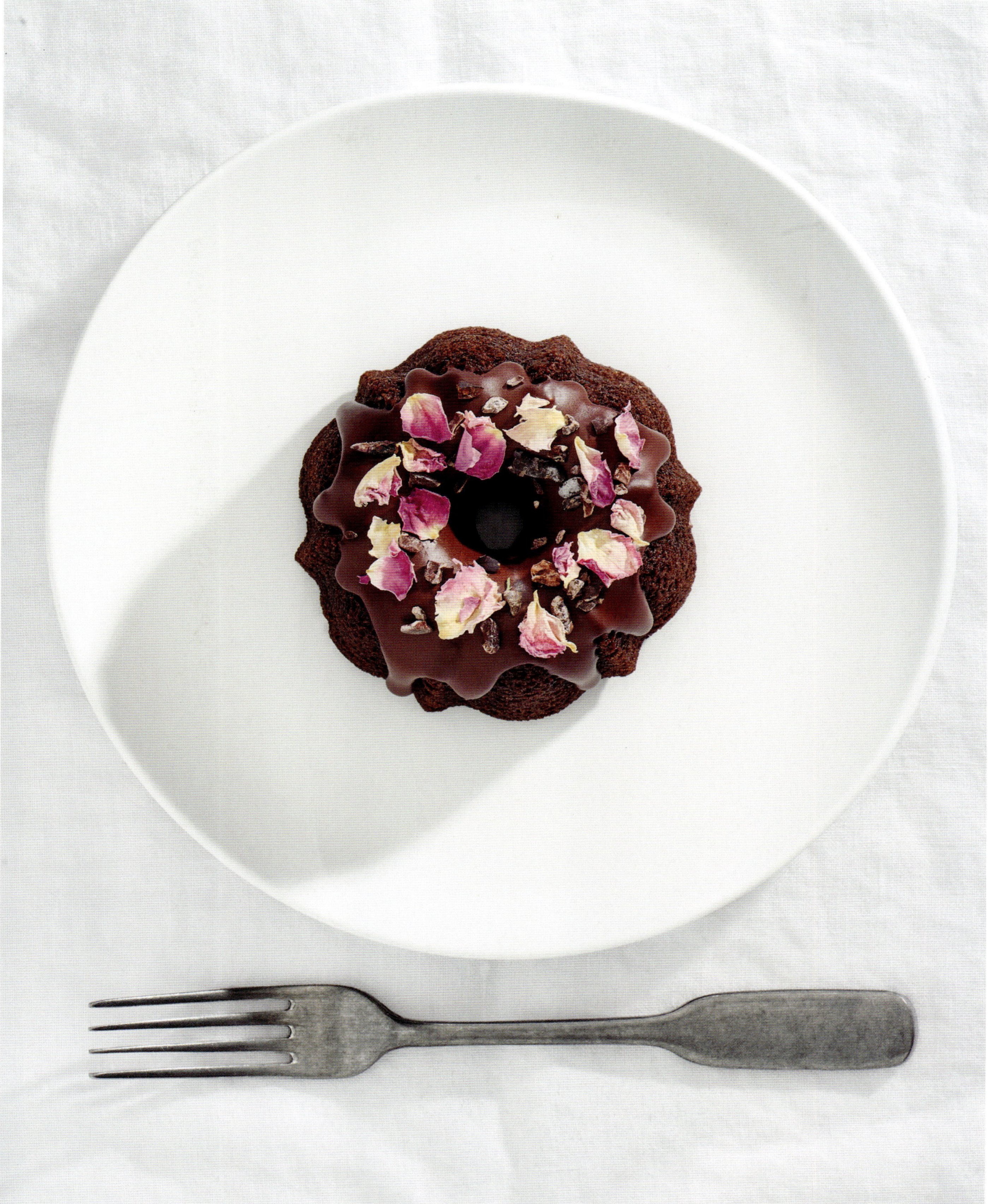

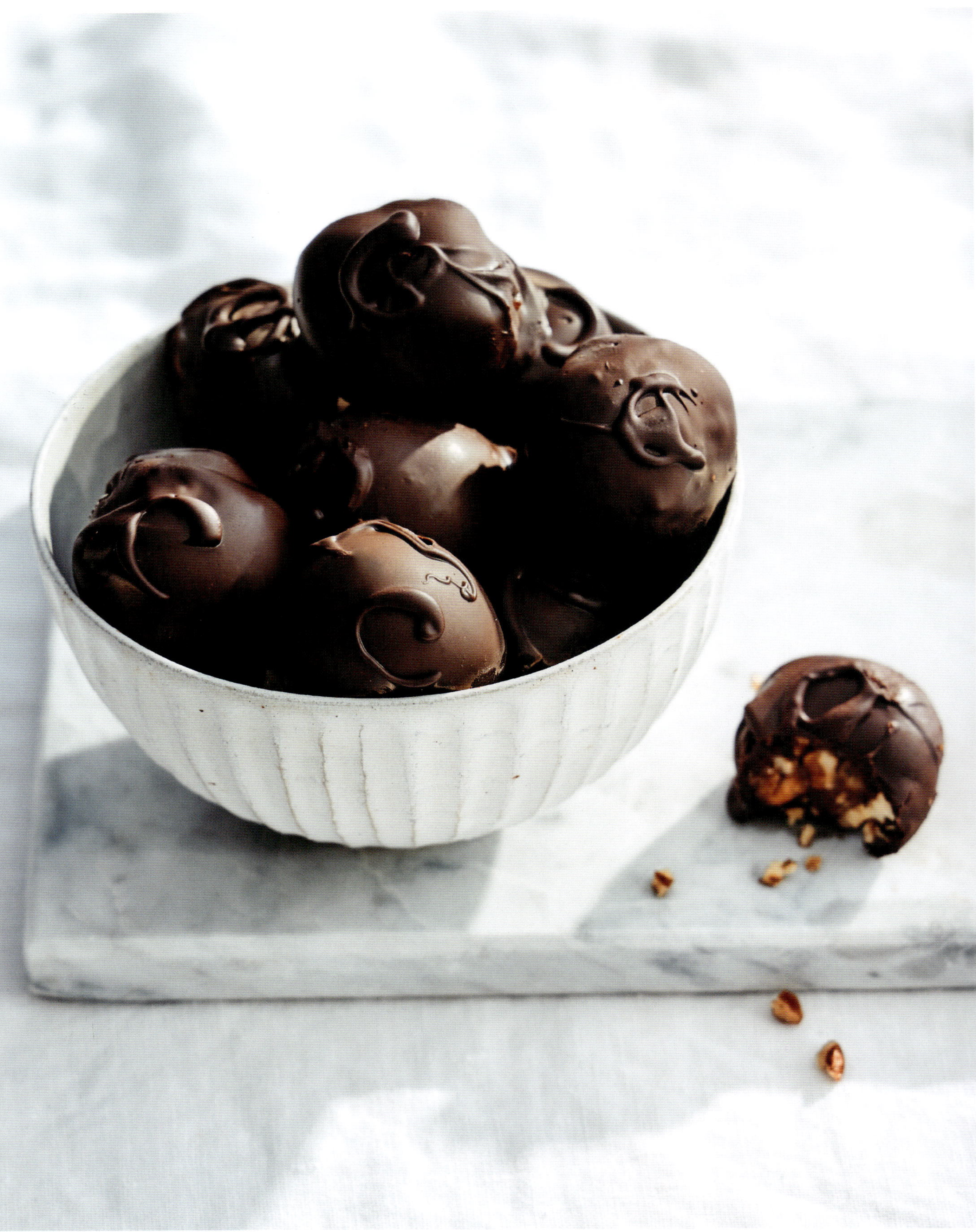

The crispy snap of the dark chocolate exterior gives way to a sweet, sumptuous center as these truffles hit all the nostalgic notes of a pecan pie, without the icky ingredients—namely high-fructose corn syrup. Toast your pecans to within an inch of their life for the best flavor and so they'll hold their crunch. But keep a watchful eye on them, because nuts can go from golden to scorched in a moment. The truffles hold up in the fridge for weeks or stored in glass jars in the freezer for even longer. You are in for a treat!

Pecan Pie Truffles with Salted Caramel + Toasted Pecans

MAKES ABOUT 24 TRUFFLES

- 6 large, soft Medjool dates, pitted
- 1/4 cup (53 g) virgin coconut oil
- 1/2 cup (157 g) pure maple syrup
- 1/2 cup (130 g) well-stirred roasted almond butter
- 1 teaspoon vanilla extract
- 3/4 teaspoon pink salt
- 1 1/4 cups (136 g) well-toasted pecans, chopped
- 9 oz (255 g) dark chocolate, chopped, for coating (see Note)

Start with room temperature ingredients. Place the truffle ingredients, except pecans and chocolate, in a food processor and process until smooth, about 2 minutes. Scrape down the sides of the bowl and give it another few pulses. Transfer the mixture to a bowl. Add the chopped pecans and use a sturdy spoon to fold the mixture until the nuts are evenly distributed. Cover with plastic wrap and freeze for 2 hours, until firm, so the balls will hold their shape when rolled.

Using a small (size 70) cookie scoop, roll mixture into balls. Freeze the balls for 30–60 minutes on a small baking sheet lined with parchment paper. This will help them to hold their shape and help the chocolate set up quickly once dipped.

Transfer the chilled balls to a plate and line the baking sheet with a fresh sheet of parchment paper.

Place chocolate in a microwave-safe bowl and microwave in 30-second intervals, stirring each time, until fully melted.

Using 2 forks, dip each ball in chocolate, making sure it's fully coated on all sides. Give each ball a shake so the excess chocolate can drip off, before placing it on the prepared baking sheet. Refrigerate until the chocolate is fully set.

Truffles can be stored for up to a month in the fridge or freezer in glass jars.

NOTE

I use the Trader Joe's Pound Plus 72% dark chocolate bar for dipping because it's economical, but it does contain some cane sugar. There are options available that are sweetened with coconut sugar, dates, or stevia.

ACKNOWLEDGMENTS

I fought nearly as hard for this book as I've had to fight for my life.

But here we are, and I'm incredibly grateful.

My husband and BFF Joe, you are the captor of my heart and the nurturer of my soul. It's only because you took such good care of me and my sick body that this book was possible.

Robert K. Naviaux, MD, PhD (University of California San Diego researcher known for his cell danger response hypothesis): Thank you for your support of this project! I'm forever grateful you trusted me as your study coordinator and, more recently, as your community liaison. My work with you gave me a sense of purpose and community as I was learning to navigate a life with ME/CFS.

Adrian Bean, you are a treasured friend, a talented practitioner, and the best kind of weirdo.

Jennifer Machian, you continued testing my recipes even after that rideshare driver plowed into your kitchen at 4 AM. Thank you for your generosity and all the deep dives!

To my friends, supporters, recipe testers, and community comrades who have contributed in ways big and small, I am deeply grateful for you.

Thank you to Brian Lexmond, Jennifer Berntsen, Sharon Spencer, Austin Kleweno, J.P. Koval, Steve Moore, Cort Johnson, Anita Enander, Tracy Masington, Justin Reilly, Janet Dafoe, Rylee Spencer, Caroline Christian, Sarah Reynolds Robbins, Carollynn Bartosh, Linda Tannenbaum, Pat Vogel, Laura Callender, Kristin Donnelly, Samantha Bishop, Rachel Liang, Garrette F. Nasworthy, Manasi Pimpley, Evelyne Parissier Lewis, Nathanael Daum, Vincent Tong, Haley and Danny McCarthy, Vanessa Keeslar, Signe Liisa Lugus, Sarah Kronzer, Jennie Spotila, Maria Berger, Lissa Nilsson, Sharon D. Greenspan, Adam Weisman, Rivka Solomon, F. Gonzalez, Lisa Edelsward, Lianne Beyerl, Angel Hayse, Kira Stoops, Sarah Ramey, Judy Machian, Jennifer Vaughn Caldwell, Fereshteh Jahanbani, Cindy Hennard, Lynn Esteban, Ed Illig, Michael Van Huffel, Cher Campbell, Karen Lubell, Barbara Kyne, Tara Hulen, Barbara Dimmick, Johanna Jones, Cynthia Uribe, Katie Bach, Dani Morsberger, Lynn and Brian Riggio, Donna Lee, Heather Howe, Lizzy Jones, Catherine Rowmatowski, Katie Highsmith, Jennifer Stitt, Melinda West Maxwell, Laura Barron Stoll, Tamara Romanuk, Katie Kerr, Karen Mann, Aaron Anderson, Gina Freize, Chloe Bridge, Susan Lasley, Sophie Kooman, David Tuller, Hannah Campion, Janet Barker, Jane Daykin, Iain Burgess, Kira Dyksta, Maren Jensen, Kaspar B. Burger, Jill Easton, Anna Stansbury, Tim and Julie Blankenship, Cathleen Jones, Lauren Saikkonen, Carol Hutton, Valerie

Mallinson, Geli Lehmann, Deborah Van Valkenburgh, Heidi St. Jean, Joan Markham, Lu Geffen, Anna Caudill, Kylie Foot, Sandra Hall, Carmen Atherton, Brianna Pogue, Matt Lazell-Fairman, Matt Cary, Clare Kane, Cheryl McPherson, Francesca Edwards, Joanne Alexander, Sandra Carroll, Elizabeth L. Tapley, Sheeri W. Wes, Mai Nguyen, Julie Lobel, Carolyn Hanes, Pamela Calderwood, Elizabeth Anderson, Brian Bindon, Lacinda Hummel, Sumit Bhagra, Kathleen Smith, Andrea Peakovic, Courtney Menzies, Brenda Stokvis, Anne Skupin, Anthea Robertson, Mary McIntyre, Catherine Suter, Penelope Holliday, Savita Nair, Larry Christensen, Ida Larsen, Mary Ross, Vivienne Gilchrist, David Lombardi, Krista Williams, Brigitte Martin, Moyna Sinnamon, Gina Kemp, Jackson Barnett, Karie Lew, Tamesin Eldredge, Claudia Person, Kim Moy, Kandice Dickinson, Anne R. Peterson, Mary Blalock, Emily Corbett, Jessica Diamond, Kathryn Joy, Caitlin Lynch, Krista Ripley, Elaine Pollack, Jeff Brody, Sandra Lubkin, Diana Rypkema Kshirsagar, Maria Lord, Christina Yesenofski, E.J. Gilbard, Susan Fischer, Judith Oversby, Charlotte Vonsalis, Zoe Thorp, Juta Lugus, Lisa La Rosa, Diane Nangeroni, Clare McHale, Tristan Crippen, Miya Komori-Glatz, Alexa Buffini, Evelyn Adams, Kwong Yuan Tew, Eric Shiels, Jess Pippen, Perry Norton, Guy Williams, Kyle Gee, Tara Gates, Gordon Prowse, Dina Guzovsky, David Hernandez, Pamuditha Mahadiulwewa, Michelle Valente, Megan Santa Ana, Kristen Constantine, Ajna Ellis, Patti Reichenecker, Rebecca Jones, Molly Greenwood, Kim Girgenti, Carrie Young, Nora Hammack, Pam Ardizzone, Niko Niedo, Quenby Morrow, Bettine Molenberg, MLD, Nancy Henson, Karen Neff, Vania Terzopoulou, Elizabeth Streckert, Jane Shiyah, Diane Bean, Karen Skoff, Susan Sikes, Ann McDonald, Denise King, Michael Sieverts, Michael Eichner, Coral Bohne, Carol Froese, Galen Warden, Donna Lutz, Victoria Bowden, Louise Blyton, Josiah Johnson, Triada Samaras, Elizabeth Kessler, R.E. Camp, Tracey Allen, Nancy Alexander, Gloria Baca, Ashley Andrews, Lisa Fennessy, Helen Perryer, Susie Mitchell, Helen Reynolds, Peggy Lami, Theresa Karnecki, Cassius C, Ruth Diver, Emily Moothart, Janis Hall, Valerie Lumsden, Anne Slifkin, Jill Leite, Nancy Mackay-Dietrich, Lori Peloquin, Katy M. Hunt, Albin Burkacki, Carol Furchner, Robert Sykes, Joyce Eslinger, Kathrin Meyer, Emily Fraser, Katharine London, Catherine Klatt, Yelena Sayko, Nancy Hornewer, Teme Ring, Anne Alexander, Lisa Zinzow, Ruth Tenenbaum, Margaret Phillips, Julie Piggott, Anne Kebler, Mark Harper, Robin Thomas, H.G. Venema, Alex Kennedy, Deborah Rose, Elizabeth Ansell, Nicole Webb, Gretchen Dawson, Isabel Burnett, Debbie Burgeson, Eileen Rosenbloom, Tamara Mathews, Peter Labor, Janice Reilly, Tess McEnulty, Elizabeth

Holloway, Jaclyn Bobich, Giselle Park, Renate Eklund, JuLee K. Dugan, Molly Freedenberg, Amanda Stephen, Michael Askren, Ilona Holewijn, Brenda Glazier, Lynisha Ramoutar, Nicole de Blois, Kym Adams, Helen Mann, Georgina Coghlan, Janet Molina, Travis Hardy, Kevin Meboe, Jane Gold, Maxine Fidler, Karin Friederic, Aiden Maguire, Patricia Wilson, Sue Dyar, Salome Hancock, Donna Chapin, Erika Edmondstone, April Flynn, Leo Rosenstein, Rebecca Sorrells, Famille Helstroffer, Laura McCall, Michael Anassori, Pamela Campos, Desirie McKinnon, Lisa Wieland, Yuriko Shotter, Sujata Sanghvi, Jane Houk, Patricia McWeeney, Liz Carlson, Brian Shanfeld, Debra Epner, Pamela Bakst, Orsi Crawford, Joan Spear, Amy Jeffreys, Paulette Johnson, Barb Crombie, Graham Sephton, Sally Lemkemeier, Deborah Eckstein, Julia Lawrence, Rebecca Edelson, Sarah Turnbull, Sandhya King, Wendy Murray, Jolie Solomon, Elizabeth Parker, Kara Sherry, and Grace Ewing.

My photography team, Marian Cooper Cairns and Colin Price: Thank you for bringing my vision to life despite a COVID scare, a hurricane (in Los Angeles no less), and a power outage!

Megan Morello, dear friend and photographer: Thanks for helping me get those last cookbook shots. You are a joy, and a rare shining example of a human. My styling inexpertise does not do your photography justice!

Jason Mraz, your spirit of generosity is contagious!

Adeena Sussman, you are so full of heart and make us all want to shop the shuk with you!

Dr. Terry Wahls, you are a true badass. Thank you for inspiring us all to dig deeper in the pursuit of better health. You have set a high bar, but I will keep reaching. In a space that often feels vapid, following your unapologetic, vanity-free posts on Instagram has been a breath of fresh air.

To my team at Figure 1—Chris, Lara, Heidi, Mark, Mélanie, Christine, Michelle, Anastasia, Iva—and Jessica + Naomi from DSGN Dept.: I couldn't have asked for a lovelier, more talented team!

INDEX

Page numbers in italics refer to photos.

A

ahi, seared, + baby bok choy salad with fish sauce dressing, 148–49, *151*

ALMOND BUTTER

- blackout cookies with 100% chocolate + flake salt, 52, *53*
- fudgy brownies with toasted almonds + flake salt, *204*, 205
- pecan pie truffles with salted caramel + toasted pecans, *210*, 211
- strawberry + almond energy balls, *44*, 45

ALMONDS

- Asian-style chicken salad + honey-lime dressing, *152*, 153
- coconut-almond snack cake + dark chocolate chunks, 178, *179*
- fresh strawberry pie + toasted almond crust, *197*, 198–99
- fudgy brownies with toasted almonds + flake salt, *204*, 205
- Pasadena chicken salad + sweet sesame dressing, 168, *169*
- seared ahi + baby bok choy salad with fish sauce dressing, 148–49, *151*
- strawberry + almond energy balls, *44*, 45
- summer kale + strawberry salad, 74, *75*
- watercress with roast chicken, tart apples + tarragon dressing, *170*, 171

anchovy + toasted walnut vinaigrette, chicory salad with, *76*, 77

APPLES

- Brussels sprouts slaw with Honeycrisp + pistachios, 82, *83*
- chicken liver mousse with apple + thyme, *58*, 59
- rutabaga mash with sage + crispy shallots, *113*, 115
- watercress with roast chicken, tart apples + tarragon dressing, *170*, 171

ARUGULA

- baby kale with roasted sweet potato, walnuts + maple-ginger dressing, 160, *161*
- bison sirloin au poivre + baby kale with maple-Dijon dressing, *154*, 155
- Mediterranean tuna + dry-cured olives with thyme vinaigrette, *162*, 163
- warm arugula vichyssoise, 96, *97*

Asian-style chicken salad + honey-lime dressing, *152*, 153

ASPARAGUS

- asparagus leek soup + spring chive blossoms, *102*, 103
- asparagus mimosa with tarragon + orange, *72*, 73
- charred asparagus + lemon-pistachio gremolata, *116*, 117
- creamy, salty + tangy tonnato sauce with grilled veg, 64, *65*
- 10-minute asparagus + rotisserie chicken bowl, 172, *173*

AVOCADO

- the Baja chop, *166*, 167
- lettuce wrapped lamb burgers + lemon aioli, 144, *145*
- Little Gem wedge salad with green goddess dressing, *80*, 81
- minty fresh + lemony salad smoothie, 34, *35*
- Pasadena chicken salad + sweet sesame dressing, 168, *169*

B

baby bok choy. *See* bok choy, baby

baby kale with roasted sweet potato, walnuts + maple-ginger dressing, 160, *161*

the Baja chop + honey-chipotle dressing, *166*, 167

BANANA

- banana + toasted walnut muffins, 68, *69*
- the everyday smoothie with wild blueberry, banana + hemp powder, *32*, 33

BEEF

- grilled flank steak, 136, *137*
- savory French onion beef, *138*, 139

Belgian endive. *See* endive
BISON
- bison meatloaf + jus, 140, *141*
- bison sirloin au poivre + baby kale with maple-Dijon dressing, *154*, 155

black cod, ginger marinated, + roasted baby bok choy, *129*, 130–31
Black Forest cake with coconut whip + fresh summer cherries, 194–95, *196*
blackberry gastrique + thyme, wild salmon with, 126–27, *128*
blackout cookies with 100% chocolate + flake salt, 52, *53*
blood oranges + roasted Brussels sprouts with sweet white balsamic, *119*, 120–21
BLUEBERRIES, WILD
- egg white omelet + wild blueberry compote, *36*, 37
- the everyday smoothie with wild blueberry, banana + hemp powder, 32, *33*
- vanilla coconut yogurt + wild blueberry compote, *40*, 41

BOK CHOY, BABY
- ginger marinated black cod + roasted baby bok choy, *129*, 130–31
- seared ahi + baby bok choy salad with fish sauce dressing, 148–49, *151*

broccoli, charred, + lemon tahini sauce, *106*, 107
brownie balls, walnut fudge, *54*, 55
brownies, fudgy, with toasted almonds + flake salt, *204*, 205
BRUSSELS SPROUTS
- Brussels sprouts slaw with Honeycrisp + pistachios, 82, *83*
- roasted Brussels sprouts + blood oranges with sweet white balsamic, *119*, 120–21

burgers, lettuce wrapped lamb, + lemon aioli, 144, *145*

C

CAKE
- Black Forest cake, 194–95, *196*
- cinnamon-walnut coffee cake, 202, *203*
- coconut-almond snack cake, 178, *179*
- dark chocolate birthday cake, *191*, 192–93
- the everyday chocolate cake, *184*, 185
- Linzer cake with hazelnut + dried raspberry, 182, *183*
- mint chocolate mini bundts, 206–7, 208–9
- morning glory muffins + breakfast cake, 38, *39*
- the signature chocolate cake + sweet raspberry filling, 188–89, *190*
- strawberry snack cake, 200, *201*

capers, in creamy, salty + tangy tonnato sauce with grilled veg, 64
caramel, salted, + toasted pecans, pecan pie truffles with, *210*, 211
CARDAMOM
- fresh cranberry relish with cherries + cardamom, 86, *87*
- strawberry snack cake, 200, *201*

CARROTS
- Asian-style chicken salad + honey-lime dressing, *152*, 153
- bison meatloaf + jus, 140, *141*
- creamy carrot tahini, 60, *61*
- creamy coconut carrot soup, 92, *93*
- Little Gem salad with grapes + za'atar dressing, *84*, 85
- morning glory muffins + breakfast cake, 38, *39*

CAULIFLOWER
- creamy cauliflower soup, *94*, 95
- garlic mashed cauliflower, 112, *113*
- tahini-charred cauliflower with dates + mint, 108, *109*

CELERY
- creamy cauliflower soup, *94*, 95
- creamy coconut carrot soup, 92, *93*

celery root + fennel mash, 114
charred asparagus + lemon-pistachio gremolata, *116*, 117
charred broccoli + lemon tahini sauce, *106*, 107

CHERRIES
Black Forest cake with coconut whip + fresh summer cherries, 194–95, *196*
fresh cranberry relish with cherries + cardamom, 86, *87*
CHICKEN
Asian-style chicken salad + honey-lime dressing, *152*, 153
baby kale with roasted sweet potato, walnuts + maple-ginger dressing, 160, *161*
the Baja chop, *166*, 167
chicken liver mousse with apple + thyme, *58*, 59
Pasadena chicken salad + sweet sesame dressing, 168, *169*
roast chicken, *134*, 135
10-minute asparagus + rotisserie chicken bowl, 172, *173*
Thai-style herb salad with chicken, strawberries + lime dressing, 164, *165*
watercress with roast chicken, tart apples + tarragon dressing, *170*, 171
chicory salad with toasted walnut + anchovy vinaigrette, *76*, 77
chipotle-honey dressing, the Baja chop +, *166*, 167
CHOCOLATE. *See also* cocoa powder
Black Forest cake, 194–95, *196*
blackout cookies with 100% chocolate + flake salt, 52, *53*
choc-a-lot muffins, 56, *57*
chocolate-dipped coconut macaroons, 186, *187*
coconut-almond snack cake + dark chocolate chunks, 178, *179*
dark chocolate birthday cake, *191*, 192–93
dark chocolate pots de crème, *180*, 181
dark chocolate tahini truffles, *176*, 177
the everyday chocolate cake, *184*, 185
fresh figs in dark chocolate, *66*, 67
fudgy brownies, *204*, 205
mint chocolate mini bundts, 206–7, 208, 209
pecan pie truffles, *210*, 211
the signature chocolate cake + sweet raspberry filling, 188–89, *190*
CINNAMON
banana + toasted walnut muffins, 68, *69*
cinnamon-walnut coffee cake, 202, *203*
fresh cranberry relish with cherries + cardamom, 86, *87*
lettuce wrapped lamb burgers + lemon aioli, 144, *145*
morning glory muffins + breakfast cake, 38, *39*
COCOA POWDER
Black Forest cake, 194–95, *196*
blackout cookies, 52, *53*
choc-a-lot muffins, 56, *57*
dark chocolate birthday cake, *191*, 192–93
dark chocolate tahini truffles, *176*, 177
the everyday chocolate cake, *184*, 185
fudgy brownies, *204*, 205
mint chocolate mini bundts, 206–7, 208, 209
the signature chocolate cake + sweet raspberry filling, 188–89, *190*
walnut fudge brownie balls, *54*, 55
COCONUT
chocolate-dipped coconut macaroons, 186, *187*
cinnamon-walnut coffee cake, 202, *203*
coconut-almond snack cake + dark chocolate chunks, 178, *179*
morning glory muffins + breakfast cake, 38, *39*
summer kale + strawberry salad, 74, *75*
Thai-style herb salad with chicken, strawberries + lime dressing, 164, *165*
COCONUT MILK
asparagus leek soup + spring chive blossoms, *102*, 103
cream of porcini mushroom soup, *90*, 91

creamy cauliflower soup, *94*, 95
creamy coconut carrot soup, 92, *93*
dark chocolate + dark chocolate birthday cake, *191*, 192–93
dark chocolate pots de crème, *180*, 181
the everyday chocolate cake, *184*, 185
garlic mashed cauliflower, 112, *113*
rustic fennel + celery root mash, *113*, 114
rutabaga mash with sage + crispy shallots, *113*, 115
the signature chocolate cake + sweet raspberry filling, 188–89, *190*
coconut whip, 194, 199
coconut yogurt, vanilla, + wild blueberry compote, *40*, 41
cold brew coffee granita, *47*, 48
compote, wild blueberry, 37, 41
COOKIES
blackout cookies with 100% chocolate + flake salt, 52, *53*
chocolate-dipped coconut macaroons, 186, *187*
CRANBERRIES
fresh cranberry relish with cherries + cardamom, 86, *87*
winter salmon salad + cranberry-lime relish, 156, *157*
cream of porcini mushroom soup, *90*, 91
creamy carrot tahini, 60, *61*
creamy cauliflower soup, *94*, 95
creamy coconut carrot soup, 92, *93*
creamy, salty + tangy tonnato sauce with grilled veg, 64, *65*
cremini mushrooms, in cream of porcini mushroom soup, 91
crispy shallots, 115
CUCUMBER
lettuce wrapped lamb burgers + lemon aioli, 144, *145*
summer salmon salad with cool, crisp veg + dilly dressing, *158*, 159
summer slushy with lime + mint, *50*, 51
CUMIN
creamy carrot tahini, 60, *61*
honey-chipotle dressing, 167
lettuce wrapped lamb burgers + lemon aioli, 144, *145*

D

dark chocolate. *See* chocolate
DATES
pecan pie truffles with salted caramel + toasted pecans, *210*, 211
strawberry + almond energy balls, *44*, 45
tahini-charred cauliflower with dates + mint, 108, *109*
walnut fudge brownie balls, *54*, 55
DIJON MUSTARD
bison sirloin au poivre + baby kale with maple-Dijon dressing, *154*, 155
pan-seared lamb lollipops with rosemary, maple + Dijon, *142*, 143
DILL
chicory salad with toasted walnut + anchovy vinaigrette, *76*, 77
summer salmon salad with cool, crisp veg + dilly dressing, *158*, 159
tahini-charred cauliflower with dates + mint, 108, *109*
wild salmon cakes + lemon aioli, *124*, 125
DIPS AND SPREADS. *See also* sauce
chicken liver mousse with apple + thyme, *58*, 59
coconut whip, 194, 199
creamy carrot tahini, 60, *61*
fresh cranberry relish with cherries + cardamom, 86, *87*
ganache, 185, 189, 192–93
lemon aioli, 125
zesty herbed tahini dip, *62*, 63
DRESSING
anchovy vinaigrette, 77
dilly dressing, 159
fish sauce dressing, 148
green goddess dressing, 81
honey-chipotle dressing, 167
honey-lime dressing, 153
lime dressing, 164
maple-Dijon dressing, 155
maple-ginger dressing, 160
sherry vinaigrette, 78
sweet sesame dressing, 168
tarragon dressing, 171
thyme vinaigrette, 163
za'atar dressing, 85

E

EGGS
- asparagus mimosa with tarragon + orange, 72, *73*
- chocolate-dipped coconut macaroons, 186, *187*
- egg white omelet + wild blueberry compote, *36*, 37
- Mediterranean tuna + dry-cured olives with thyme vinaigrette, *162*, 163
- warm arugula vichyssoise, 96, *97*

ENDIVE
- chicory salad with toasted walnut + anchovy vinaigrette, *76*, 77
- creamy, salty + tangy tonnato sauce with grilled veg, 64, *65*

energy balls, strawberry + almond, *44*, 45
the everyday chocolate cake, *184*, 185
the everyday smoothie with wild blueberry, banana + hemp powder, *32*, 33
everything seasoning encrusted halibut + horseradish aioli, 132, *133*

F

FENNEL
- lemon-scented fennel soup + grilled salmon, *99*, 100–101
- rustic fennel + celery root mash, *113*, 114

FIGS
- fresh figs in dark chocolate, *66*, 67
- radicchio + fig salad with sherry vinaigrette, 78, *79*

fish sauce dressing, seared ahi + baby bok choy salad with, 148–49, *151*
flank steak, grilled, 136, *137*
French beans, in haricots verts with hazelnuts + orange, 111
fresh cranberry relish with cherries + cardamom, 86, *87*
fresh figs in dark chocolate, *66*, 67
fresh strawberry pie + toasted almond crust, *197*, 198–99
frisée, in chicory salad with toasted walnut + anchovy vinaigrette, 77
fudge brownie balls, walnut, *54*, 55
fudgy brownies with toasted almonds + flake salt, *204*, 205

G

ganache, 185, 189, 192–93
garlic mashed cauliflower, 112, *113*

GINGER
- ginger marinated black cod + roasted baby bok choy, *129*, 130–31
- maple-ginger dressing, 160

GRANITA
- cold brew coffee granita, *47*, 48
- watermelon + lime granita, *47*, 49

grapes + za'atar dressing, Little Gem salad with, *84*, 85
green beans, in haricots verts with hazelnuts + orange, 111
gremolata, lemon-pistachio, + charred asparagus, *116*, 117
grilled flank steak, 136, *137*
grilled veg, creamy, salty + tangy tonnato sauce with, 64, *65*

H

halibut, everything seasoning encrusted, + horseradish aioli, 132, *133*
haricots verts with hazelnuts + orange, *110*, 111

HAZELNUTS
- haricots verts with hazelnuts + orange, *110*, 111
- Linzer cake with hazelnut + dried raspberry, 182, *183*

hemp powder, wild blueberry + banana, the everyday smoothie with, *32*, 33

HONEY
- Asian-style chicken salad + honey-lime dressing, *152*, 153
- the Baja chop + honey-chipotle dressing, *166*, 167

horseradish aioli, 132

J

jicama, in the Baja chop, 167

K

KALE
- baby kale with maple-ginger dressing, 160
- bison sirloin au poivre + baby kale, 155

summer kale + strawberry salad, *74*, *75*

L

LAMB
- lettuce wrapped lamb burgers + lemon aioli, 144, *145*
- pan-seared lamb lollipops with rosemary, maple + Dijon, *142*, 143

LEEKS
- asparagus leek soup + spring chive blossoms, *102*, 103
- cream of porcini mushroom soup, *90*, 91
- warm arugula vichyssoise, 96, *97*

LEMON
- charred asparagus + lemon-pistachio gremolata, *116*, 117
- charred broccoli + lemon tahini sauce, *106*, 107
- lemon-scented fennel soup + grilled salmon, *99*, 100–101
- lettuce wrapped lamb burgers + lemon aioli, 144, *145*
- minty fresh + lemony salad smoothie, 34, *35*
- wild salmon cakes + lemon aioli, *124*, 125

lettuce wrapped lamb burgers + lemon aioli, 144, *145*

LIME
- Asian-style chicken salad + honey-lime dressing, *152*, 153
- summer slushy with lime + mint, *50*, 51
- Thai-style herb salad with chicken, strawberries + lime dressing, 164, *165*
- watermelon + lime granita, *47*, 49
- winter salmon salad + cranberry-lime relish, 156, *157*

Linzer cake with hazelnut + dried raspberry, 182, *183*

LITTLE GEM LETTUCE
- Little Gem salad with grapes + za'atar dressing, *84*, 85
- Little Gem wedge salad with green goddess dressing, *80*, 81
- summer salmon salad with cool, crisp veg + dilly dressing, *158*, 159

liver, chicken, mousse with apple + thyme, *58*, 59

M

macaroons, chocolate-dipped coconut, 186, *187*

mango, in the Baja chop, 167

MAPLE
- baby kale with roasted sweet potato, walnuts + maple-ginger dressing, 160, *161*
- bison sirloin au poivre + baby kale with maple-Dijon dressing, *154*, 155
- pan-seared lamb lollipops with rosemary, maple + Dijon, *142*, 143

MASH
- garlic mashed cauliflower, 112, *113*
- rustic fennel + celery root mash, *113*, 114
- rutabaga mash with sage + crispy shallots, *113*, 115

meatloaf, bison, + jus, 140, *141*

Mediterranean tuna + dry-cured olives with thyme vinaigrette, *162*, 163

MINT
- lettuce wrapped lamb burgers, 144, *145*
- mint chocolate mini bundts, 206–7, 208–9
- minty fresh + lemony salad smoothie, 34, *35*
- summer slushy with lime + mint, *50*, 51
- tahini-charred cauliflower with dates + mint, 108, *109*
- Thai-style herb salad with chicken + strawberries, 164, *165*

morning glory muffins + breakfast cake, 38, *39*

mousse, chicken liver, with apple + thyme, *58*, 59

MUFFINS
- banana + toasted walnut muffins, *68*, *69*
- choc-a-lot muffins, 56, *57*
- coconut-almond muffins, 178
- morning glory muffins + breakfast cake, 38, *39*

mushroom soup, cream of porcini, *90*, 91

N

Napa cabbage, in Asian-style chicken salad, 153

nectarine, in the Baja chop, 167

O

olives, dry-cured, + Mediterranean tuna with thyme vinaigrette, *162*, 163
omelet, egg white, + wild blueberry compote, 36, *37*
onion beef, savory French, *138*, 139. *See also* red onion
ORANGE
- asparagus mimosa with tarragon + orange, *72*, 73
- fresh strawberry pie + toasted almond crust, *197*, 198–99
- haricots verts with hazelnuts + orange, *110*, 111
- roasted Brussels sprouts + blood oranges with sweet white balsamic, *119*, 120–21

P

pan-seared lamb lollipops with rosemary, maple + Dijon, *142*, 143
Pasadena chicken salad + sweet sesame dressing, 168, *169*
peach, in the Baja chop, 167
pecan pie truffles with salted caramel + toasted pecans, *210*, 211
PISTACHIOS
- Brussels sprouts slaw with Honeycrisp + pistachios, 82, *83*
- charred asparagus + lemon-pistachio gremolata, *116*, 117

porcini mushroom soup, cream of, *90*, 91
pots de crème, dark chocolate, *180*, 181

R

RADICCHIO
- chicory salad with toasted walnut + anchovy vinaigrette, *76*, 77
- creamy, salty + tangy tonnato sauce with grilled veg, 64, *65*
- radicchio + fig salad with sherry vinaigrette, 78, *79*

RADISHES
- creamy, salty + tangy tonnato sauce with grilled veg, 64, *65*
- Little Gem wedge salad with green goddess dressing, *80*, 81
- summer salmon salad with cool, crisp veg + dilly dressing, *158*, 159

raisins, in morning glory muffins + breakfast cake, 38
RASPBERRIES
- dark chocolate pots de crème, *180*, 181
- Linzer cake with hazelnut + dried raspberry, 182, *183*
- the signature chocolate cake + sweet raspberry filling, 188–89, *190*

red cabbage, in Asian-style chicken salad, 153
RED ONION
- baby kale with roasted sweet potato, walnuts + maple-ginger dressing, 160, *161*
- the Baja chop, 167
- creamy, salty + tangy tonnato sauce with grilled veg, 64, *65*
- lettuce wrapped lamb burgers + lemon aioli, 144, *145*
- Little Gem salad with grapes + za'atar dressing, *84*, 85
- savory French onion beef, *138*, 139
- winter salmon salad + cranberry-lime relish, 156, *157*

RELISH
- cranberry-lime relish, 156
- fresh cranberry relish with cherries + cardamom, 86, *87*

roast chicken, *134*, 135
roasted Brussels sprouts + blood oranges with sweet white balsamic, *119*, 120–21
ROMAINE LETTUCE
- the Baja chop + honey-chipotle dressing, *166*, 167
- Little Gem salad with grapes + za'atar dressing, *84*, 85
- Little Gem wedge salad with green goddess dressing, *80*, 81
- minty fresh + lemony salad smoothie, 34, *35*
- Pasadena chicken salad + sweet sesame dressing, 168, *169*

rosemary, maple + Dijon, pan-seared lamb lollipops with, *142*, 143
rustic fennel + celery root mash, *113*, 114
rutabaga mash with sage + crispy shallots, *113*, 115

S

sage + crispy shallots, rutabaga mash with, *113*, 115

SALAD

- Asian-style chicken salad + honey-lime dressing, *152*, 153
- asparagus mimosa with tarragon + orange, *72*, 73
- baby kale with roasted sweet potato, walnuts + maple-ginger dressing, 160, *161*
- the Baja chop + honey-chipotle dressing, *166*, 167
- bison sirloin au poivre + baby kale with maple-Dijon dressing, *154*, 155
- Brussels sprouts slaw with Honeycrisp + pistachios, 82, *83*
- chicory salad with toasted walnut + anchovy vinaigrette, *76*, 77
- Little Gem salad with grapes + za'atar dressing, *84*, 85
- Little Gem wedge salad with green goddess dressing, *80*, 81
- minty fresh + lemony salad smoothie, 34, *35*
- Pasadena chicken salad + sweet sesame dressing, 168, *169*
- radicchio + fig salad with sherry vinaigrette, *78*, 79
- seared ahi + baby bok choy salad with fish sauce dressing, 148–49, *151*
- summer kale + strawberry salad, 74, *75*
- summer salmon salad with cool, crisp veg + dilly dressing, *158*, 159
- Thai-style herb salad with chicken, strawberries + lime dressing, 164, *165*
- watercress with roast chicken, tart apples + tarragon dressing, *170*, 171
- winter salmon salad + cranberry-lime relish, 156, *157*

SALMON

- lemon-scented fennel soup + grilled salmon, *99*, 100–101
- summer salmon salad with cool, crisp veg + dilly dressing, *158*, 159
- wild salmon cakes + lemon aioli, *124*, 125
- wild salmon with blackberry gastrique + thyme, 126–27, *128*
- winter salmon salad + cranberry-lime relish, 156, *157*

SAUCE. *See also* dips and spreads; dressing

- horseradish aioli, 132
- lemon aioli, 144
- lemon tahini sauce, 107
- lemon-pistachio gremolata, 117
- tonnato sauce, 64
- wild blueberry compote, 37, 41

savory French onion beef, *138*, 139

seared ahi + baby bok choy salad with fish sauce dressing, 148–49, *151*

the signature chocolate cake + sweet raspberry filling, 188–89, *190*

slaw, Brussels sprouts, with Honeycrisp + pistachios, 82, *83*

slushy, summer, with lime + mint, *50*, 51

SMOOTHIES

- the everyday smoothie with wild blueberry, banana + hemp powder, *32*, 33
- minty fresh + lemony salad smoothie, 34, *35*

SOUPS

- asparagus leek soup + spring chive blossoms, *102*, 103
- cream of porcini mushroom soup, *90*, 91
- creamy cauliflower soup, *94*, 95
- creamy coconut carrot soup, 92, *93*
- lemon-scented fennel soup + grilled salmon, *99*, 100–101
- warm arugula vichyssoise, 96, *97*

spreads. *See* dips and spreads

steak, grilled flank, 136, *137*

STRAWBERRIES

- fresh strawberry pie + toasted almond crust, *197*, 198–99
- strawberry + almond energy balls, *44*, 45
- strawberry snack cake, 200, *201*

summer kale + strawberry salad, *74*, *75*
Thai-style herb salad with chicken, strawberries + lime dressing, 164, *165*
summer kale + strawberry salad, *74*, *75*
summer salmon salad with cool, crisp veg + dilly dressing, *158*, 159
summer slushy with lime + mint, *50*, 51
SWEET POTATOES
baby kale with roasted sweet potato, walnuts + maple-ginger dressing, 160, *161*
warm arugula vichyssoise, 96, *97*

T

TAHINI
charred broccoli + lemon tahini sauce, *106*, 107
creamy carrot tahini, 60, *61*
dark chocolate tahini truffles, *176*, 177
tahini-charred cauliflower with dates + mint, 108, *109*
zesty herbed tahini dip, *62*, 63
TARRAGON
asparagus mimosa with tarragon + orange, *72*, 73
Little Gem wedge salad with green goddess dressing, *80*, 81
watercress with roast chicken, tart apples + tarragon dressing, *170*, 171
10-minute asparagus + rotisserie chicken bowl, 172, *173*
Thai-style herb salad with chicken, strawberries + lime dressing, 164, *165*
THYME
charred asparagus + lemon-pistachio gremolata, *116*, 117
chicken liver mousse with apple + thyme, *58*, 59
cream of porcini mushroom soup, *90*, 91
Mediterranean tuna + dry-cured olives with thyme vinaigrette, *162*, 163
wild salmon with blackberry gastrique + thyme, 126–27, *128*
tonnato sauce, 64, *65*
truffles, pecan pie, *210*, 211
TUNA
creamy, salty + tangy tonnato sauce with grilled veg, 64, *65*
Mediterranean tuna + dry-cured olives with thyme vinaigrette, *162*, 163
seared ahi + baby bok choy salad with fish sauce dressing, 148–49, *151*

V

vanilla coconut yogurt + wild blueberry compote, *40*, 41
vichyssoise, warm arugula, 96, *97*

W

WALNUTS
baby kale with roasted sweet potato + walnuts, 160, *161*
banana + toasted walnut muffins, 68, *69*
chicory salad with toasted walnut + anchovy vinaigrette, *76*, 77
cinnamon-walnut coffee cake, 202, *203*
morning glory muffins + breakfast cake, 38, *39*
radicchio + fig salad with sherry vinaigrette, 78, *79*
walnut fudge brownie balls, *54*, 55
warm arugula vichyssoise, 96, *97*
watercress with roast chicken, tart apples + tarragon dressing, *170*, 171
watermelon + lime granita, *47*, 49
white balsamic, sweet, roasted Brussels sprouts + blood oranges with, *119*, 120–21
wild blueberry. *See* blueberries, wild
wild salmon. *See* salmon
winter salmon salad + cranberry-lime relish, 156, *157*

Y

yogurt, vanilla coconut, + wild blueberry compote, *40*, 41

Z

ZA'ATAR
Little Gem salad with grapes + za'atar dressing, *84*, 85
roast chicken, *134*, 135
zesty herbed tahini dip, *62*, 63

ABOUT THE AUTHOR

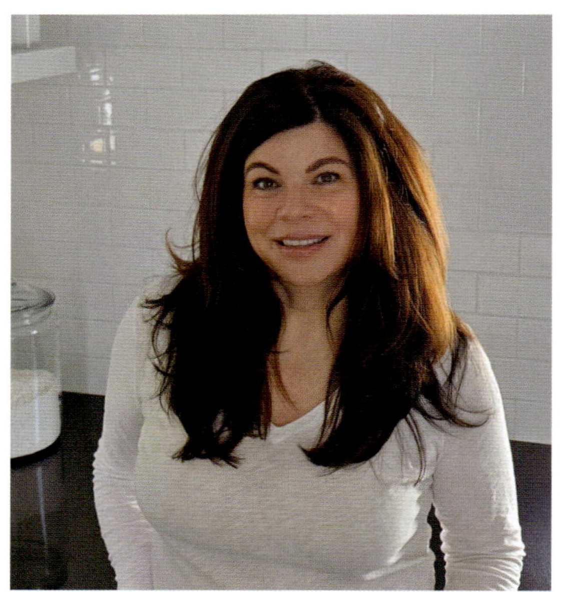

Rachel Riggs is a former specialty food shop owner and business development consultant who has written for *Bon Appétit* and Camille Styles. After her life was upended by illness, she made a paradigm shift to her diet and now develops nutrient-dense, allergen-aware recipes that appeal to her California sensibilities. She lives in San Diego with her husband.

Instagram: @the.rachel.riggs
www.RachRiggs.com

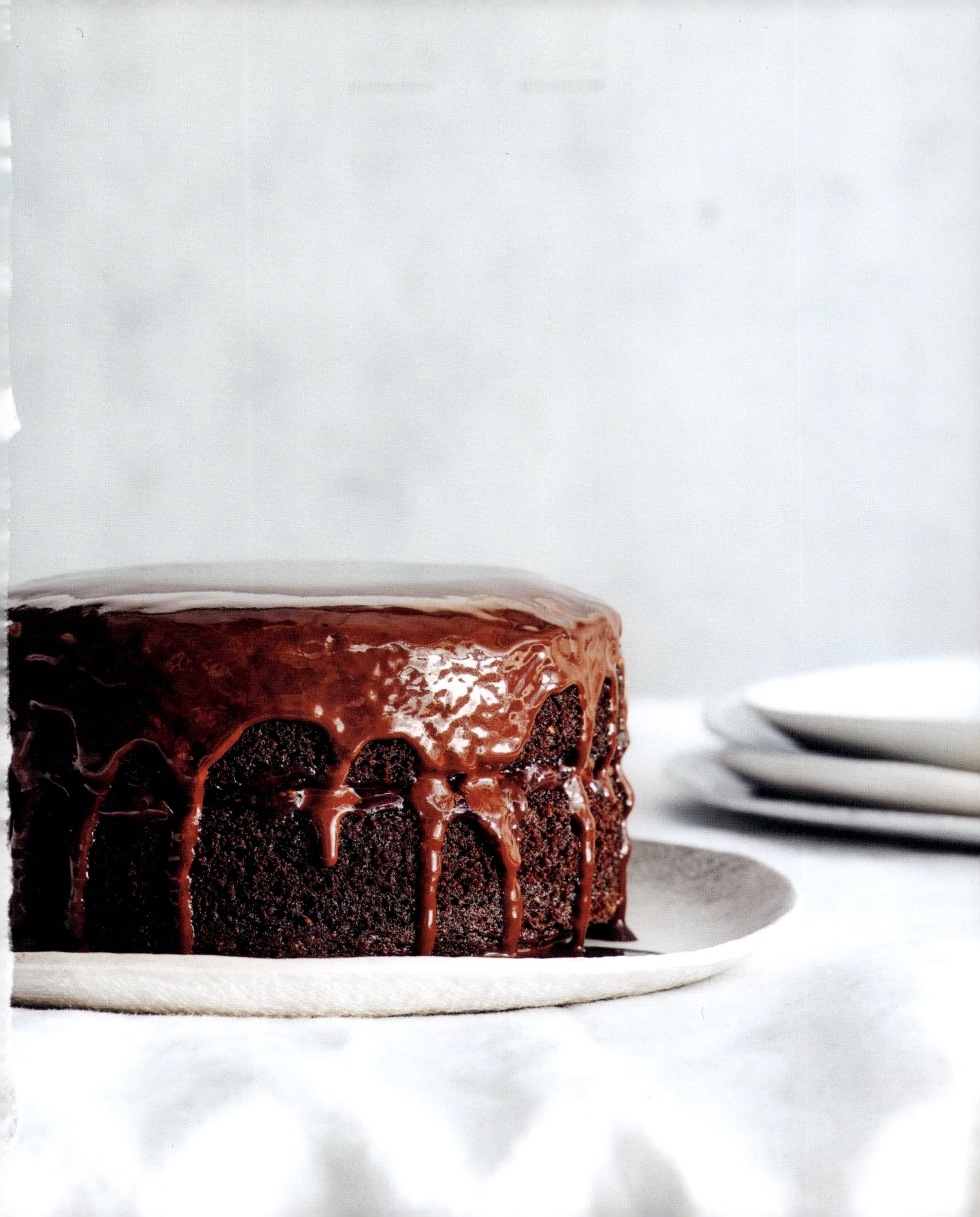

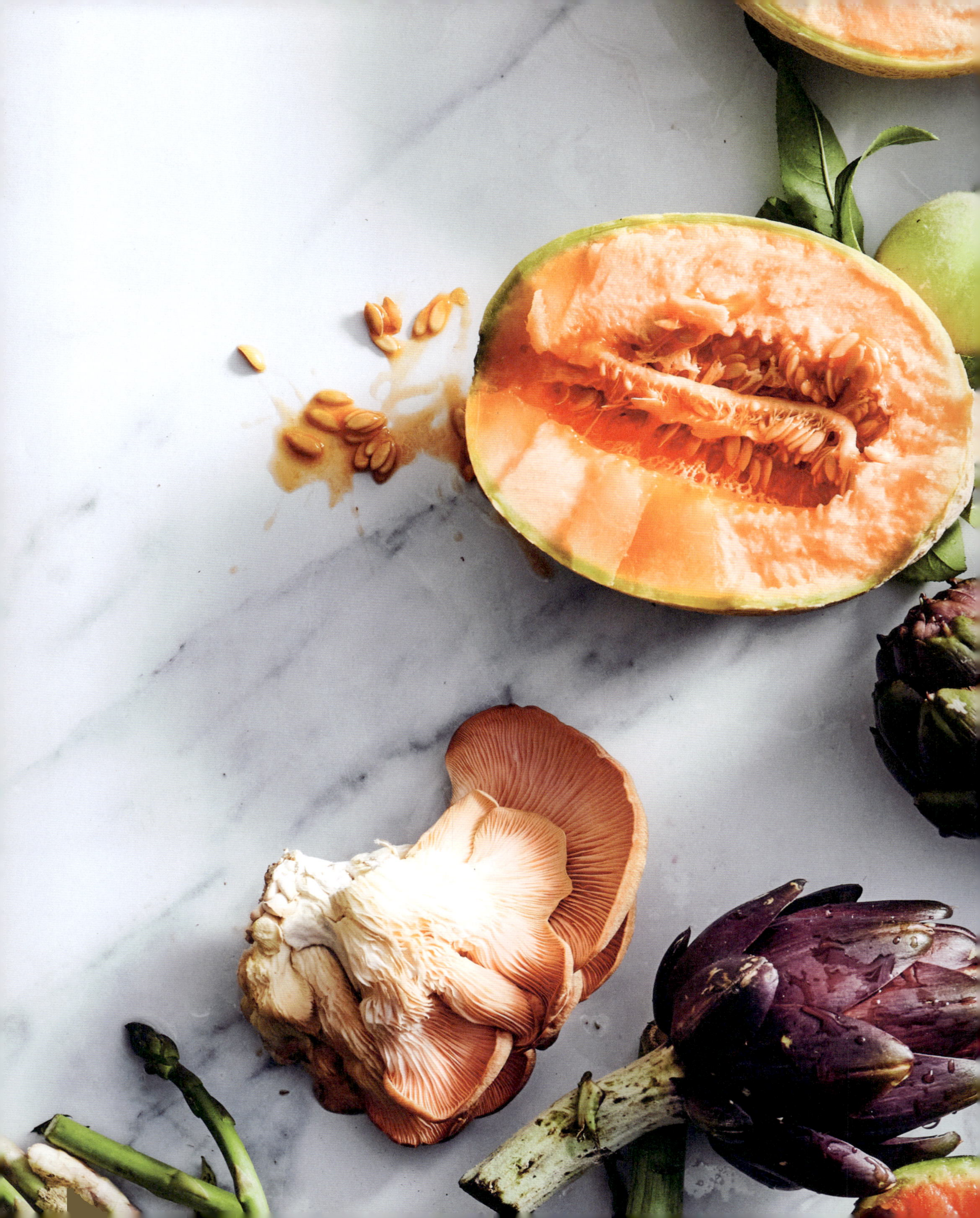